Advances in Viral Hepatitis B and D: Moving Toward the Goals of Elimination

Editor

ROBERT G. GISH

CLINICS IN LIVER DISEASE

www.liver.theclinics.com

Consulting Editor
NORMAN GITLIN

November 2023 • Volume 27 • Number 4

ELSEVIER

1600 John F. Kennedy Boulevard • Suite 1800 • Philadelphia, Pennsylvania, 19103-2899

http://www.theclinics.com

CLINICS IN LIVER DISEASE Volume 27, Number 4
November 2023 ISSN 1089-3261, ISBN-13: 978-0-323-93947-8

Editor: Kerry Holland
Developmental Editor: Akshay Samson

Clinics in Liver Disease (ISSN 1089-3261) is published quarterly by Elsevier Inc., 360 Park Avenue South, New York, NY 10010-1710. Months of issue are February, May, August, and November. Business and Editorial Offices: 1600 John F. Kennedy Blvd., Ste. 1800, Philadelphia, PA 19103-2899. Customer Service Office: 3251 Riverport Lane, Maryland Heights, MO 63043. Periodicals postage paid at New York, NY and additional mailing offices. Subscription prices are $339.00 per year (U.S. individuals), $100.00 per year (U.S. student/resident), $674.00 per year (U.S. institutions), $434.00 per year (international individuals), $200.00 per year (international student/resident), $837.00 per year (international instituitions), $393.00 per year (Canadian individuals), $100.00 per year (Canadian student/resident), and $837.00 per year (Canadian institutions). Foreign air speed delivery is included in all *Clinics* subscription prices. All prices are subject to change without notice. **POSTMASTER:** Send address changes to *Clinics in Liver Disease*, Elsevier Health Sciences Division, Subscription Customer Service, 3251 Riverport Lane, Maryland Heights, MO 63043. **Customer Service: Telephone: 1-800-654-2452 (U.S. and Canada); 314-447-8871 (outside U.S. and Canada). Fax: 314-447-8029. E-mail: journalscustomer service-usa@elsevier.com (for print support); journalsonlinesupport-usa@elsevier.com (for online support).**

Reprints. For copies of 100 or more of articles in this publication, please contact the Commercial Reprints Department, Elsevier Inc., 360 Park Avenue South, New York, NY 10010-1710. Tel.: 212-633-3874; Fax: 212-633-3820; E-mail: reprints@elsevier.com.

Clinics in Liver Disease is covered in *MEDLINE/PubMed (Index Medicus)*, Science Citation Index Expanded, Journal Citation Reports/Science Edition, and Current Contents/Clinical Medicine.

Contributors

CONSULTING EDITOR

NORMAN GITLIN, MD, FRCP (LONDON), FRCPE (EDINBURGH), FAASLD, FACP, FACG
Head of Hepatology, Southern California Liver Centers, San Clemente, California, USA

EDITOR

ROBERT G. GISH, MD
Medical Director, Hepatitis B Foundation, Doylestown, Pennsylvania, USA; Adjunct Professor of Medicine, University of Nevada, Reno, Reno, Nevada, USA; Adjunct Professor of Medicine, University of Nevada, Las Vegas, Las Vegas, Nevada, USA; Adjunct Professor of Pharmacy, Skaggs School of Pharmacy and Pharmaceutical Sciences, University of California, San Diego, La Jolla, California, USA; Clinical Professor, Loma Linda University, Loma Linda, California, USA

AUTHORS

KOSH AGARWAL, B Med Sci (Hons), MBBS, MRCP, MD
Consultant, Institute of Liver Studies, King's College Hospital, London, United Kingdom

HAROUT AJOYAN, BSc
Storr Liver Centre, The Westmead Institute for Medical Research, The University of Sydney at Westmead Hospital, Westmead, New South Wales, Australia

LITAL ALIASI-SINAI, BSc
Sackler School of Medicine, Tel Aviv University, Tel Aviv, Israel

JOSEPH J. ALUKAL, MD
Professor, University of California, School of Medicine, Riverside, California, USA

TARIK ASSELAH, MD, PhD
Professor of Medicine, Université Paris-Cité, Hôpital Beaujon, AP-HP & INSERM UMR1149, Clichy, France

PABLO BARREIRO, MD, PhD
Associate Professor, Public Health Regional Laboratory, Hospital Isabel Zendal, Universidad Rey Juan Carlos, Madrid, Spain

CAMILLA CECCATELLI BERTI, PhD
Department of Medicine and Surgery, University of Parma, Parma, Italy

CAROLINA BONI, MD
Adjunct Professor, Unit of Infectious Diseases and Hepatology, Azienda Ospedaliero-Universitaria di Parma, Parma, Italy

CAROL BROSGART, MD
Clinical Professor, Medicine, Biostatistics, and Epidemiology, University of California, San Francisco, San Francisco, California, USA

JONGGI CHOI, MD, PhD
Professor, Department Gastroenterology, Asan Medical Center, University of Ulsan College of Medicine, Seoul, Republic of Korea

WON-MOOK CHOI, MD, PhD
Professor, Department of Gastroenterology, Asan Medical Center, University of Ulsan College of Medicine, Seoul, Republic of Korea

SARA DOSELLI, BSc
Department of Medicine and Surgery, University of Parma, Parma, Italy

ZAHRA DOSSAJI, DO
Resident, Internal Medicine, Kirk Kerkorian School of Medicine at the University of Nevada, Las Vegas, Las Vegas, Nevada, USA

PAOLA FISICARO, PhD
Unit of Infectious Diseases and Hepatology, Azienda Ospedaliero-Universitaria di Parma, Parma, Italy

JACOB GEORGE, MBBS, FRACP, PhD, FAASLD
Director, Storr Liver Centre, The Westmead Institute for Medical Research, The University of Sydney at Westmead Hospital, Westmead, New South Wales, Australia

ROBERT G. GISH, MD
Medical Director, Hepatitis B Foundation, Doylestown, Pennsylvania, USA; Adjunct Professor of Medicine, University of Nevada, Reno, Reno, Nevada, USA; Adjunct Professor of Medicine, University of Nevada, Las Vegas, Las Vegas, Nevada, USA; Adjunct Professor of Pharmacy, Skaggs School of Pharmacy and Pharmaceutical Sciences, University of California, San Diego, La Jolla, California, USA; Clinical Professor, Loma Linda University, Loma Linda, California, USA

MARIA FERNANDA GUERRA VELOZ, MD, PhD
Institute of Liver Studies, King's College Hospital, London, United Kingdom

JULIO GUTIERREZ, MD
Associate Professor, Center for Organ Transplant, Scripps Clinic, Scripps MD Anderson Center, Scripps Green Hospital, La Jolla, California, USA

LUBABA HAQUE, DO
Resident, Internal Medicine, Kirk Kerkorian School of Medicine at the University of Nevada, Las Vegas, Las Vegas, Nevada, USA

REX WAN-HIN HUI, MBBS
Clinical Practitioner, Department of Medicine, School of Clinical Medicine State Key Laboratory of Liver Research, The University of Hong Kong, Pokfulam, Hong Kong

IRA M. JACOBSON, MD, FACP, FAGA, FAASLD, FACG
Director, Professor, Department of Medicine, NYU Grossman School of Medicine, New York, New York, USA

TATYANA KUSHNER, MD, MSCE
Assistant Professor, Division of Liver Diseases, Icahn School of Medicine at Mount Sinai, New York, New York, USA

DILETTA LACCABUE, BSc
Department of Medicine and Surgery, University of Parma, Parma, Italy

TOOBA LAEEQ, MD
Resident, Internal Medicine, Kirk Kerkorian School of Medicine at the University of Nevada, Las Vegas, Las Vegas, Nevada, USA

MARCIA LANGE, BSc
Research student, Icahn School of Medicine at Mount Sinai, New York, New York, USA

YOUNG-SUK LIM, MD, PhD
Professor, Department of Gastroenterology, Asan Medical Center, University of Ulsan College of Medicine, Seoul, Republic of Korea

JAMES LOK, MA, MBBS, MRCP
Institute of Liver Studies, King's College Hospital, London, United Kingdom

LUNG-YI MAK, MD
Assistant Professor, Department of Medicine, School of Clinical Medicine, State Key Laboratory of Liver Research, The University of Hong Kong, Pokfulam, Hong Kong

GABRIELE MISSALE, MD
Unit of Infectious Diseases and Hepatology, Azienda Ospedaliero-Universitaria di Parma, Department of Medicine and Surgery, University of Parma, Parma, Italy

ANNA MONTALI, PhD
Department of Medicine and Surgery, University of Parma, Parma, Italy

ILARIA MONTALI, PhD
Postdoctoral Researcher, Department of Medicine and Surgery, University of Parma, Parma, Italy

KEVIN PAK, MD
Assistant Professor, Naval Medical Center, San Diego, California, USA

AMALIA PENNA, PhD
Unit of Infectious Diseases and Hepatology, Azienda Ospedaliero-Universitaria di Parma, Parma, Italy

ZOË POST, MD
Gastroenterology and Hepatology Fellow, Rush University Medical Center, Chicago, Illinois, USA

NANCY REAU, MD
Professor of Medicine, Richard B. Capps Chair of Hepatology, Chief, Section of Hepatology, Associate Director, Solid Organ Transplantation, Rush University Medical Center, Chicago, Illinois, USA

VALENTINA REVERBERI, BSc
Unit of Infectious Diseases and Hepatology, Azienda Ospedaliero-Universitaria di Parma, Parma, Italy

KATERINA ROMA, DO
Physician, Internal Medicine, Kirk Kerkorian School of Medicine at the University of Nevada, Las Vegas, Las Vegas, Nevada, USA

MARZIA ROSSI, PhD
Department of Medicine and Surgery, University of Parma, Parma, Italy

SIMONA SCHIVAZAPPA, MD
Unit of Infectious Diseases and Hepatology, Azienda Ospedaliero-Universitaria di Parma, Parma, Italy

WAI-KAY SETO, MD
Consultant, Department of Medicine, School of Clinical Medicine, State Key Laboratory of Liver Research, The University of Hong Kong, Pokfulam, Hong Kong

KENNETH E. SHERMAN, MD, PhD
Director, Clinical Trials Development, Gastroenterology Division, Massachusetts General Hospital/Harvard Medical School, Boston, Massachusetts, USA

VICENTE SORIANO, MD, PhD
Full Professor, Health Sciences School and Medical Center, Universidad Internacional La Rioja (UNIR), Madrid, Spain

FENG SU, MD MSCR
Department of Medicine, NYU Grossman School of Medicine, NYU Langone Transplant Institute, New York, New York, USA

CAMILLA TIEZZI, BSc
Department of Medicine and Surgery, University of Parma, Parma, Italy

THOMAS TU, PhD
Group Leader, Storr Liver Centre, The Westmead Institute for Medical Research, Centre for Infectious Diseases and Microbiology, Sydney Infectious Diseases Institute, The University of Sydney at Westmead Hospital, The University of Sydney School of Medicine and Health, Westmead, New South Wales, Australia

EMUEJEVUOKE UMUKORO, DO
Scripps Mercy Hospital, Chula Vista, California, USA

ANDREA VECCHI, BSc
Unit of Infectious Diseases and Hepatology, Azienda Ospedaliero-Universitaria di Parma, Parma, Italy

THERESA WORTHINGTON, BSBA
Division of Liver Diseases, Icahn School of Medicine at Mount Sinai, New York, New York, USA

DEBRA W. YEN, MD
Clinical Instructor, Division of Digestive Diseases, University of Cincinnati College of Medicine, Cincinnati, Ohio, USA

MAN-FUNG YUEN, DSc, MD, PhD
Professor, Department of Medicine, School of Clinical Medicine, State Key Laboratory of Liver Research, The University of Hong Kong, Pokfulam, Hong Kong

HENRIK ZHANG, BSc
The Westmead Institute for Medical Research, The University of Sydney School of Medicine and Health, Westmead, New South Wales, Australia

Contents

The main aim of antiviral therapy in patients with chronic hepatitis B (CHB) is to prevent disease progression and reduce the risk of hepatocellular carcinoma (HCC). In general, treatment is recommended for select patient groups viewed as being at higher risk of developing adverse outcomes from CHB. However, patients who do not meet treatment criteria under current international guidelines may still benefit from antiviral therapy to reduce CHB-related complications. Moreover, well-tolerated antiviral drugs that are highly effective at suppressing viral replication are now widely available, and withholding therapy from patients with viremia is increasingly controversial. In this article, we review traditional treatment paradigms and argue the merits of expanding treatment eligibility to patients with CHB who do not meet current treatment criteria.

In treatment-naïve patients with chronic hepatitis B virus (HBV) infection, entecavir (ETV), tenofovir disoproxil fumarate (TDF), and tenofovir alafenamide have a minimal or no risk of drug-resistance. These 3 nucleos(t)ide analog agents are highly potent inducing high rate of virologic response (reducing serum HBV DNA to levels undetectable by polymerase chain reaction assays) in most treatment-naïve patients. Our randomized trials have demonstrated that monotherapy with TDF can provide a successful virological response in most of the heavily pretreated patients with multidrug resistance to ETV or adefovir.

The natural history of hepatitis B virus (HBV) infection is closely dependent on the dynamic interplay between the host immune response and viral replication. Spontaneous HBV clearance in acute self-limited infection is the result of an adequate and efficient antiviral immune response. Instead, it is widely recognized that in chronic HBV infection, immunologic dysfunction contributes to viral persistence. Long-lasting exposure to high viral antigens, upregulation of multiple co-inhibitory receptors, dysfunctional intracellular signaling pathways and metabolic alterations, and intrahepatic regulatory mechanisms have been described as features ultimately leading to a hierarchical loss of effector functions up to full T-cell exhaustion.

Chronic infection with Hepatitis B is a common, incurable, and deadly infection. Despite inexpensive laboratory tests for diagnosis and management that have been established for decades, the worldwide rate of diagnosis is only ~10%, and ~5% of people are under treatment. Novel assays have been developed to improve linkage to care by providing more flexible approaches to determine a patient's health status. Other assays have been established to better investigate intrahepatic host-virus interactions to support clinical trials for cure research. This review outlines the clinical and scientific challenges still to be solved and the upcoming methods used to address them.

Nucleos(t)ide analogs are the cornerstone of treatment against hepatitis B virus; however, they have no direct effect on its transcriptional template (ie, covalently closed circular DNA) and so functional cure is rarely achieved. Over recent years, there has been a significant improvement in our understanding of the viral life cycle and its mechanisms of immune evasion. In this review article, we will explore novel therapeutic targets, discuss the latest data from clinical trials, and highlight future research priorities.

Currently approved treatment of patients with chronic hepatitis B infection is insufficient to achieve functional cure. Numerous new compounds are identified, and among many, capsid assembly modulators (CAMs) and nucleic acid polymers (NAPs) are 2 classes of virus-directing agents in clinical development. CAMs interfere with viral pregenomic RNA encapsidation and are effective in viral load reduction but have limited effects on hepatitis B surface antigen (HBsAg). NAPs prevent HBsAg release from hepatocytes and induce intracellular degradation, leading to potent suppression of serum HBsAg when combined with nucleoside analogues and pegylated interferon demonstrated by initial data, but awaiting further confirmation studies.

Chronic hepatitis B virus (HBV) infection is a serious disease that currently has no cure. Key forms of HBV include covalently closed circular DNA, which mediates chronic persistence, and integrated DNA, which contributes to immune evasion and carcinogenesis. These forms are not targeted by current therapies; however, gene editing technologies have emerged as promising tools for disrupting HBV DNA. Gene editor-induced double-stranded breaks at precise locations within the HBV genome can induce effects ranging from inactivation of target genes to complete degradation of the target genome. Although promising, several challenges remain in efficacy and safety that require solutions.

Delta Hepatitis

Maternal-to-child transmission of hepatitis B virus (HBV) and hepatitis delta virus (HDV) can lead to the risk of progressive liver disease in infants, but fortunately effective interventions exist to decrease transmission. Counseling on the risk of maternal-to-child transmission, care pathways to decrease transmission, and the implications of HBV and HDV on pregnancy outcomes are the key components of caring for pregnant people living with HBV and HDV.

Diagnosis of HDV exposure is based on clinical assays of anti-hepatitis D antibody and current infection with hepatitis D RNA PCR. The role of hepatitis D antigen testing is not yet defined. RT-qPCR is the gold standard for measuring HDV RNA viral load, which is used to assess response to the treatment of HDV infection. Gaps in testing include poor sensitivity of antigen testing and quantitative HDV RNA accuracy can be affected by the genotypic variability of the virus and variation in laboratory techniques. There is also a limitation in HDV testing due to access, cost, and limited knowledge of testing indications. Droplet digital PCR promises to be a more accurate method to quantify HDV RNA. Also, the recent development of a rapid HDV detection test could prove useful in resource-limited areas.

Hepatitis delta virus (HDV) only infects patients with hepatitis B virus (HBV) due to its reliance on HBV surface proteins to form its envelope. With shared routes of transmission, HDV coinfection is estimated to occur in 15% of patients with HIV and HBV. However, HDV is often underdiagnosed and may be missed particularly in people living with HIV (PLWH) who are already on antiretroviral therapy with anti-HBV activity and coincidental HBV suppression. At the same time, HDV causes the most severe form of chronic viral hepatitis and leads to faster progression of liver disease and hepatocellular carcinoma. Thus, increased recognition and effective treatment are paramount, and as novel treatment options approach global markets, the study of their efficacy in PLWH should be pursued.

The disease burden of HDV is poorly understood. Our review identified multiple reasons: (1) HDV infection rates are overestimated in the general population due to limited sample sizes, sampling high-risk populations, and significant regional variations, (2) estimates are based on chronic HBV populations, but HBV burden itself is uncertain, (3) there is a lack of testing in at-risk populations, (4) prevalence testing is based on HDV antibody testing and not HDV RNA, which distinguishes between active infection versus prior exposure, (5) older studies used less reliable testing and (6) HBV vaccination programs have affected HDV prevalence, but is often not accounted for.

HDV use the cell enzymes for its own replication, and the HBsAg as an envelope. There is an urgent need to develop new drugs for chronic hepatitis D (CHD). Pegylated interferon alpha (PEG-IFNα) (direct-antiviral and immune modulator) has been used and recommended by scientific guidelines, although not approved, with moderate efficacy and poor tolerability. There are several drugs in development which target the host: bulevirtide (BLV), lonafarnib (LNF), nucleic acid polymer, and others.

Back to "B"

Hepatitis B infection affects approximately 262 million people worldwide and is responsible for 900,000 deaths annually. This article reviews the major factors limiting HBV elimination, which includes limited linkage to care and complicated HBV testing and treatment guidelines. The article then provides solutions to these pressing issues.

CLINICS IN LIVER DISEASE

SERIES OF RELATED INTEREST

Gastroenterology Clinics of North America
https://www.gastro.theclinics.com

THE CLINICS ARE AVAILABLE ONLINE!
Access your subscription at:
www.theclinics.com

Preface

The "B and D" Times, They Are A-Changin'

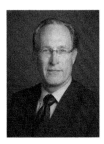

Robert G. Gish, MD
Editor

The state of hepatitis B and delta infection is changing rapidly. Since the advent 1 year ago of the Advisory Committee on Immunization Practices' recommendation to vaccinate all adults for hepatitis B, we have met other milestones. This great advance was followed in the spring of 2023 by the Centers for Disease Control and Prevention's recommendation to test all adults for hepatitis B with the hepatitis B virus (HBV) triple panel. More recently, in June of 2023, the European Association for the Study of the Liver (EASL)'s guidelines came out with the recommendation to test all HBsAg-positive individuals for delta infection. Bookending this very exciting time is the development of a wide variety of new technologies to test for hepatitis B before and during treatment, using new biomarkers as well as a deeper understanding of the immunovirology of hepatitis B. The data behind this enhanced understanding have helped—along with patient advocacy from the Hepatitis B Foundation, the American Association for the Study of Liver Diseases (AASLD), EASL, Asian Pacific Association for the Study of the Liver, and many others, and with investment from the pharmaceutical industry—to develop new treatment strategies. Overall, I have counted 16 different HBV "targets" or "tools" that could be used as part of a hepatitis B cure.

We can also talk about the great advances in delta diagnosis and treatment. There is a World Health Organization standard to evaluate new tests for hepatitis D virus (HDV). We also have two medications that are approaching regulatory approval and one medication already approved under conditional use in the European Union. We can't talk about the delta cure until we can fully control and cure hepatitis B, but from my optimistic perspective, I think this is on the horizon. Control or suppression of HDV RNA is an intermediate step to improve the prognosis of patients with HDV. I do believe that there needs to be "4 pillars" of treatment for hepatitis B functional cure to reach 30% to 40% and that this is achievable with the next wave of treatment options. A

Clin Liver Dis 27 (2023) xiii–xiv
https://doi.org/10.1016/j.cld.2023.07.011
1089-3261/23/© 2023 Published by Elsevier Inc.

liver.theclinics.com

cornerstone of this treatment, of course, will be moderating the immune system. It's very likely that nucleoside or nucleotide analogues will be a cornerstone for the near term with a variety of other technologies that include interfering with RNA expression and ultimately gene editing to reach this next goal. The treatment endpoints article published in June of 2023 from EASL and AASLD will help keep the pace toward realistic treatment goals in the near term.

The articles in this issue of *Clinics in Liver Disease* provide state-of-the-art clinical summaries of the advances in Hepatitis B and D, with emphasis on HBV viro-immunology, novel assays, new targets, and tests for HBV and HDV, to name a few. Readers will come away with the clinical information they need to better manage and improve outcomes for these patients. Keep an eye out for two additional articles on organ transplantation and tests for HDV that are planned for online publication in the coming months to continue this discussion.

DISCLOSURES

Disclosures found at www.robertgish.com.

Robert G. Gish, MD
Medical Director
Hepatitis B Foundation
Doylestown, PA, USA

Adjunct Professor of Medicine
University of Nevada, Reno
Reno, NV, USA

Adjunct Professor of Medicine
University of Nevada, Las Vegas
Las Vegas, NV, USA

Adjunct Professor of Pharmacy
Skaggs School of Pharmacy and Pharmaceutical Sciences
University of California, San Diego
La Jolla, CA, USA

Clinical Professor
Loma Linda University
Loma Linda, CA, USA

Robert G. Gish Consultants, LLC
6022 La Jolla Mesa Drive
San Diego, CA 92037, USA

E-mail address:
rgish@robertgish.com

Hepatitis B

Chronic Hepatitis B
Treat all Who Are Viremic?

Feng Su, MD, MSCr[a,b,*], Ira M. Jacobson, MD, FAGA, FAASLD, FACG[a]

KEYWORDS

- Hepatitis B • Antiviral • Viremia • Immune tolerant • Chronic infection
- Hepatocellular carcinoma • Treatment criteria • Treatment guidelines

KEY POINTS

- Many patients with chronic hepatitis B (CHB) fall short of international guideline criteria for antiviral therapy. However, patients who do not meet current treatment criteria may still be at risk for adverse outcomes of CHB including hepatocellular carcinoma (HCC) or end-stage liver disease.
- The association between hepatitis B viral load and HCC risk is well described, due in part to viral integration into the host genome.
- Accumulating evidence indicates that antiviral therapy can reduce viral integration.
- We propose a simplified approach to CHB treatment that expands treatment eligibility.
- Expanding treatment eligibility has been shown to be cost effective, has the potential to increase treatment coverage, and may offer important ancillary benefits such as improved patient-reported outcomes and quality of life.

INTRODUCTION

The goals of antiviral therapy in patients with chronic hepatitis B (CHB) are to prevent disease progression and reduce the risk of hepatocellular carcinoma (HCC).[1–3] Treatment criteria set forth by international guidelines identify patient groups at the highest risk of adverse outcomes to target for treatment. In general, treatment is recommended for individuals with CHB with immune active disease or cirrhosis with detectable viremia, whereas it is not recommended in individuals with hepatitis B e antigen (HBeAg) positive chronic infection (otherwise known as "immune tolerant" disease) or in patients in the inactive carrier state.[1–3] The rationale for current treatment criteria is that antiviral therapy is thought to be unnecessary for nonprogressive or "benign" phases of disease and may not change the natural history of infection in patients with HBeAg-positive chronic infection. However, the perception that some phases

[a] Department of Medicine, New York University Grossman School of Medicine, 150 East 32nd Street, Suite 101, New York, NY 10016, USA; [b] New York University Langone Transplant Institute, 317 East 34th Street, 8th Floor, New York, NY 10016, USA
* Corresponding author
E-mail address: feng.su@nyulangone.org

Clin Liver Dis 27 (2023) 791–808
https://doi.org/10.1016/j.cld.2023.06.001
1089-3261/23/© 2023 Elsevier Inc. All rights reserved.
liver.theclinics.com

of CHB are "benign" has been challenged in recent years.[4,5] There is also longstanding recognition that viremia contributes to HCC risk independently of inflammation and fibrosis.[6] Plausible mechanistic explanations for this observation have now been proposed through research on HBV DNA integration and clonal hepatocyte expansion.[4,7] CHB is additionally associated with well-described extrahepatic manifestations that may be mitigated by viral suppression, and we should not discount the ancillary benefits of viral suppression including preventing transmission, improving quality of life, and reducing the stigma and discrimination associated with active HBV infection. Given the availability of well-tolerated antiviral drugs that are highly effective at suppressing viral replication and have high barriers to resistance, withholding therapy from patients with viremia is increasingly controversial. The current debate over existing treatment paradigms is timely, and the merits of a "treat all" approach are worth contemplating.

NATURAL HISTORY OF CHRONIC HEPATITIS B

The defining feature of hepatitis B pathophysiology is that the virus itself is not cytopathic, and liver damage is incurred by host immune activity directed at virus-infected hepatocytes.[1–3] Disease activity over time is a reflection of the interaction between the virus and a poorly regulated host immune response, leading to periods of inflammation and liver injury resulting in fibrosis, cirrhosis, and HCC. Additionally, due to the persistence of HBV covalently closed circular DNA and HBV DNA integration into the host genome, it is not yet possible to fully eradicate the virus after initial infection. Instead, the best resolution currently achievable is a "functional cure" defined by clearance of hepatitis B surface antigen (HBsAg) and undetectable HBV DNA, which is typically accompanied by the appearance of hepatitis B surface antibody (anti-HBs). While most healthy adults who are exposed to hepatitis B will spontaneously resolve their infection, the majority of individuals exposed to hepatitis B perinatally or at an early age go on to develop chronic infection. The rate of spontaneous HBsAg loss is extremely low among patients with CHB, estimated at 1% per year.[1]

CHB is traditionally separated into four phases–the immune tolerant phase, hepatitis B e antigen (HBeAg) positive immune active disease, the inactive carrier state, and HBeAg-negative immune active disease.[1] In an update to traditional terminology, the European Association for the Study of the Liver (EASL) coined the synonymous terms HBeAg-positive chronic infection, HBeAg-positive chronic hepatitis, HBeAg-negative chronic infection, and HBeAg-negative chronic hepatitis to more accurately reflect the underlying disease activity.[2] The HBeAg-positive chronic infection phase (ie, immune tolerant phase) is characterized by the presence of HBeAg, active viral replication leading to high viral loads, and normal ALT associated with no or minimal necroinflammation on liver biopsy. While there is no widely accepted HBV DNA cut-off that identifies this phase, viral loads are quite high (typically > 8 $\log_{10}$ IU/mL).[8] Patients with HBeAg-positive chronic infection may later progress to HBeAg-positive chronic hepatitis (ie, immune active disease) and develop elevated ALT levels, histologic evidence of active inflammation and progressive fibrosis. The HBeAg-negative chronic infection phase is characterized by seroconversion to positive e antibody (anti-HBe), low virus levels (<2000 IU/mL), and normal ALT; this phase represents the end of host immune activity and patients in this stage are generally considered at very low risk of liver complications. And lastly, some patients who lose HBeAg may have periods of "immune escape," or HBeAg-negative chronic hepatitis. Patients have negative HBeAg, elevated ALT, and virus levels that are higher than typical for eAg-negative patients (>2000 IU/mL). Patients may transition between phases over time–or never go through certain phases-depending on the age at initial infection and the interplay of the virus and the host immune response.

Importantly, hepatitis B is a dynamic virus and these discrete "phases" do not adequately capture the complexity of the host-virus interaction, nor do they reflect other factors that affect the risk of long-term outcomes in an individual with CHB. The main concerns for patients with CHB are HCC and progression to cirrhosis. The risk of progression is highly variable and depends on disease activity, patient demographics (increased risk with older age and male sex), and antiviral therapy. A critical determinant of disease progression and HCC risk among untreated patients is the circulating virus level. The REVEAL-HBV study was a large, prospective cohort study that enrolled untreated HBsAg-positive patients in several townships in Taiwan in the early 1990s.[6] Routine laboratory parameters were measured at study entry, including HBV DNA level. Over a 13-year follow-up period, investigators ascertained study participants for the development of HCC. Results demonstrated a strong association between HBV DNA level and HCC risk, with a stepwise gradient of risk with increasing baseline viral loads. This association persisted regardless of HBeAg status, ALT level, and presence or absence of cirrhosis. The importance of viral load as a driver of CHB outcomes is further demonstrated by the benefit of long-term viral suppression, which has been shown to improve clinical outcomes.[9–15]

Treatment criteria proposed by guidelines

Current international guidelines agree that treatment is indicated in patients who clearly have HBeAg-positive or negative chronic hepatitis and in patients with cirrhosis who have detectable virus.[1–3,16] However, there are differences in the restrictiveness of treatment recommendations and in specific ALT and HBV DNA cut-offs proposed as treatment thresholds (**Table 1**). Current frontline antiviral drugs include the nucleo(s)tide analogues entecavir, tenofovir disoproxil, and tenofovir alafenamide. These agents are highly effective at suppressing viral replication but are not able to completely eradicate the hepatitis B virus. Pegylated interferon alpha remains on the list of frontline treatment in the guidelines, but is seldom used in the United States.

Patients with HBeAg-positive chronic infection are a key group for whom guideline recommendations differ, although none advocate universal treatment of all such patients (**Table 2**). The American Association for the Study of Liver Disease (AASLD) advises against therapy for these individuals, using an ALT upper limit of normal (ULN) of 35 U/L for males and 25 U/L for females.[1] Asian Pacific Association for the Study of the Liver (APASL) guidelines also do not recommend treatment.[3] Both the AASLD and APASL guidelines allow for the treatment of patients with HBeAg-positive chronic infection if a liver biopsy shows histologic inflammation or fibrosis, but this begs the question of whether and when to biopsy these patients. The AASLD suggests close monitoring of ALT levels and-in those with persistent borderline or slightly elevated ALT-performing a liver biopsy or noninvasive fibrosis testing.[1] There is an emphasis on considering biopsy or noninvasive fibrosis assessment in patients over the age of 40 in particular. Patients with moderate-to-severe inflammation and/or fibrosis can be considered for therapy. APASL guidelines recommend noninvasive fibrosis assessment in all patients with HBeAg-positive chronic infection and obtaining biopsy if noninvasive tests suggest fibrosis.[3] If there is a family history of HCC or cirrhosis, biopsy is also recommended. In contrast, a more expansive perspective was offered in EASL guidelines, which suggested that treatment can be considered in patients with HBeAg-positive chronic infection older than 30 years *regardless* of the severity of biopsy findings.[2] Recent Chinese Society of Infectious Disease and Society of

Table 1
Summary of chronic hepatitis B treatment guidelines for patients with immune active disease and cirrhosis

	No Cirrhosis		Cirrhosis
	HBeAg positive	**HBeAg-negative**	
AASLD[a] 2018	Treat if ALT $\geq$ 2X ULN and HBV DNA > 20,000[b]	Treat if ALT $\geq$ 2X ULN and HBV DNA > 2000	Treat if any detectable HBV DNA regardless of ALT level
APASL[c] 2015	Treat if ALT > 2X ULN and HBV DNA > 20,000	Treat if ALT > 2X ULN and HBV DNA > 2000	Treat if HBV DNA > 2000 regardless of ALT level
	HBeAg-positive or negative		
EASL[d] 2017	Treat if ALT > 2X ULN and HBV DNA > 20,000		Treat if any detectable HBV DNA regardless of ALT level
WHO[e] 2015	Treat if ALT > ULN, HBV DNA > 20,000, and age > 30. If HBV DNA testing not available, consider treatment if ALT > ULN		Treat regardless of HBV DNA or ALT
Chinese Societies of Infectious Disease and Hepatology 2021[f]	Treat if ALT > ULN and HBV DNA is detectable		Treat if any detectable HBV DNA regardless of ALT level
Martin et al[g] 2021	Treat if ALT > ULN and HBV DNA > 2000		Treat regardless of HBV DNA or ALT
Dieterich et al[h] 2023	Age > 30: Treat all with HBV DNA > 2000. Age < 30: Treat all with HBV DNA > 2000 and ALT > ULN		Treat regardless of HBV DNA or ALT

Abbreviations: AASLD, American Association for the Study of Liver Disease; APASL, Asian Pacific Association for the Study of the Liver; EASL, European Association for the Study of the Liver; WHO, World Health Organization; HBeAg, hepatitis B e antigen; ALT, alanine aminotransferase; HBV, hepatitis B virus; ULN, upper limit of normal.
[a] AASLD: ALT upper limit of normal defined as 35 U/L for males and 25 U/L for females
[b] HBV DNA is expressed in IU/mL.
[c] APASL: ALT upper limit of normal defined as 40 U/L.
[d] EASL: ALT upper limit of normal defined as 40 U/L.
[e] WHO: ALT upper limit of normal defined as 30 U/L for males and 19 U/L for females
[f] ALT upper limit of normal not specified.
[g] Martin et al: ALT upper limit of normal defined as 30 U/L for males and 19 U/L for females
[h] Dieterich et al: ALT upper limit of normal defined as 30 U/L for males and 19 U/L for females

Table 2
Treatment guidelines for patients with "indeterminate" chronic hepatitis B and patients with HBeAg-positive chronic infection

| | Indeterminate | | HBeAg-Positive Chronic Infection |
	HBeAg positive	HBeAg-negative	
AASLD[a] 2018	ALT ≥ 2X ULN HBV DNA 2000–20,000[b] or ALT > ULN and < 2X ULN HBV DNA > 20,000 or ALT > ULN and < 2X ULN HBV DNA 2000–20,000 Recommendations: Treat if ≥ F2 or ≥ A3, or if persistent ALT > ULN and other causes excluded, especially if age > 40	ALT ≥ 2X ULN HBV DNA < 2000 or ALT > ULN and < 2X ULN Any HBV DNA or ALT normal HBV DNA ≥ 2000 Recommendations: If ALT ≤ ULN, monitor. If ALT > ULN, treat if ≥ F2 or ≥ A3, or if persistent ALT > ULN and other causes excluded, especially if age > 40.	Do not treat; can be considered in adults > 40 year old with liver biopsy showing significant inflammation or fibrosis
APASL[c] 2015	ALT 1-2X ULN HBV DNA > 20,000 or Any ALT HBV DNA 2000–20,000 or Any ALT HBV DNA < 2000 Recommendations: Assess fibrosis noninvasively, biopsy if evidence of fibrosis or ALT persistently > ULN or age > 35 or family hx HCC/cirrhosis, treat if moderate-severe inflammation or significant fibrosis	ALT 1-2X ULN HBV DNA > 2000 or ALT normal HBV DNA > 2000 or ALT normal or > ULN HBV DNA < 2000 Recommendations: Assess fibrosis noninvasively, biopsy if evidence of fibrosis or ALT persistently > ULN or age > 35 or family hx HCC/cirrhosis, treat if moderate-severe inflammation or significant fibrosis	Assess fibrosis noninvasively, biopsy if evidence of fibrosis or family history of HCC or cirrhosis, treat if moderate to severe inflammation or fibrosis
EASL[d] 2017	Treat if ALT > ULN, HBV DNA > 2,000, and biopsy shows moderate inflammation or fibrosis		Consider treatment if age > 30 regardless of severity of histology
WHO[e] 2015	Age > 30: ALT > ULN but HBV DNA < 20,000: Defer treatment and monitor ALT intermittently > ULN, any HBV DNA: Defer treatment and monitor		

(continued on next page)

Table 2
(continued)

	Indeterminate		HBeAg-Positive Chronic Infection
	HBeAg positive	*HBeAg-negative*	
Chinese Societies of Infectious Disease and Hepatology 2021[f]	Age < 30: ALT persistently normal, HBV DNA > 20,000: Defer treatment and monitor	ALT > ULN and HBV DNA is detectable: Treat ALT normal and HBV DNA is detectable: Treat if moderate inflammation or moderate fibrosis on biopsy, family history of cirrhosis or liver cancer and age > 30, or HBV-related extrahepatic manifestations	
Martin et al[g] 2021	ALT > ULN and HBV DNA > 2000: Treat ALT normal and HBV DNA ≥ 2000: HBeAg-negative: Treat if fibrosis present HBeAg-positive: Consider treatment based on risk factors for HCC, age, lifestyle, patient preference		
Dieterich et al[h] 2023	Age > 30: Treat all with HBV DNA > 2000 Age < 30: ALT > ULN and HBV DNA > 2000: Treat ALT normal and HBV DNA > 2000: Defer treatment and monitor		

Abbreviations: AASLD, american association for the study of liver disease; APASL, asian pacific association for the study of the liver; CHB, Chronic Hepatitis B; WHO, world health organization; EASL, european association for the study of the liver; HBeAg, hepatitis B e antigen; ALT, alanine aminotransferase; HBV, hepatitis B virus; ULN, upper limit of normal.

[a] AASLD: ALT upper limit of normal defined as 35 U/L for males and 25 U/L for females
[b] HBV DNA is expressed in IU/mL.
[c] APASL: ALT upper limit of normal defined as 40 U/L.
[d] EASL: ALT upper limit of normal defined as 40 U/L.
[e] WHO: ALT upper limit of normal defined as 30 U/L for males and 19 U/L for females
[f] ALT upper limit of normal not specified.
[g] Martin et al: ALT upper limit of normal defined as 30 U/L for males and 19 U/L for females
[h] Dieterich et al: ALT upper limit of normal defined as 30 U/L for males and 19 U/L for females

Hepatology guidelines do not explicitly advise antiviral treatment in patients with HBeAg-positive chronic infection, but suggest that treatment be considered selectively in patients aged greater than 30 years with a family history of HBV related cirrhosis or liver cancer[17] (see **Table 2**). In treatment algorithms outlined by expert panels, antiviral therapy is recommended in patients with normal ALT and HBV DNA level greater than 2000 IU/mL on a selective basis, depending on age, HCC risk factors, and patient preference[18,19] (see **Table 2**).

A large proportion of patients with CHB do not fit the traditional phases of infection and fall short of guideline criteria for antiviral therapy (see **Table 2**). The terminology used for these patients in the literature is variable, and they are sometimes referred to as patients with "gray zone" or "indeterminate" CHB. Specific ALT thresholds and HBV DNA levels used to define such patients vary across guidelines and across studies. Additionally, some authors include patients with HBeAg-positive CHB in this group[20] whereas others restrict this group to HBeAg-negative patients.[21,22] In the AASLD guidelines, patients in the gray zone are defined as those with HBeAg-negative CHB who have ALT ≥ 2X ULN but HBV DNA less than 2000 IU/mL, ALT that is elevated but < 2X ULN, or normal ALT but HBV DNA greater than 2000 IU/mL(1). The AASLD recommends pursuing non-invasive tests or liver biopsy to assess for fibrosis and/or inflammation in these patients, and in those with evidence of at least moderate fibrosis or inflammation, treatment is advised. Patients with persistently elevated ALT > ULN are also advised to be treated if they are greater than 40 year old. Patients with HBeAg-positive CHB may also fall short of treatment criteria. In current AASLD guidelines, HBeAg-positive patients with ALT ≥ 2X ULN but HBV DNA less than 20,000 – uncommon, to be sure-and patients with ALT that is elevated but < 2X ULN are advised to undergo non-invasive tests or liver biopsy, and to be treated if these demonstrate moderate-severe inflammation or fibrosis.[1] APASL guidelines are similar and recommend assessing these patients for other causes of elevated liver enzymes, assessing fibrosis noninvasively, and selectively pursuing liver biopsy in patients with fibrosis or risk factors for disease progression and HCC(3). Treatment is recommended in the setting of moderate to severe inflammation or fibrosis. EASL treatment guidelines take a more simplified approach and recommend non-invasive testing and/or liver biopsy in those with elevated ALT > ULN and HBV DNA greater than 2000 IU/mL regardless of HBeAg status, and offering treatment if there is at least moderate inflammation or moderate fibrosis.[2] Simplified treatment recommendations are also proposed by Chinese treatment guidelines and expert panels (see **Table 2**).[17–19]

Treatment of patients with HBeAg-positive chronic infection

Historically, treatment has not been advocated for patients with HBeAg-positive chronic infection, despite their very high HBV DNA levels. There are several arguments proposed. First, this phase is generally considered benign, with no inflammation or fibrosis histologically, which is thought to translate to a low risk of HCC and a low risk of disease progression while patients remain in this phase.[8] This is attributed to a tolerogenic host immune environment resulting in minimal immune response directed against HBV. Second, the treatment of patients with HBeAg-positive chronic infection is thought to be ineffective and unlikely to alter the natural history of CHB.[23] And third, there is concern that the treatment of such patients–who are usually young– necessitates long term, perhaps indefinite therapy, which sets the stage for treatment nonadherence, antiviral resistance, and treatment-related toxicities.

Several lines of evidence have led us to reconsider the notion that the HBeAg-positive chronic infection phase is benign.[24–27] Kennedy and colleagues challenged whether a state of immunologic tolerance is an accurate characterization of this phase of CHB in the first place.[5] They demonstrated that patients with HBeAg-positive infection possess peripheral HBV-specific T-cells with the capacity to expand and produce antiviral cytokines, and that the response of these T cells is in fact more robust than that of older individuals with CHB(5). Additionally, it is well known that HBV can cause liver cancer even in the absence of cirrhosis, likely because the virus itself has oncogenic potential. It has long been established that HBV DNA integrates into the host genome, which contributes to hepatic carcinogenesis through insertional mutagenesis and chromosomal alterations.[28] Insertion of viral DNA proximate to tumor promoter or suppressor genes may also disrupt the regulation of gene expression conducive to oncogenesis. And liver cancers with a high number of HBV integrations have been associated with poorer prognosis.[28] These integration events have been shown to occur in patients with HBeAg-positive infection to a similar degree as patients with HBeAg-positive chronic hepatitis (ie, immune active phase).[4] HBeAg-positive infection patients may also have more clonal hepatocyte expansion than expected from normal liver cell turnover, which could promote tumor formation.[4] Patients often stay in this phase for decades, during which such potentially oncogenic events have the ability to accumulate.

It is often assumed that the HBeAg-positive chronic infection phase is nonprogressive based on studies such as that by Hui and colleagues, who followed patients over a relatively short period of a few years.[29] However, these studies do not capture the natural history of HBV infection over decades. There are unlikely to be large studies of patients with HBeAg-positive chronic infection with sufficiently long follow-up to characterize their natural history over several decades, nor are there likely to be studies that assess the impact of viral integration on outcomes many years later. The lack of such long-term studies notwithstanding, we can still ask the question of whether, with earlier treatment initiation, we might be able to avoid the cumulative effects of HBV DNA integration and clonal hepatocyte expansion. In a study by Hsu and colleagues, data and specimens were leveraged from a randomized controlled trial that allocated treatment-naïve patients with minimally active CHB to tenofovir disoproxil versus placebo in order to determine the effect of antiviral therapy on disease progression.[30] Patients in the study underwent paired liver biopsies before treatment initiation and after receiving 3 years of treatment. The investigators quantified HBV DNA integration in the genome of 119 patients with paired liver biopsies. Several findings were noteworthy. First, the number of HBV DNA integrations appeared to correlate with markers of active viral transcription including viral RNA and quantitative HBsAg. Second, the number of integrations also correlated with the degree of viremia. And third, patients treated with tenofovir had a significantly greater reduction in the number of integrations after 3 years of treatment compared to patients treated with placebo. In vitro data has shown that tenofovir cannot directly block de novo HBV DNA integration in hepatocytes,[31] hence the authors hypothesized that their findings may be mediated by sustained inhibition of viral replication. A separate study by Chow and colleagues involved 28 patients with CHB who received nucleo(s)tide analogs and underwent liver biopsy at baseline and during follow-up.[7] The authors demonstrated that HBV DNA integration was present in all patients at baseline. The median integration frequency per liver was lower after 1 year of treatment, and was further reduced in the subset of 7 patients who had liver biopsies after 10 years of treatment. The median hepatocyte clone size was also progressively lower at 1 year and 10 years after treatment, and the median number of detectable clones also declined. These findings require further study, and the mechanisms by which nucleo(s)tide analogs lead to reduced HBV DNA integration and clonal expansion require further exploration.

However, these two studies provide a plausible scientific basis for speculating that earlier antiviral therapy may reduce the long-term risk of cancer in patients with CHB, including those with HBeAg-positive chronic infection.

A persistent concern with offering treatment to individuals with HBeAg-positive chronic infection is that treatment is ineffective when it comes to HBeAg seroconversion or HBsAg loss. A study of 162 HBeAg-positive patients with high viral load and normal ALT who received tenofovir disoproxil or tenofovir + emtricitabine showed that antiviral therapy resulted in very low rates of HBeAg seroconversion and HBsAg loss.[32] An extension of this study demonstrated a high rate of virologic relapse when antiviral therapy was stopped.[33] Prompted by the modest success of combined nucleo(s)tide analogue + interferon therapy in children with CHB,[34,35] a recent study by the Hepatitis B Research Network sought to determine the efficacy of finite duration, combination therapy in adult patients with HBeAg-positive chronic infection.[36] Patients received 8 weeks of entecavir, followed by 40 weeks of entecavir plus pegylated interferon. Treatment was discontinued after 48 weeks and patients were followed for another 48 weeks from the end of treatment. Of the 29 patients enrolled, none achieved the primary endpoint of combined HBeAg seroconversion and viral suppression at the end of the follow-up period, and nearly all had rebound in viral levels to baseline.[36]

The results of studies that demonstrate low rates of treatment-induced HBeAg seroconversion or HBsAg loss in patients without "active" liver disease-combined with the slow rate of disease progression during this phase-have led to the perpetuation of recommendations not to treat such patients. To some extent, such positions are a "holdover" from an era of finite therapy with interferon or earlier antiviral agents with poor resistance profiles. The modern perspective places greater focus on the pathogenicity of the virus and our ability to effect profound viral suppression with remarkably safe drugs and virtually no risk of emergent resistance with tenofovir or entecavir.[37] The ability to confer such profound suppression of viral replication, despite the absence of HBeAg loss, was clearly shown years ago by Chan and colleagues. In this study, 55% of patients on tenofovir and 76% of patients on tenofovir + emtricitabine achieved HBV DNA less than 69 IU/mL with over 6 $\log_{10}$ HBV DNA reductions in both treatment groups.[32] Moreover, no cases of resistance emerged during NA treatment after long-term follow-up. Similarly, in the study from the Hepatitis B Research Network, all patients who completed 48 weeks of therapy achieved HBV DNA less than 1000 IU/mL at the end of treatment.[36] Given the potential for NAs to reduce long-term cancer risk by preventing HBV DNA integration, achieving long term viral suppression seems a worthwhile endpoint irrespective of HBeAg seroconversion. In accordance with these principles, the current EASL guidelines advocate that viral suppression be considered the main endpoint for all treatment strategies.[2]

Clinical studies suggest that the biological effects of antiviral therapy outlined above may indeed translate into lower risks of adverse outcomes. Data from an observational study in Korea point to the potential risk of leaving patients with HBeAg-positive chronic infection untreated.[38] Kim and colleagues demonstrated that untreated patients in this phase had a 2- to 3-fold higher risk of HCC compared to their treated HBeAg-positive chronic hepatitis (immune active) counterparts. The cumulative incidence of HCC at 10 years was also surprisingly high at 12.7%. Notably, subsequent studies have not come to the same conclusion[39–41] and the study by Kim and colleagues has been criticized for insufficiently stringent inclusion criteria for the HBeAg-positive chronic infection group. In other words, perhaps not all patients were truly "immune tolerant" and therefore had higher HCC risk than was apparent.[42]

However, these arguments raise the question of whether there may be important practical benefits to liberalizing treatment thresholds. In real-world practice, it can be difficult to determine whether an individual has "true" HBeAg-positive infection versus HBeAg-positive hepatitis. Biochemical parameters like the ALT are only surrogate markers of underlying disease activity and the appropriate upper limit of normal is subject to debate. There is no widely agreed upon HBV DNA level to distinguish HBeAg-positive chronic infection patients. Frequent monitoring over time is challenging, and noninvasive methods of fibrosis assessment and liver biopsy are not easily accessible for all patients. A cohort of 2338 patients with CHB enrolled in the Chronic Hepatitis Cohort study was followed to determine the frequency with which they received routine monitoring laboratory tests.[43] A majority (78%) of patients had at least one ALT checked per year of follow-up, but only a minority (37%) of patients had an annual HBV DNA level assessed and a sizable proportion (18%) never had an HBV DNA checked after cohort entry. Among patients with an elevated ALT during follow-up, in only 57% of instances of elevated ALT was an HBV DNA level checked within 60 days. In an ideal setting, patients with presumed HBeAg-positive chronic infection are closely followed and have ready access to noninvasive tests or liver biopsy to ensure they do not have significant inflammation or fibrosis. This often does not occur in practice and offering antiviral therapy as the "default" approach avoids the risks associated with misclassifying patients as having HBeAg-positive chronic infection when they may actually have more active disease.

Treatment of patients with "indeterminate (gray zone)" chronic hepatitis B

Following HBeAg seroconversion, patients may enter the inactive carrier phase (ie, HBeAg-negative chronic infection).[1-3] This phase is characterized by persistently normal ALT, very low HBV DNA levels, and absence of hepatic inflammation. It is considered the end of immune-mediated liver damage and is generally associated with good prognosis. As such, antiviral therapy is typically not recommended. However, there is a risk of reactivation and patients have variable degrees of fibrosis depending on the duration and severity of liver injury that occurred during the preceding phases.[1,44] In some patients with HBeAg-negative CHB, ALT or HBV DNA may fluctuate over time and reach levels that are borderline between the HBeAg-negative chronic infection phase (ie, inactive carrier phase) and HBeAg-negative chronic hepatitis phase (ie, HBeAg-negative immune active phase). These patients are in the "gray zone" or referred to as having "indeterminate" CHB. Often lumped into the "indeterminate" nomenclature are patients with HBeAg-positive CHB who have elevated ALT but less than the threshold for treatment (typically 2X ULN by the main international guidelines) or viral levels less than the threshold for treatment. Several lines of evidence demonstrate that patients with indeterminate CHB are at risk of adverse outcomes including HCC. Expanding treatment eligibility to these patients has the potential to prevent complications in patients outside of traditional treatment criteria, who constitute a large proportion of patients with CHB.

Two cohort studies examined the distribution of phases among non-cirrhotic, treatment-naive CHB patients and found that nearly 40% patients were "indeterminate" based on ALT and HBV DNA parameters in the AASLD treatment guidelines.[20,45] Follow-up of these patients demonstrated that most remain indeterminate over time, but a substantial proportion transitioned to a different phase, including over 20% who eventually transitioned to the immune active phase warranting antiviral therapy.[20,45] In an exploratory analysis, indeterminate patients with normal ALT but high viral load had the highest likelihood of transitioning to a different phase.[45]

Studies of patients with CHB undergoing liver biopsies suggest that patients in the gray zone may also have more significant underlying liver disease than apparent based on biochemical parameters.[46–51] A study of 101 treatment naïve patients with CHB and high viral loads (>100,000 IU/mL for HBeAg-positive patients and > 10,000 IU/mL for HBeAg-negative patients) but mostly normal ALT (ULN defined as 40 U/L) demonstrated that 30% had significant histologic disease on liver biopsy, defined as stage 2 or greater fibrosis, or grade 2 or higher inflammation with stage 1 fibrosis.[46] Patients with fluctuating ALT (ie, intermittent ALT elevation to > ULN) were more likely to have a significant histologic disease than patients with persistently normal ALT levels. Similarly, Kumar and colleagues demonstrated that approximately 1/3 of patients with HBeAg-negative or HBeAg-positive CHB and intermittently elevated ALT (ULN defined as 40 U/L) had at least F2 fibrosis on liver biopsy.[48] A recent study of 242 patients in China with CHB in the gray zone demonstrated that a surprisingly high proportion (75%) of patients had a significant histologic disease, defined as at least grade 2 inflammation or stage 2 or greater fibrosis.[50] In another large cohort study from China of over 4000 patients with treatment naïve CHB, 28% of patients were classified as "gray zone" because they did not fit the typical phases of CHB as defined by the AASLD. The proportion of patients with advanced fibrosis or cirrhosis was particularly high (33%) in gray zone patients who were HBeAg-positive with elevated ALT levels but viral load less than 20,000 IU/mL.

Recognizing that many patients with indeterminate CHB can have significant underlying histologic disease, it is not surprising that long-term risks of adverse outcomes are also elevated in these patients.[20,52–54] The risk of HCC has been shown to be significant in untreated patients with indeterminate CHB and approaches the 0.2% annualized incidence agreed upon as the threshold at which HCC screening is considered cost effective.[1,20,53] In a multicenter consortium study by Huang and colleagues, the 10-year cumulative HCC incidence was 4.6% (95% CI 3.0%–7.2%) in the "indeterminate" group, compared to 0.5% (95% 0.2–1.3) in the inactive carrier group. The indeterminate phase was independently associated with a higher risk of HCC development compared to the inactive phase, with an adjusted hazard ratio of 14.1 (95% CI 1.3–153.3). A large Korean-based cohort study reported an annualized HCC incidence of 0.92% per year in untreated HBeAg-negative, non-cirrhotic patients with CHB with a viral load ≥ 2000 IU/mL and normal ALT.[53] In multivariable analysis, these patients had a higher risk of HCC compared to patients with active disease who were treated with NAs.[53] A separate Korean multicenter study reported HCC incidence rates in patients with CHB who did not meet current international guideline-based treatment recommendations.[52] The 5-year cumulative incidence of HCC was 2.1% in patients who did not meet AASLD, APASL, or EASL recommendations for treatment. Notably, of 161 incident HCCs that occurred in their cohort, 33.5% developed in patients who did not meet treatment criteria by any of these guidelines. In contrast, Bonacci and colleagues evaluated predominantly Caucasian patients with HBeAg-negative CHB who were in the gray zone and reported that only 6.3% of patients developed active disease requiring treatment, and only 1 case of HCC occurred out of 150 patients.[22] The explanation for the difference in outcomes between studies is unclear, but may be related to differences in study design such as inclusion criteria and sample size, or related to viral and patient factors such as genotype and natural history.[21]

Proposed approach to treatment

For HBeAg-positive or HBeAg-negative patients with ALT > ULN and HBV DNA greater than 2000 IU/mL, our suggestion is to offer treatment (**Fig. 1**). In those with an ALT > ULN but low HBV DNA levels less than 2000 IU/mL without another cause of elevated liver enzymes–an exceedingly rare clinical scenario in our experience–treatment can be considered. Recently, a panel of clinical experts proposed an

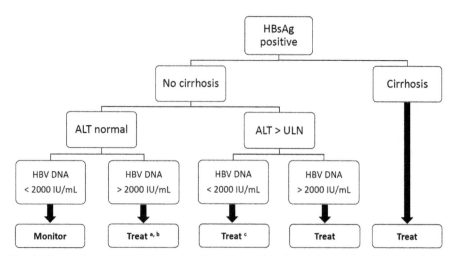

Fig. 1. Proposed approach to treatment in patients with chronic hepatitis B. [a] Includes but is not restricted to patients with HBeAg positive chronic infection (i.e., immune tolerant patients) [b] Treatment decisions should take into consideration patient preference after discussion of international guideline recommendations regarding treatment and the limitations and benefits of treatment. [c] Treat if other causes of elevated ALT have been excluded.

algorithm in which patients with HBV DNA greater than 2000 IU/mL should be treated even if ALT levels are normal[19] (see **Tables 1** and **2**), extrapolating from studies such as REVEAL in which the inflection point for HBV DNA levels correlating with long term risk of HCC was 2000 IU/mL in a population that consisted predominantly of patients with normal ALT levels at the time of enrollment into the cohort.[6] We concur to the extent that, as we propose for patients with HBeAg-positive chronic infection, HBeAg-negative patients with normal ALT levels can be apprised of the benefits and limitations of treatment and participate in informed decision-making. Patients who are not treated should have ALT levels monitored closely and should undergo non-invasive testing or liver biopsy to evaluate for fibrosis, and treatment should be considered if ALT levels become elevated or if fibrosis is present.

BENEFITS OF EXPANDING TREATMENT ELIGIBILITY

Due to the high burden of morbidity and mortality associated with viral hepatitis worldwide, there is renewed focus on hepatitis B from international organizations. The World Health Organization (WHO) has set ambitious goals of reducing new cases of viral hepatitis by 90% and reducing deaths due to viral hepatitis by 65% by the year 2030. At present, no country is on track to meet these targets.[55] While meeting viral elimination targets requires a multi-faceted approach including increased birth-dose and infant vaccination uptake along with improvements in HBV screening and linkage to care, simplifying treatment eligibility criteria and lowering treatment thresholds may go a long way toward improving treatment coverage.[19,56]

Among patients with CHB, only a minority are treatment-eligible by current international guidelines and only a fraction of those who are treatment eligible go on to receive therapy. A study utilizing data from a commercial insurance database in the United States found that in a large cohort of relatively well-educated and higher income patients with CHB, only about 50% received the necessary laboratory evaluation (ALT, HBV DNA levels, and HBeAg) to determine treatment eligibility.[57] Among those who underwent the requisite testing, only 11.2% were treatment eligible by AASLD guidelines. And of treatment eligible patients, only 65.2% actually received antiviral therapy.

The gap between treatment eligibility and actual receipt of treatment is magnified in areas that are resource poor but where there tends to be high HBV endemicity. A study by the Polaris Observatory collaborators estimated that of the 292 million HBsAg-positive individuals globally in the year 2016, 32% were treatment eligible (by WHO guidelines, see **Tables 1** and **2**) but only 5% of treatment eligible individuals actually received treatment.[58] In high-income countries (as designated by the World Bank), where the prevalence of positive HBsAg was 0.9%, only an estimated 24% of treatment eligible patients were treated. In low-income countries, where the prevalence of HBsAg positivity was 6.2%, less than 1% of treatment eligible patients were treated. The lack of screening programs contributes to these discouraging numbers, as do policies that restrict access to antiviral drugs.[59] An equally important barrier is a lack of access to routine testing. Laboratory assays required to determine treatment eligibility based on current guidelines are not widely available in many endemic areas.[59] Given these constraints, simplified approaches to treatment based on simple parameters may improve treatment coverage.[19,56,59]

Studies demonstrate that expanding treatment coverage may, in fact, be more cost-effective than more restrictive treatment criteria. A study evaluating the cost-effectiveness of treating HBeAg-positive chronic infection patients in Korea found that treatment is more cost-effective than no treatment.[60] There was improved cost-effectiveness particularly with higher HCC incidence rates and decreasing drug costs.[60] Another study from Korea evaluated the cost-effectiveness of progressively less restrictive treatment criteria.[61] The base scenario was based on Korean treatment reimbursement criteria, which covers treatment for patients with decompensated cirrhosis with any detectable viremia, compensated cirrhosis if HBV DNA is greater than 2000 IU/mL, and noncirrhotic immune active patients defined as ALT > 2X ULN or significant fibrosis or inflammation in addition to viral load requirements of greater than equal to 2000 IU/mL for HBeAg-negative individuals and greater than or equal to 20,000 IU/mL for HBeAg-positive individuals. The cost-effectiveness of changes in treatment criteria was assessed, including removing viral load restrictions for patients with cirrhosis, lowering the ALT threshold for the treatment of noncirrhotic patients to > ULN, and lastly removing ALT and HBeAg restrictions altogether and treating all patients with HBV DNA greater than 2000. IU/mL. The least restrictive scenario resulted in the greatest reduction in the incidence of decompensated cirrhosis, HCC, and liver-related death. All three scenarios were cost-effective and far below the Korean threshold for willingness to pay.

The benefits of more expansive treatment criteria extend beyond improved cost-effectiveness and reductions in the hepatic manifestations of CHB. Increasing the pool of patients who are eligible for treatment also has the potential to prevent viral transmission, all the more so in patients with HBeAg-positive chronic infection who have amongst the highest levels of viremia of any HBV-infected population. Additionally, HBV is known to be associated with several extrahepatic conditions including polyarteritis nodosa, glomerulonephritis, non-Hodgkin lymphoma, and cryoglobuline-mia.[62,63] It is generally recommended that patients with extrahepatic manifestations of CHB be treated with antiviral agents regardless of the severity of liver disease.[1] Viral suppression with antiviral agents has been proposed as a key component of treatment success in patients with autoimmune manifestations of CHB.[64,65] Among patients with HBV-related lymphoma, antivirals are essential to prevent viral flares in the setting of immunosuppressive therapy. Lastly, the expansion of treatment eligibility also has the potential to address overlooked aspects of HBV care. The burden of CHB is often measured in survival, liver-related outcomes, or cost-effectiveness, whereas the impact on patient-reported outcomes including health-related quality of life and stigma is only now being quantified.[66,67] A qualitative analysis involving individuals affected by HBV identified fear of transmission to others as a common concern, as well as experiences with stigma and discrimination in the workplace, school, or in relationships.[68] Lowering treatment thresholds could go a long way toward better addressing these important aspects of patient-centered care.

CONCLUSION-IS IT TIME TO ADOPT A TREAT ALL APPROACH?

It is our view that lowering treatment thresholds for patients with CHB is an approach that has merit. This is based on accumulating evidence linking viremia to oncogenesis in patients with CHB, the potential for nucleo(s)tide analogs to interfere with this process, and multiple cohort studies demonstrating a significant risk of long-term complications in patients who fall outside of traditional treatment criteria. Patients with HBeAg-positive chronic infection ought to be considered for treatment, or at the very least understand that this is an option. In addition to reducing the risk of HCC and decompensated liver disease, expanding treatment coverage may also reduce viral transmission and improve patient-reported outcomes related to CHB. Patients who fall short of current treatment criteria should be treated if they have an elevated ALT greater than the upper limit normal and a viral load greater than 2000 IU/mL, irrespective of histology. For patients with a normal ALT but viral load greater than 2000 IU/mL, treatment should be considered after a discussion of the benefits and limitations of treatment. Patients who are not treated need close monitoring, an assessment for fibrosis, and providers should have a low threshold to initiate treatment if fibrosis is present.

One challenge to a treat all approach is that endpoints for finite treatment duration are not widely agreed upon, and the ideal endpoint of treatment–HBsAg loss–is a rare clinical event. As such, many patients may require consideration of indefinite treatment with currently available antiviral medications. While the low risk of adverse effects and high barrier to resistance of front-line antiviral therapy makes this a palatable approach in many patients, establishing safe thresholds to stop therapy will be important, as are multiple current efforts to develop novel therapies that can effect much higher rates of HBsAg clearance ("functional cure") than are currently attainable.

In conclusion, greater consideration should be given to expanding antiviral treatment eligibility in order to reduce the overall burden of CHB.

CLINICS CARE POINTS

- The possibility of antiviral therapy should be discussed with patients with HBeAg-positive chronic infection (i.e. "immune tolerant" patients), including the potential benefits, limitations, and areas of uncertainty. There should be shared decision-making regarding whether to initiate antiviral therapy or monitor without therapy.

- Patients with an elevated ALT and a hepatitis B viral load > 2000 IU/mL should be considered for antiviral therapy.

- All patients who are not offered treatment or choose to be monitored without treatment should have ALT checked serially and should undergo periodic noninvasive testing to evaluate for fibrosis. Treatment should be considered if ALT becomes elevated after excluding other causes, or if fibrosis is present.

DECLARATION OF FUNDING SOURCES

F. Su–None, I. Jacobson–None.

DECLARATION OF PERSONAL INTERESTS

F. Su–None. I. Jacobson-Consulting: Aligos, Arbutus, Eiger, Gilead Sciences, Janssen, Roche. Research funding: Assembly, Janssen, Roche; Data Monitoring Committee: GSK.

AUTHORS' CONTRIBUTIONS AND AUTHORSHIP STATEMENT

F. Su–drafting and critical revision, I.M. Jacobson–drafting and critical revision.

REFERENCES

1. Terrault NA, Lok ASF, McMahon BJ, et al. Update on prevention, diagnosis, and treatment of chronic hepatitis B: AASLD 2018 hepatitis B guidance. Hepatology 2018;67:1560–99.
2. European Association for the Study of the Liver. Electronic address eee, European association for the study of the L. EASL 2017 clinical practice guidelines on the management of hepatitis B virus infection. J Hepatol 2017;67:370–98.
3. Sarin SK, Kumar M, Lau GK, et al. Asian-Pacific clinical practice guidelines on the management of hepatitis B: a 2015 update. Hepatol Int 2016;10:1–98.
4. Mason WS, Gill US, Litwin S, et al. HBV DNA integration and clonal hepatocyte expansion in chronic hepatitis B patients considered immune tolerant. Gastroenterology 2016;151:986–998 e984.
5. Kennedy PTF, Sandalova E, Jo J, et al. Preserved T-cell function in children and young adults with immune-tolerant chronic hepatitis B. Gastroenterology 2012; 143:637–45.
6. Chen CJ, Yang HI, Su J, et al. Risk of hepatocellular carcinoma across a biological gradient of serum hepatitis B virus DNA level. JAMA 2006;295:65–73.
7. Chow N, Wong D, Lai CL, et al. Effect of antiviral treatment on hepatitis B virus integration and hepatocyte clonal expansion. Clin Infect Dis 2023;76:e801–9.
8. Tseng TC, Kao JH. Treating immune-tolerant hepatitis B. J Viral Hepat 2015;22: 77–84.
9. Papatheodoridis GV, Chan HL, Hansen BE, et al. Risk of hepatocellular carcinoma in chronic hepatitis B: assessment and modification with current antiviral therapy. J Hepatol 2015;62:956–67.
10. Okada M, Enomoto M, Kawada N, et al. Effects of antiviral therapy in patients with chronic hepatitis B and cirrhosis. Expert Rev Gastroenterol Hepatol 2017;11: 1095–104.
11. Lok AS, McMahon BJ, Brown RS Jr, et al. Antiviral therapy for chronic hepatitis B viral infection in adults: a systematic review and meta-analysis. Hepatology 2016; 63:284–306.
12. Liaw YF, Sung JJ, Chow WC, et al. Lamivudine for patients with chronic hepatitis B and advanced liver disease. N Engl J Med 2004;351:1521–31.
13. Zoutendijk R, Reijnders JG, Zoulim F, et al. Virological response to entecavir is associated with a better clinical outcome in chronic hepatitis B patients with cirrhosis. Gut 2013;62:760–5.
14. Wu CY, Lin JT, Ho HJ, et al. Association of nucleos(t)ide analogue therapy with reduced risk of hepatocellular carcinoma in patients with chronic hepatitis B: a nationwide cohort study. Gastroenterology 2014;147:143–151 e145.

15. Kim SS, Hwang JC, Lim SG, et al. Effect of virological response to entecavir on the development of hepatocellular carcinoma in hepatitis B viral cirrhotic patients: comparison between compensated and decompensated cirrhosis. Am J Gastroenterol 2014;109:1223–33.

16. (WHO) WHO. Guidelines for the prevention, care and treatment of persons with chronic hepatitis B infection.

17. Wang G, Duan Z. Guidelines for prevention and treatment of chronic hepatitis B. J Clin Transl Hepatol 2021;9:769–91.

18. Martin P, Nguyen MH, Dieterich DT, et al. Treatment algorithm for managing chronic hepatitis B virus infection in the United States: 2021 update. Clin Gastroenterol Hepatol 2022;20:1766–75.

19. Dieterich DT, Graham C, Wang S, et al. It is time for a simplified approach to hepatitis B elimination. Gastro Hep Advances 2023;2:209–18.

20. Huang DQ, Li X, Le MH, et al. Natural history and hepatocellular carcinoma risk in untreated chronic hepatitis B patients with indeterminate phase. Clin Gastroenterol Hepatol 2022;20:1803–1812 e1805.

21. Bonacci M, Forns X, Lens S. The HBeAg-negative "gray zone" phase: a frequent condition with different outcomes in western and asian patients? Clin Gastroenterol Hepatol 2020;18:263–4.

22. Bonacci M, Lens S, Marino Z, et al. Anti-viral therapy can be delayed or avoided in a significant proportion of HBeAg-negative Caucasian patients in the Grey Zone. Aliment Pharmacol Ther 2018;47:1397–408.

23. Wong GL. Management of chronic hepatitis B patients in immunetolerant phase: what latest guidelines recommend. Clin Mol Hepatol 2018;24:108–13.

24. Dolman GE, Koffas A, Mason WS, et al. Why, who and when to start treatment for chronic hepatitis B infection. Curr Opin Virol 2018;30:39–47.

25. Howell J, Chan HLY, Feld JJ, et al. Closing the stable door after the horse has bolted: should we Be treating people with immune-tolerant chronic hepatitis B to prevent hepatocellular carcinoma? Gastroenterology 2020;158:2028–32.

26. Koffas A, Mak LY, Gill US, et al. Early Treatment Consideration in Patients with Hepatitis B 'e' Antigen-Positive Chronic Infection: is It Time for a Paradigm Shift? Viruses 2022;14.

27. Koffas A, Petersen J, Kennedy PT. Reasons to consider early treatment in chronic hepatitis B patients. Antiviral Res 2020;177:104783.

28. Peneau C, Imbeaud S, La Bella T, et al. Hepatitis B virus integrations promote local and distant oncogenic driver alterations in hepatocellular carcinoma. Gut 2022;71:616–26.

29. Hui CK, Leung N, Yuen ST, et al. Natural history and disease progression in Chinese chronic hepatitis B patients in immune-tolerant phase. Hepatology 2007;46:395–401.

30. Hsu YC, Suri V, Nguyen MH, et al. Inhibition of viral replication reduces transcriptionally active distinct hepatitis B virus integrations with implications on host gene dysregulation. Gastroenterology 2022;162:1160–1170 e1161.

31. Tu T, Budzinska MA, Vondran FWR, et al. Hepatitis B virus DNA integration occurs early in the viral life cycle in an in vitro infection model via sodium taurocholate cotransporting polypeptide-dependent uptake of enveloped virus particles. J Virol 2018;92.

32. Chan HL, Chan CK, Hui AJ, et al. Effects of tenofovir disoproxil fumarate in hepatitis B e antigen-positive patients with normal levels of alanine aminotransferase and high levels of hepatitis B virus DNA. Gastroenterology 2014;146:1240–8.

33. Wong VW, Hui AJ, Wong GL, et al. Four-year outcomes after cessation of tenofovir in immune-tolerant chronic hepatitis B patients. J Clin Gastroenterol 2018;52: 347–52.

34. D'Antiga L, Aw M, Atkins M, et al. Combined lamivudine/interferon-alpha treatment in "immunotolerant" children perinatally infected with hepatitis B: a pilot study. J Pediatr 2006;148:228–33.

35. Poddar U, Yachha SK, Agarwal J, et al. Cure for immune-tolerant hepatitis B in children: is it an achievable target with sequential combo therapy with lamivudine and interferon? J Viral Hepat 2013;20:311–6.

36. Feld JJ, Terrault NA, Lin HS, et al. Entecavir and Peginterferon Alfa-2a in Adults With Hepatitis B e Antigen-Positive Immune-Tolerant Chronic Hepatitis B Virus Infection. Hepatology 2019;69:2338–48.

37. Martin P. Immune-tolerant hepatitis B: maybe a misnomer but still hard to treat. Hepatology 2019;69:2315–7.

38. Kim GA, Lim YS, Han S, et al. High risk of hepatocellular carcinoma and death in patients with immune-tolerant-phase chronic hepatitis B. Gut 2018;67:945–52.

39. Jeon MY, Kim BK, Lee JS, et al. Negligible risks of hepatocellular carcinoma during biomarker-defined immune-tolerant phase for patients with chronic hepatitis B. Clin Mol Hepatol 2021;27:295–304.

40. Lee HA, Lee HW, Kim IH, et al. Extremely low risk of hepatocellular carcinoma development in patients with chronic hepatitis B in immune-tolerant phase. Aliment Pharmacol Ther 2020;52:196–204.

41. Lee HW, Chon YE, Kim BK, et al. Negligible HCC risk during stringently defined untreated immune-tolerant phase of chronic hepatitis B. Eur J Intern Med 2021; 84:68–73.

42. Zhou K, Terrault N. Immune tolerant HBV and HCC: time to revise our tolerance levels for therapy? AME Med J 2018;3.

43. Spradling PR, Xing J, Rupp LB, et al. Infrequent clinical assessment of chronic hepatitis B patients in United States general healthcare settings. Clin Infect Dis 2016;63:1205–8.

44. Koffas A, Kumar M, Gill US, et al. Chronic hepatitis B: the demise of the 'inactive carrier' phase. Hepatol Int 2021;15:290–300.

45. Di Bisceglie AM, Lombardero M, Teckman J, et al. Determination of hepatitis B phenotype using biochemical and serological markers. J Viral Hepat 2017;24: 320–9.

46. Nguyen MH, Garcia RT, Trinh HN, et al. Histological disease in Asian-Americans with chronic hepatitis B, high hepatitis B virus DNA, and normal alanine aminotransferase levels. Am J Gastroenterol 2009;104:2206–13.

47. Lai M, Hyatt BJ, Nasser I, et al. The clinical significance of persistently normal ALT in chronic hepatitis B infection. J Hepatol 2007;47:760–7.

48. Kumar M, Sarin SK, Hissar S, et al. Virologic and histologic features of chronic hepatitis B virus-infected asymptomatic patients with persistently normal ALT. Gastroenterology 2008;134:1376–84.

49. Ren S, Wang W, Lu J, et al. Effect of the change in antiviral therapy indication on identifying significant liver injury among chronic hepatitis B virus infections in the grey zone. Front Immunol 2022;13:1035923.

50. Wang J, Yan X, Zhu L, et al. Significant histological disease of patients with chronic hepatitis B virus infection in the grey zone. Aliment Pharmacol Ther 2023;57:464–74.

51. Yao K, Liu J, Wang J, et al. Distribution and clinical characteristics of patients with chronic hepatitis B virus infection in the grey zone. J Viral Hepat 2021;28: 1025–33.
52. Sinn DH, Kim SE, Kim BK, et al. The risk of hepatocellular carcinoma among chronic hepatitis B virus-infected patients outside current treatment criteria. J Viral Hepat 2019;26:1465–72.
53. Choi GH, Kim GA, Choi J, et al. High risk of clinical events in untreated HBeAg-negative chronic hepatitis B patients with high viral load and no significant ALT elevation. Aliment Pharmacol Ther 2019;50:215–26.
54. Lee HW, Kim SU, Park JY, et al. Prognosis of untreated minimally active chronic hepatitis B patients in comparison with virological responders by antivirals. Clin Transl Gastroenterol 2019;10:e00036.
55. Blach S, Razavi-Shearer D, Mooneyhan E, et al. Updated evaluation of global progress towards HBV and HCV elimination, preliminary data through 2021. Hepatology 2022;76:S1–1564.
56. Hsu YC, Huang DQ, Nguyen MH. Global burden of hepatitis B virus: current status, missed opportunities and a call for action. Nat Rev Gastroenterol Hepatol 2023. https://doi.org/10.1038/s41575-023-00760-9.
57. Ye Q, Kam LY, Yeo YH, et al. Substantial gaps in evaluation and treatment of patients with hepatitis B in the US. J Hepatol 2022;76:63–74.
58. Polaris Observatory C. Global prevalence, treatment, and prevention of hepatitis B virus infection in 2016: a modelling study. Lancet Gastroenterol Hepatol 2018;3: 383–403.
59. Lemoine M, Thursz MR. Battlefield against hepatitis B infection and HCC in africa. J Hepatol 2017;66:645–54.
60. Kim HL, Kim GA, Park JA, et al. Cost-effectiveness of antiviral treatment in adult patients with immune-tolerant phase chronic hepatitis B. Gut 2021;70:2172–82.
61. Lim YS, Ahn SH, Shim JJ, et al. Impact of expanding hepatitis B treatment guidelines: a modelling and economic impact analysis. Aliment Pharmacol Ther 2022; 56:519–28.
62. Cacoub P, Asselah T. Hepatitis B virus infection and extra-hepatic manifestations: a systemic disease. Am J Gastroenterol 2022;117:253–63.
63. Mazzaro C, Adinolfi LE, Pozzato G, et al. Extrahepatic manifestations of chronic HBV infection and the role of antiviral therapy. J Clin Med 2022;11.
64. Guillevin L, Mahr A, Callard P, et al. Hepatitis B virus-associated polyarteritis nodosa: clinical characteristics, outcome, and impact of treatment in 115 patients. Medicine (Baltim) 2005;84:313–22.
65. Mazzaro C, Bomben R, Visentini M, et al. Hepatitis B virus-infection related cryoglobulinemic vasculitis. Clinical manifestations and the effect of antiviral therapy: a review of the literature. Front Oncol 2023;13:1095780.
66. Younossi ZM, Stepanova M, Younossi I, et al. Development and validation of a hepatitis B-specific health-related quality-of-life instrument: CLDQ-HBV. J Viral Hepat 2021;28:484–92.
67. Yendewa GA, Sellu EJ, Kpaka RA, et al. Measuring stigma associated with hepatitis B virus infection in Sierra Leone: validation of an abridged Berger HIV stigma scale. J Viral Hepat 2023;30:621–9.
68. Freeland C, Racho R, Kamischke M, et al. Health-related quality of life for adults living with hepatitis B in the United States: a qualitative assessment. J Patient Rep Outcomes 2021;5:121.

Are the New Nucleos(t)ide Analogs Better than the Old Nucleos(t)ide Analogs?

Jonggi Choi, MD, PhD[1], Won-Mook Choi, MD, PhD[1],
Young-Suk Lim, MD, PhD*

KEYWORDS

- Lamivudine • Adefovir • Entecavir • Tenofovir • Hepatitis B
- Hepatocellular carcinoma

KEY POINTS

- The absolute number of liver cancer cases due to hepatitis B virus (HBV) increased by 106.6% between 1990 and 2016 at the global level; at this rate, global deaths from hepatocellular carcinoma (HCC) due to HBV are projected to double by 2040.
- Since lamivudine (LAM) was first introduced for the treatment of CHB, several additional nucleos(t)ide analog agents (NUCs), namely, adefovir, clevudine, telbivudine, entecavir (ETV), besifovir dipivoxil maleate, tenofovir disoproxil fumarate (TDF), and tenofovir alafenamide (TAF) have been approved.
- Intermediate surrogate endpoints, such as virological, biochemical, and serological biomarkers, that are easy to assess, occur frequently, and are considered to correlate with clinical outcomes, have been used for the evaluation of treatment efficacy and approval of the drugs.
- The aim of this narrative review is to comprehensively compare the effectiveness of different NUCs in terms of the virological response, risk of death or transplantation and HCC in patients with chronic HBV infection.

INTRODUCTION

An estimated 262 million individuals worldwide have chronic hepatitis B virus (HBV) infection (CHB), which is the most common cause of hepatocellular carcinoma (HCC).[1–3] HCC is the most common form of primary liver cancer, which is the third leading cause of cancer-related death. The absolute number of liver cancer cases due to HBV increased by 106.6% between 1990 and 2016 at the global level[4]; at this rate, global deaths from HCC due to HBV are projected to double by 2040.[1,5]

Department Gastroenterology, Asan Medical Center, University of Ulsan College of Medicine, 88, Olympic-ro 43-gil, Songpa-gu, Seoul 05505, Republic of Korea
[1] Equally contributed to this study and deserve cofirst authorship.
* Corresponding author.
E-mail address: limys@amc.seoul.kr

Clin Liver Dis 27 (2023) 809–818
https://doi.org/10.1016/j.cld.2023.05.005
1089-3261/23/© 2023 Elsevier Inc. All rights reserved.

liver.theclinics.com

Although HCC develops in up to 25% of patients with CHB without antiviral treatment,[6] long-term antiviral treatment with oral nucleos(t)ide analog agents (NUCs) can reduce the risk of HCC by 50% in immune-active patients with CHB.[7] Nonetheless, on-treatment HCC risk persists,[8] thus making it important to identify the factors associated with on-treatment HCC risk in patients with CHB.

Since lamivudine (LAM) was first introduced for the treatment of CHB, several additional NUCs, namely, adefovir, clevudine, telbivudine, entecavir (ETV), besifovir dipivoxil maleate, tenofovir disoproxil fumarate (TDF), and tenofovir alafenamide (TAF) have been approved. Among the NUCs, the use of adefovir is associated with potential nephrotoxicity and bone toxicity. Clevudine and telbivudine have potential muscle toxicity and have not been widely used. Furthermore, clevudine and besifovir are approved only in a few countries, such as Korea and the Phillipines. Consequently, most of the data have been accumulated for the long-term use of LAM, ETV, TDF, and TAF. A randomized placebo-controlled trial showed that when compared with no treatment, LAM significantly reduces mortality and prevents HCC in patients with CHB and advanced liver disease.[9] However, ETV, TDF, and TAF are more potent than LAM in terms of suppressing HBV replication with a minimal risk of resistance. Thus, ETV and tenofovir have been recommended as first-line agents for CHB by most clinical practice guidelines during the last several decades.[10–12]

Ideally, for hepatitis B therapies to be approved, they should demonstrate efficacy in preventing HCC and liver-related deaths. However, these clinical endpoints evolve over years or decades. Therefore, intermediate surrogate endpoints, such as virological, biochemical, and serological biomarkers, that are easy to assess, occur frequently, and are considered to correlate with clinical outcomes, have been used for the evaluation of treatment efficacy and approval of the drugs. Consequently, the question whether LAM, ETV, TDF, and TAF have different effects on reducing the clinical events, such as death or HCC, has remained unanswered until recently. Randomized controlled trials may provide the highest level of evidence to address this topic. However, they are unlikely to be conducted given the length of follow-up time and number of patients required. Therefore, comparative effectiveness studies based on large-scale historical cohorts may be the only realistic way on this topic if biases and confounders are adequately controlled. In fact, historical cohort studies from clinical databases may better reflect real-world practice.

Therefore, the aim of this narrative review is to comprehensively compare the effectiveness of different NUCs in terms of the virological response, risk of death or transplantation and HCC in patients with CHB.

VIROLOGICAL RESPONSE AND DRUG-RESISTANCE

In treatment-naïve patients with CHB, ETV, TDF, and TAF have a minimal or no risk of drug-resistance. These 3 NUCs are highly potent inducing high rate of virologic response (reducing serum HBV DNA to levels undetectable by polymerase chain reaction assays) in most treatment-naïve patients.[13–18] However, in patients who were refractory to an earlier LAM treatment, the rate of ETV-resistance increases up to 51% after 5 years of ETV treatment, which is in striking contrast to a 1.2% resistance rate in NUC-naive patients.[19,20] This difference is because the ETV resistance barrier is lowered by the initial selection of the LAM-resistant HBV mutation, rtM204V/I.[21] In contrast, there has been virtually no case who developed clinically meaningful resistance to TDF or TAF so far.[15,22] Furthermore, our randomized trials have demonstrated that monotherapy with TDF can provide a successful virological response in most of the heavily pretreated patients with multidrug resistance to ETV or adefovir.[23–26]

TAF has also demonstrated high anti-HBV efficacy similar to TDF in randomized trials of treatment-naïve and treatment-experienced patients with CHB.[16,17,27] Additionally, we reproduced the effect of TAF in multidrug-resistant patients by a randomized trial.[28,29] In the patients with resistance to ETV and/or adefovir, switching to TAF from TDF maintained a high rate of virological response (99%), which was comparable to the continuation of TDF during a 48-week treatment period,[28] and was maintained during 3-years of TAF treatment.[29]

ALT NORMALIZATION

Considerable attention has been given to on-treatment alanine aminotransferase (ALT) normalization because several recent studies have shown that the rate of ALT normalization would be different among patients using different NUCs, and that early on-treatment ALT normalization is associated with clinical outcomes.

In two phase 3 trials comparing TAF with TDF,[16–18] the rate of ALT normalization was significantly higher in the TAF group than in the TDF group at all time points. Even after excluding the risk factors for metabolic syndrome in the analysis, the TAF group still had a significantly higher ALT normalization rate than the TDF group (57% vs 42%, respectively).[17,18] Interestingly, in our recent historical cohort study, TDF treatment was associated with a significantly higher rate of ALT normalization at 1 year of treatment and a significantly lower risk of HCC compared with ETV treatment.[30]

A large-scale cohort study from Hong Kong suggested that ALT normalization at 1 year of NUC treatment was associated with a lower risk of liver-related events in patients with CHB.[31] Our study from Korea confirmed the importance of earlier ALT normalization upon NUC treatment initiation. Earlier on-treatment ALT normalization was independently associated with incrementally decreased HCC risk in patients with CHB who received treatment with either ETV or TDF, irrespective of baseline fatty liver or cirrhosis and achievement of virologic response during treatment.[32] Compared with ALT normalization within 6 months of treatment, delayed ALT normalization at 6 to 12 (adjusted hazard ratio [aHR]: 1.40, $P < .001$), 12 to 24 (aHR: 1.74, $P < .001$), and greater than 24 months (aHR: 2.45, $P < .001$) was associated with incrementally increased on-treatment HCC risk.

Whether the difference in the rate of on-treatment ALT normalization among NUCs is directly linked with lower HCC incidence should be explored by further studies.

LONG-TERM SAFETY OF NUCLEOS(T)IDE ANALOG AGENT TREATMENTS

TAF is a prodrug of tenofovir, exhibits higher stability in plasma than TDF. Therefore, treatment with TAF has demonstrated lower renal and bone toxicity than TDF in randomized trials of patients with CHB.[16,17] Switching to TAF from TDF was associated with a reduced decline in renal function and reduced loss of bone mineral density compared with the continuation of TDF.[27,28,33] However, increases in body weight and cholesterol levels with TAF treatment after switching from TDF were reported by short-term studies.[33–35] Thus, longer term research was required to investigate the impact of these complex safety signals with TAF treatment in the patients with CHB.

In our recent 3-year trial with TAF in CHB patients with multidrug-resistant HBV, the early increases in body weight (median 1.1 kg) and cholesterol levels during the first 48 weeks after switching to TAF from TDF were not progressive during 144 weeks of continued TAF treatment, which was consistent with the findings of the previous observational studies.[35] Furthermore, the total/high-density lipoprotein (HDL) cholesterol ratio decreased after the switch to TAF from TDF. Notably, the total/HDL cholesterol ratio is considered a better cardiovascular disease predictor than a single lipid profile, such as total and LDL cholesterol.[36]

Previous trials reported that TDF treatment caused decreases in total, HDL, LDL cholesterol, and triglyceride levels compared with TAF treatment.[16,17,27,28] A recent observational study also found that a significant decrease in the total cholesterol level was noted at 48 weeks with TDF treatment.[37,38] However, no significant difference in the cholesterol levels was identified between the TAF-treated group and no-treatment control groups at 48 weeks in these studies. Therefore, the differences in lipid profiles between the TAF-treatment and TDF-treatment are thought to be due to a lipid-lowering effect of TDF rather than the lipid-raising effect of TAF.[27,39] It is unclear whether TAF has weight-gaining effect or TDF has weight-losing effect, and the underlying mechanisms and long-term clinical outcomes associated with the changes in body weight with TAF treatment require additional study. The association between metabolic changes with TAF treatment and the risk of cardiovascular events may have to be verified in a large-scale longer-term study in the future.

ECOLOGICAL STUDIES FOR THE MORTALITY BY LIVER DISEASE AND LIVER CANCER

A population-based study conducted in Korea where HBV is endemic revealed that liver disease mortality has fallen by about 65% during the previous 2 decades.[40] In contrast, liver cancer mortality has increased for 18% throughout the same period as measured by crude death rate and the absolute number of death by HCC. This divergence between liver disease and liver cancer mortality coincided with the sharp increase in annual prescriptions of NUCs, especially LAM and ETV, and the increasing life expectancy of patients with liver disease.[40] Marked reduction in liver disease mortality by widespread use of NUCs against HBV may increase the life expectancy and number of patients at risk of developing liver cancer, inadvertently leading to an increased burden of liver cancer in a HBV-endemic population. The competing nature between death from liver disease and that from liver cancer should be carefully considered in establishing a health-care policy.

HEPATOCELLULAR CARCINOMA RISK: ENTECAVIR VERSUS LAMIVUDINE OR ADEFOVIR (ADV)

Our large-scale cohort study including 5374 patients with CHB showed that, compared with LAM treatment, ETV therapy was associated with a significantly lower risk of death or transplantation, which was well expected considering the higher virologic response by ETV.[41] By contrast, unexpectedly, ETV was no better than LAM at reducing the risk of HCC. A randomized controlled trial including 12,378 patients with CHB also demonstrated no significant difference in HCC incidence between ETV and non-ETV (71.7% adefovir) therapies during 10 years of follow-up evaluation.[42]

HEPATOCELLULAR CARCINOMA RISK: ENTECAVIR VERSUS TENOFOVIR DISOPROXIL FUMARATE

Our study using the nationwide cohort and the large-scale single-center validation cohort first reported that TDF is superior to ETV in preventing HCC.[30] Since then, a heated debate has erupted over which drug is superior for preventing HCC. Of note, all studies that have compared the risk of HCC between the 2 drugs have either supported TDF[43,44] or found no discernible differences.[45–47] No study has shown the opposite direction of favoring ETV over TDF. Even the studies reporting no statistical difference in HCC risk between the treatments showed a lower hazard ratio for HCC with TDF. This suggests the presence of a beta error, likely due to small number of HCC events, in those studies.

Yet, the debate has expanded to the meta-analyses. Eighteen meta-analyses have been published between December 2019 and February 2023. Although the meta-analyses included similar primary studies, their statistical significance and clinical interpretation differed. Whereas most meta-analyses, including ours, suggested that TDF is better than ETV in preventing HCC and should be the preferred option for CHB,[48–56] others concluded that there is no difference between the 2 drugs.[57] Although randomized-controlled trials are considered the highest standard of evidence for evaluating treatment efficacy, it is not feasible to address this topic, making it heavily reliant on data from observational studies. However, observational studies can be constrained by heterogeneous methodologies and patient populations, resulting in within-study and between-study heterogeneities that may lead to varying conclusions in previous meta-analyses. In light of this, individual patient data (IPD) meta-analyses could provide a solution to the difficulties faced by aggregate data meta-analyses by using a consistent methodological approach across data from multiple studies.[58] Our recent IPD meta-analysis, which collected IPD from 11 studies including 42,939 patients from Korea, Hong Kong, and Taiwan, confirmed that TDF-treated patients have a significantly lower risk of HCC than ETV-treated patients (aHR, 0.77; 95% confidence interval, 0.61–0.98). The HCC incidence started to diverge after 2.5 years of follow-up between the 2 treatment groups in this study.[59]

HEPATOCELLULAR CARCINOMA RISK: TENOFOVIR ALAFENAMIDE VERSUS TENOFOVIR DISOPROXIL FUMARATE

Pooled data from global and Chinese phase 3 trials with more than 1600 patients suggested that TAF seemed to have a lower HCC risk as well as earlier ALT normalization than TDF during treatment.[60] We and others using real-world data found no significant difference in HCC risk between TDF and TAF treatment.[61,62] However, considering the risk of beta error in those studies caused by small number of HCC events, further larger scale and longer follow-up studies are warranted in the near future to determine whether there is a difference in the risk of HCC between TAF and TDF.

HEPATOCELLULAR CARCINOMA RECURRENCE: ENTECAVIR VERSUS TENOFOVIR DISOPROXIL FUMARATE

Several studies have addressed the different effects of NUCs for the tertiary prevention of HCC after curative-intent treatment. Our recent study, which included 1695 patients with very early or early HBV-associated HCC, showed that TDF treatment is associated with a lower risk of HCC recurrence after curative-intent surgical resection than ETV treatment.[63] Intriguingly, the difference in risk for late recurrence (occurring 2 or more years after resection; hazard ratio, 0.68) was more prominent than that for early recurrence (occurring within 2 years after resection; hazard ratio, 0.79). It is generally accepted that most early recurrence within 2 years of hepatectomy results from dissemination of the primary tumor, whereas most late recurrence after 2 years of hepatectomy stems from de novo recurrence of tumors spontaneously originating in the remaining liver.[64,65] Therefore, the more prominent differences in recurrence rates after 2 years of hepatectomy between the 2 treatment groups might stem from their differences in the preventive effect on de novo HCC recurrence. Although some studies supported the findings of our study,[66,67] others found no differences between the 2 drugs.[68,69] A recent meta-analysis on this topic concluded that TDF treatment is associated with a 27% lower risk of HCC recurrence than ETV treatment after curative-intent treatment of HCC.[70] Of note, TDF reduces the risk of late recurrence (aHR, 0.73; 95% confidence interval, 0.65–0.81) but not early recurrence (aHR, 0.88; 95% confidence interval, 0.76–1.02).[70]

SUMMARY

Conducting randomized-controlled trials to evaluate the different effects of various NUCs on hard clinical outcomes such as HCC development would be practically impossible due to the substantial amount of time and resources required. Therefore, we must rely on well-designed, high-quality observational studies with minimized potential bias to address these issues. In the current landscape, where the use of old NUCs has become less prevalent and is not recommended by clinical practice guidelines, it may not be clinically meaningful to compare the different effects on HCC prevention between old and new NUCs. Instead, it would be more important to perform studies on the differences in HCC prevention among the new NUCs. Interestingly, it should be noted that observational studies comparing TDF and ETV in both secondary and tertiary preventive settings so far have indicated one direction favoring TDF over ETV or no direction. Virtually, no high-quality studies have indicated the opposite direction, favoring ETV over TDF. TAF seems to perform at least as well as TDF in HCC risk reduction.

CONFLICT OF INTERESTS

Y-S. Lim is an advisory board member of Gilead Sciences. All other authors have declared that no conflict of interest exists.

ROLE OF FUNDING SOURCE

This study was supported by grants from the Patient-Centered Clinical Research Coordinating Center (PACEN; grant number HC20C0062) of the National Evidence-based Healthcare Collaborating Agency and the National R&D Program for Cancer Control through the National Cancer Center (grant number: HA21C0110), funded by the Ministry of Health & Welfare, Republic of Korea. The funding sources had no role in the design of this study, its execution, analyses, interpretation of the data, or decision to submit the results.

REFERENCES

1. Dusheiko G, Agarwal K, Maini MK. New approaches to chronic hepatitis B. N Engl J Med 2023;388:55–69.
2. Cui F, Blach S, Manzengo Mingiedi C, et al. Global reporting of progress towards elimination of hepatitis B and hepatitis C. Lancet Gastroenterol Hepatol 2023;8: 332–42.
3. Luxenburger H, Neumann-Haefelin C. Liver-resident CD8+ T cells in viral hepatitis: not always good guys. J Clin Invest 2023;133:e165033.
4. Liu Z, Jiang Y, Yuan H, et al. The trends in incidence of primary liver cancer caused by specific etiologies: results from the global burden of disease study 2016 and implications for liver cancer prevention. J Hepatol 2019;70:674–83.
5. European Association for the Study of the Liver. EASL clinical practice guidelines: management of hepatocellular carcinoma. J Hepatol 2018;69:182–236.
6. Nordenstedt H, White DL, El-Serag HB. The changing pattern of epidemiology in hepatocellular carcinoma. Dig Liver Dis 2010;42:S206–14.

7. Lok AS, McMahon BJ, Brown RS Jr, et al. Antiviral therapy for chronic hepatitis B viral infection in adults: a systematic review and meta-analysis. Hepatology 2016; 63:284–306.
8. Papatheodoridis GV, Chan HL, Hansen BE, et al. Risk of hepatocellular carcinoma in chronic hepatitis B: assessment and modification with current antiviral therapy. J Hepatol 2015;62:956–67.
9. Liaw YF, Sung JJ, Chow WC, et al. Lamivudine for patients with chronic hepatitis B and advanced liver disease. N Engl J Med 2004;351:1521–31.
10. Lampertico P, Agarwal K, Berg T, et al. EASL 2017 clinical practice guidelines on the management of hepatitis B virus infection. J Hepatol 2017;67:370–98.
11. Terrault NA, Lok ASF, McMahon BJ, et al. Update on prevention, diagnosis, and treatment of chronic hepatitis B: AASLD 2018 hepatitis B guidance. Hepatology 2018;67:1560–99.
12. Korean Association for the Study of the L. KASL clinical practice guidelines for management of chronic hepatitis B. Clin Mol Hepatol 2019;25:93–159.
13. Kitrinos KM, Corsa A, Liu Y, et al. No detectable resistance to tenofovir disoproxil fumarate after 6 years of therapy in patients with chronic hepatitis B. Hepatology 2014;59:434–42.
14. Chang TT, Lai CL, Kew Yoon S, et al. Entecavir treatment for up to 5 years in patients with hepatitis B e antigen-positive chronic hepatitis B. Hepatology 2010;51: 422–30.
15. Cathcart AL, Chan HL, Bhardwaj N, et al. No resistance to tenofovir alafenamide detected through 96 weeks of treatment in patients with chronic hepatitis B infection. Antimicrob Agents Chemother 2018;62. 010644-18.
16. Agarwal K, Brunetto M, Seto WK, et al. 96weeks treatment of tenofovir alafenamide vs. tenofovir disoproxil fumarate for hepatitis B virus infection. J Hepatol 2018;68:672–81.
17. Chan HLY, Fung S, Seto WK, et al. Tenofovir alafenamide versus tenofovir disoproxil fumarate for the treatment of HBeAg-positive chronic hepatitis B virus infection: a randomised, double-blind, phase 3, non-inferiority trial. Lancet Gastroenterol Hepatol 2016;1:185–95.
18. Buti M, Gane E, Seto WK, et al. Tenofovir alafenamide versus tenofovir disoproxil fumarate for the treatment of patients with HBeAg-negative chronic hepatitis B virus infection: a randomised, double-blind, phase 3, non-inferiority trial. Lancet Gastroenterol Hepatol 2016;1:196–206.
19. Tenney DJ, Rose RE, Baldick CJ, et al. Two-year assessment of entecavir resistance in Lamivudine-refractory hepatitis B virus patients reveals different clinical outcomes depending on the resistance substitutions present. Antimicrob Agents Chemother 2007;51:902–11.
20. Tenney DJ, Rose RE, Baldick CJ, et al. Long-term monitoring shows hepatitis B virus resistance to entecavir in nucleoside-naive patients is rare through 5 years of therapy. Hepatology 2009;49:1503–14.
21. Tenney DJ, Levine SM, Rose RE, et al. Clinical emergence of entecavir-resistant hepatitis B virus requires additional substitutions in virus already resistant to Lamivudine. Antimicrob Agents Chemother 2004;48:3498–507.
22. Liu Y, Corsa AC, Buti M, et al. No detectable resistance to tenofovir disoproxil fumarate in HBeAg+ and HBeAg- patients with chronic hepatitis B after 8 years of treatment. J Viral Hepat 2017;24:68–74.
23. Lim YS, Byun KS, Yoo BC, et al. Tenofovir monotherapy versus tenofovir and entecavir combination therapy in patients with entecavir-resistant chronic hepatitis B with multiple drug failure: results of a randomised trial. Gut 2016;65:852–60.

24. Lim YS, Yoo BC, Byun KS, et al. Tenofovir monotherapy versus tenofovir and entecavir combination therapy in adefovir-resistant chronic hepatitis B patients with multiple drug failure: results of a randomised trial. Gut 2016;65:1042–51.

25. Lim YS, Lee YS, Gwak GY, et al. Monotherapy with tenofovir disoproxil fumarate for multiple drug-resistant chronic hepatitis B: 3-year trial. Hepatology 2017;66: 772–83.

26. Lim YS, Gwak GY, Choi J, et al. Monotherapy with tenofovir disoproxil fumarate for adefovir-resistant vs. entecavir-resistant chronic hepatitis B: a 5-year clinical trial. J Hepatol 2019;71:35–44.

27. Lampertico P, Buti M, Fung S, et al. Switching from tenofovir disoproxil fumarate to tenofovir alafenamide in virologically suppressed patients with chronic hepatitis B: a randomised, double-blind, phase 3, multicentre non-inferiority study. Lancet Gastroenterol Hepatol 2020;5:441–53.

28. Byun KS, Choi J, Kim JH, et al. Tenofovir alafenamide for drug-resistant hepatitis B: a randomized trial for switching from tenofovir disoproxil fumarate. Clin Gastroenterol Hepatol 2022;20:427–437 e5.

29. Choi J, Lim YS, Kim JH, et al. Tenofovir alafenamide for multiple drug-resistant chronic hepatitis B: a 3-year clinical trial. Clin Gastroenterol Hepatol 2023. Online ahead of print.

30. Choi J, Kim HJ, Lee J, et al. Risk of hepatocellular carcinoma in patients treated with entecavir vs tenofovir for chronic hepatitis B: a Korean nationwide cohort study. JAMA Oncol 2019;5:30–6.

31. Wong GL, Chan HL, Tse YK, et al. Normal on-treatment ALT during antiviral treatment is associated with a lower risk of hepatic events in patients with chronic hepatitis B. J Hepatol 2018;69:793–802.

32. Choi J, Kim GA, Han S, et al. Earlier alanine aminotransferase normalization during antiviral treatment is independently associated with lower risk of hepatocellular carcinoma in chronic hepatitis B. Am J Gastroenterol 2020;115:406–14.

33. Lim YS, Seto WK, Kurosaki M, et al. Review article: switching patients with chronic hepatitis B to tenofovir alafenamide-a review of current data. Aliment Pharmacol Ther 2022;55:921–43.

34. Surial B, Mugglin C, Calmy A, et al. Weight and metabolic changes after switching from tenofovir disoproxil fumarate to tenofovir alafenamide in people living with HIV : a cohort study. Ann Intern Med 2021;174:758–67.

35. Ogawa E, Nakamuta M, Koyanagi T, et al. Switching to tenofovir alafenamide for nucleos(t)ide analogue-experienced patients with chronic hepatitis B: week 144 results from a real-world, multi-centre cohort study. Aliment Pharmacol Ther 2022;56:713–22.

36. Quispe R, Elshazly MB, Zhao D, et al. Total cholesterol/HDL-cholesterol ratio discordance with LDL-cholesterol and non-HDL-cholesterol and incidence of atherosclerotic cardiovascular disease in primary prevention: the ARIC study. Eur J Prev Cardiol 2020;27:1597–605.

37. Lin HY, Tseng TC. Dyslipidemia in chronic hepatitis B patients on tenofovir alafenamide: Facts and puzzles. Clin Mol Hepatol 2022;28:181–2.

38. Jeong J, Shin JW, Jung SW, et al. Tenofovir alafenamide treatment may not worsen the lipid profile of chronic hepatitis B patients: a propensity score-matched analysis. Clin Mol Hepatol 2022;28:254–64.

39. Arribas JR, Thompson M, Sax PE, et al. Brief report: randomized, double-blind comparison of tenofovir alafenamide (TAF) vs tenofovir disoproxil fumarate (TDF), each coformulated with elvitegravir, cobicistat, and emtricitabine (E/C/F)

for Initial HIV-1 treatment: week 144 results. J Acquir Immune Defic Syndr 2017; 75:211–8.

40. Choi J, Han S, Kim N, et al. Increasing burden of liver cancer despite extensive use of antiviral agents in a hepatitis B virus-endemic population. Hepatology 2017;66:1454–63.

41. Lim YS, Han S, Heo NY, et al. Mortality, liver transplantation, and hepatocellular carcinoma among patients with chronic hepatitis B treated with entecavir vs lamivudine. Gastroenterology 2014;147:152–61.

42. Hou JL, Zhao W, Lee C, et al. Outcomes of long-term treatment of chronic HBV infection with entecavir or other agents from a randomized trial in 24 countries. Clin Gastroenterol Hepatol 2020;18:457–67.

43. Yip TC, Wong VW, Chan HL, et al. Tenofovir is associated with lower risk of hepatocellular carcinoma than entecavir in patients with chronic HBV infection in China. Gastroenterology 2020;158:215–25.e6.

44. Ha Y, Chon YE, Kim MN, et al. Hepatocellular carcinoma and death and transplantation in chronic hepatitis B treated with entecavir or tenofovir disoproxil fumarate. Sci Rep 2020;10:13537.

45. Kim SU, Seo YS, Lee HA, et al. A multicenter study of entecavir vs. tenofovir on prognosis of treatment-naive chronic hepatitis B in South Korea. J Hepatol 2019; 71:456–64.

46. Lee SW, Kwon JH, Lee HL, et al. Comparison of tenofovir and entecavir on the risk of hepatocellular carcinoma and mortality in treatment-naive patients with chronic hepatitis B in Korea: a large-scale, propensity score analysis. Gut 2020;69: 1301–8.

47. Papatheodoridis GV, Dalekos GN, Idilman R, et al. Similar risk of hepatocellular carcinoma during long-term entecavir or tenofovir therapy in Caucasian patients with chronic hepatitis B. J Hepatol 2020;73:1037–45.

48. Choi WM, Choi J, Lim YS. Effects of tenofovir vs entecavir on risk of hepatocellular carcinoma in patients with chronic HBV infection: a systematic review and meta-analysis. Clin Gastroenterol Hepatol 2021;19:246–58.e9.

49. Dave S, Park S, Murad MH, et al. Comparative effectiveness of entecavir versus tenofovir for preventing hepatocellular carcinoma in patients with chronic hepatitis B: a systematic review and meta-Analysis. Hepatology 2021;73:68–78.

50. Jeong S, Cho Y, Park SM, et al. Differential effectiveness of tenofovir and entecavir for prophylaxis of hepatocellular carcinoma in chronic hepatitis B patients depending on coexisting cirrhosis and prior exposure to antiviral therapy: a systematic review and meta-analysis. J Clin Gastroenterol 2021;55:e77–86.

51. Teng YX, Li MJ, Xiang BD, et al. Tenofovir may be superior to entecavir for preventing hepatocellular carcinoma and mortality in individuals chronically infected with HBV: a meta-analysis. Gut 2020;69:1900–2.

52. Liu H, Shi Y, Hayden JC, et al. Tenofovir treatment has lower risk of hepatocellular carcinoma than entecavir treatment in patients with chronic hepatitis B: a systematic review and meta-analysis. Liver Cancer 2020;9:468–76.

53. Li M, Lv T, Wu S, et al. Tenofovir versus entecavir in lowering the risk of hepatocellular carcinoma development in patients with chronic hepatitis B: a critical systematic review and meta-analysis. Hepatol Int 2020;14:105–14.

54. Gu L, Yao Q, Shen Z, et al. Comparison of tenofovir versus entecavir on reducing incidence of hepatocellular carcinoma in chronic hepatitis B patients: a systematic review and meta-analysis. J Gastroenterol Hepatol 2020;35:1467–76.

55. Cheung KS, Mak LY, Liu SH, et al. Entecavir vs tenofovir in hepatocellular carcinoma prevention in chronic hepatitis B infection: a systematic review and meta-analysis. Clin Transl Gastroenterol 2020;11:e00236.
56. Zhang Z, Zhou Y, Yang J, et al. The effectiveness of TDF versus ETV on incidence of HCC in CHB patients: a meta analysis. BMC Cancer 2019;19:511.
57. Tseng CH, Hsu YC, Chen TH, et al. Hepatocellular carcinoma incidence with tenofovir versus entecavir in chronic hepatitis B: a systematic review and meta-analysis. Lancet Gastroenterol Hepatol 2020;5:1039–52.
58. Choi WM, Yip TC, Lim YS, et al. Methodological challenges of performing meta-analyses to compare the risk of hepatocellular carcinoma between chronic hepatitis B treatments. J Hepatol 2022;76:186–94.
59. Choi WM, Yip TC, Wong GL, et al. Hepatocellular carcinoma risk in patients with chronic hepatitis B receiving tenofovir- vs. entecavir-based regimens: individual patient data meta-analysis. J Hepatol 2023;78:534–42.
60. Lim Y, Chan HLY, Seto W, et al. Impact of treatment with Tenofovir Alafenamide (Taf) or Tenofovir Disoproxil fumarate (Tdf) on hepatocellular carcinoma (Hcc) incidence in patients with chronic hepatitis B (Chb), In The 70th Annual Meeting of the American Association for the Study of Liver Diseases (AASLD): The Liver Meeting 2019, John Wiley & Sons, Inc. The Journal's web site is located at http://www..., 2019.
61. Lim J, Choi WM, Shim JH, et al. Efficacy and safety of tenofovir alafenamide versus tenofovir disoproxil fumarate in treatment-naive chronic hepatitis B. Liver Int 2022;42:1517–27.
62. Lee HW, Cho YY, Lee H, et al. Effect of tenofovir alafenamide vs. tenofovir disoproxil fumarate on hepatocellular carcinoma risk in chronic hepatitis B. J Viral Hepat 2021;28:1570–8.
63. Choi J, Jo C, Lim YS. Tenofovir versus entecavir on recurrence of hepatitis B virus-related hepatocellular carcinoma after surgical resection. Hepatology 2021;73:661–73.
64. Imamura H, Matsuyama Y, Tanaka E, et al. Risk factors contributing to early and late phase intrahepatic recurrence of hepatocellular carcinoma after hepatectomy. J Hepatol 2003;38:200–7.
65. Chen YJ, Yeh SH, Chen JT, et al. Chromosomal changes and clonality relationship between primary and recurrent hepatocellular carcinoma. Gastroenterology 2000;119:431–40.
66. Tsai MC, Wang CC, Lee WC, et al. Tenofovir is superior to entecavir on tertiary prevention for BCLC Stage 0/A hepatocellular carcinoma after curative resection. Liver Cancer 2022;11:22–37.
67. Qi W, Shen J, Dai J, et al. Comparison of nucleoside and nucleotide analogs in the recurrence of hepatitis B virus-related hepatocellular carcinoma after surgical resection: a multicenter study. Cancer Med 2021;10:8421–31.
68. Lee JH, Kim BK, Park SY, et al. The efficacies of entecavir and tenofovir in terms of enhancing prognosis after curative treatment of hepatitis B virus-related hepatocellular carcinoma. Eur J Intern Med 2021;89:48–55.
69. Wang XH, Hu ZL, Fu YZ, et al. Tenofovir vs. entecavir on prognosis of hepatitis B virus-related hepatocellular carcinoma after curative resection. J Gastroenterol 2022;57:185–98.
70. Giri S, Agrawal D, Afzalpurkar S, et al. Tenofovir versus entecavir for tertiary prevention of hepatocellular carcinoma in chronic hepatitis B infection after curative therapy: a systematic review and meta-analysis. J Viral Hepat 2023;30:108–15.

What Is the Current Status of Hepatitis B Virus Viro-Immunology?

Carolina Boni, MD[a,1,*], Marzia Rossi, PhD[b,1], Ilaria Montali, PhD[b,1],
Camilla Tiezzi, BSc[b], Andrea Vecchi, BSc[a], Amalia Penna, PhD[a],
Sara Doselli, BSc[b], Valentina Reverberi, BSc[a],
Camilla Ceccatelli Berti, PhD[b], Anna Montali, PhD[b],
Simona Schivazappa, MD[a], Diletta Laccabue, BSc[b],
Gabriele Missale, MD[a,b], Paola Fisicaro, PhD[a,*]

KEYWORDS

- Chronic HBV infection • T-cell exhaustion • Antigen load • HBsAg level
- Checkpoint inhibitors

KEY POINTS

- Adaptive immune responses play a crucial role in antiviral protection during the resolution of acute hepatitis B.
- The natural course of hepatitis B virus (HBV) infection is associated with the evolution of the host immune response.
- In the context of the recently reviewed stages of chronic HBV infection, the previously called "immune tolerant" phase has been renamed "HBeAg + chronic infection," because HBV patients in this phase have been shown to be immune active.
- In patients with chronic HBV infection, virus-specific T and B cells are dysfunctional.
- Different factors contribute to the immunologic impairment in chronic HBV infection including the prolonged exposure to viral antigens, upregulation of co-inhibitory receptors, T-cell intracellular pathways defects, and the multiple regulatory mechanisms active within the liver.

Funding: This work was supported by a grant from the Italian Ministry of Health (Ricerca Finalizzata RF 2013-02359333), by a PRIN project from the Italian Ministry of the University and Research (protocol code n. 2017MPCWPY), and by a grant from the European Union's Horizon 2020 research and innovation programme (grant agreement no. 848223).
[a] Unit of Infectious Diseases and Hepatology, Azienda Ospedaliero-Universitaria di Parma, Parma, Italy; [b] Department of Medicine and Surgery, University of Parma, Parma, Italy
[1] These authors contributed equally to this work.
* Corresponding authors. Laboratory of Viral Immunopathology, Unit of Infectious Diseases and Hepatology, Azienda Ospedaliero-Universitaria di Parma, Via Gramsci 14, Parma 43126, Italy.
E-mail addresses: cboni@ao.pr.it (C.B.); pfisicaro@ao.pr.it (P.F.)

Clin Liver Dis 27 (2023) 819–836
https://doi.org/10.1016/j.cld.2023.05.001
1089-3261/23/© 2023 Elsevier Inc. All rights reserved.

INTRODUCTION

Chronic hepatitis B (CHB) is a major global public problem because at least 262 million people are chronically infected with hepatitis B virus (HBV).[1] There is therefore an increasing need to develop new curative therapeutic strategies as solicited by the World Health Organization, which has set a goal of eliminating hepatitis B and C by 2030.[2] Acute HBV infection acquired in adults is generally self-limited and in most cases asymptomatic, although the risk of chronic persistence of the virus is very high when the infection is contracted at birth or in the perinatal period.[3] The resolution of acute hepatitis B is strongly associated with maximal efficiency of HBV-specific T-cell responses, whereas at the early stage of infection, the innate immune response is poorly activated. Viral clearance involves a robust and efficient adaptive T-cell response immediately after the onset of active viral replication predominantly sustained by early non-cytolytic clearance of HBV.[4,5] When the acute infection evolves into chronicity, HBV-specific T cells are defective in their antiviral activity, with typical functional defects of HBV-specific T cells undergoing T-cell exhaustion up to physical deletion.[6] Also, natural killer (NK) cell function seems to be impaired showing a functional dichotomy because in most of the reports NK cell cytotoxicity results to be preserved, whereas NK cell capacity to produce IFN-γ and TNF-α has been described as defective, making NK cells more pathogenic than protective in chronic HBV infection.[7] More recently, hepatitis B surface antigen (HBsAg)-specific B cells from chronic patients have been studied and characterized by an "atypical" memory B-cell phenotype, with a reduced functionality and failure to mature in anti-HBs-producing cells in vitro.[8,9]

THE NATURAL HISTORY OF HEPATITIS B VIRUS INFECTION IS CLOSELY DEPENDENT ON THE DYNAMIC INTERPLAY BETWEEN THE HOST IMMUNE RESPONSE AND VIRAL REPLICATION

The natural course of chronic HBV infection reflects the dynamic interplay between the host immune response and the viral replication.[10] Chronic HBV infection advances through different clinical phases based on the serum HBV-DNA, alanine aminotransferase (ALT) levels, and HBsAg and HBeAg condition until achieving functional cure with undetectable circulating HBsAg and HBV-DNA, which happens rarely in the natural history of infection either spontaneously or induced by current therapy. However, even after recovery from acute or chronic HBV infection, minute amounts of virus persists within the liver which are probably responsible for long-lasting T-cell responses and the persistence of anti-HBs antibodies.[11,12] The classical segregation of the natural history phases of chronic HBV infection is entirely based on virological and biochemical profiles and still retains important clinical implications for the management of patients and for choosing the most appropriate treatment.[3,13] However, the strength and quality of HBV-specific T-cell response in CHB patients is not clearly associated with the schematic CHB classification likely due to the high heterogeneity of HBV-specific T cells.[14–18]

The early phase, named HBeAg-positive chronic infection and previously termed "immune tolerant," is connoted by HBeAg positivity, high levels of HBV-DNA and HBsAg, and normal ALT. HBV-specific responses have been always assumed to be heavily inhibited in this phase, but recent data challenge this concept showing that HBV-specific T-cell responses can be comparable to those detected in the immune active phase of infection.[19,20] Finally, also the concept of the benign nature of this phase has been called into question showing that HBV-DNA integration and clonal hepatocyte expansion can already occur early in infection and start at this stage predisposing infected patients to severe evolutions of infection, such as cirrhosis and hepatocellular carcinoma (HCC).[21] For all these reasons, time for starting antiviral therapy should be reconsidered and immune modulatory interventions should be taken into account also in young patients with HBeAg + chronic infection.

The HBeAg-positive chronic hepatitis stage, also called "Immune active," is characterized by HBeAg positivity and high HBV-DNA and ALT levels and represents the natural transition from the previous immuno-tolerance phase. During this period, most patients can present HBeAg seroconversion and continue toward the inactive carrier phase or can directly progress to HBeAg-negative chronic hepatitis.

The inactive carrier phase, now named HBeAg-negative chronic infection, is typically defined by the presence of serum anti-hepatitis B e-antigen (HBe) antibodies and persistently low viral and antigen load associated with normal transaminase values. Interestingly, in the setting of natural human HBV infection, a hierarchy of T-cell functional efficiency was described in different conditions of HBV control in relation to serum HBsAg concentrations. For example, maximal T-cell functional efficiency was observed in the resolution phase of an acute self-limited hepatitis, associated with complete control of infection and lack of HBsAg in the serum, followed by intermediate levels of T-cell functionality in chronic inactive carriers with partial control of infection and low levels of HBsAg.[22]

Instead, maximal impairment of T-cell responses was detected in patients during the HBeAg-negative chronic hepatitis phase characterized by high or fluctuating levels of viremia and ALT. In this patient population with persistent viremia and liver inflammation, exhausted HBV-specific CD8 T cells are broadly heterogeneous.[22] Characterization of their functional impairment allows distinguishing patients with different capacity to control infection and likely to respond to immune modulatory compounds in vitro.[14] This observation implies that the management of chronic patients and their selection for possible immunomodulatory therapy is complex given the heterogeneity of exhausted HBV-specific CD8 T cells and highlights the importance of identifying T cell-based predictors of response to immune reconstitution therapies.[23]

VIRAL FEATURES AND GENOTYPES

The HBV is a noncytopathic, hepatotropic, DNA virus, targeting hepatocytes through attachment to the sodium taurocholate-cotransporting peptide receptor.[24] Virions consist of a lipid bilayer, including the HBsAg antigenic component and an icosahedral nucleocapsid, composed of the hepatitis B core (HBc) protein, which encloses the viral polymerase and the partially double-stranded genomic DNA (HBV-DNA). Besides virions, a large excess of incomplete, spherical, or filamentous noninfectious subviral particles are secreted into the patient's serum, as a likely viral strategy to divert and exhaust the host immune response. HBV genome codes for four partially overlapping open reading frames, corresponding to the structural and nonstructural proteins of the virion. The S gene, comprising the pre-S1, pre-S2, and S regions, encodes for the three envelope proteins (large, middle, and small) from three different translation start codons, all containing the S sequence, which is referred to as the S domain (HBsAg).[25] HBsAg detection is routinely tested for the diagnosis of HBV infection and for monitoring patients undergoing nucleos(t)ide analog therapy (NUC). The C gene, comprising the precore/core gene, encodes for the nucleocapsid protein and the secretory antigen HBeAg. The precore sequence contains a 29-amino acid peptide which gives rise to a 22-kDa precore-derivative protein (p22) following removal of the first 19 amino acids. The simultaneous detection of serum HBcAg, HBeAg, and p22 proteins, all sharing an identical 149-amino acid sequence, is referred to as

HBc-related antigen (HBcrAg). Elevated serum HBcrAg levels have been found associated with viral transcriptional activity in the liver.[26,27] Finally, the P and X genes code, respectively, for the viral polymerase, which represents the largest viral protein and displays reverse transcriptase activity and for the X protein (HBx), with regulatory functions of viral replication and transcription.

HBV shows wide genetic plasticity mainly due to the absence of reverse transcriptase proofreading capacity resulting in the high occurrence of mutations and high replicative activity. Analysis of genetic variability of HBV reveals the presence of nine genotypes distributed worldwide ranging from A to J, in turn containing different subgenotypes.[28] Although the real impact on the disease outcome still remains unclear, the main clinical relevance of HBV genotypes lies in the different response to treatments and in the clinical course. Pegylated-interferon-alfa therapy has been reported to show more efficacies in CHB patients infected with genotype A as indicated by the higher probability to achieve HBsAg loss.[29,30] Moreover, patients infected with genotypes A and D undergoing nucleo(s)tide analogs suspension display higher rate of HBsAg clearance.[31] HBV genotypes are also associated with clinical factors because genotype C has been linked with HCC.[32]

IMMUNOLOGIC IMPAIRMENT IN CHRONIC HEPATITIS B VIRUS INFECTION

"Functional cure" is defined as a sustained loss of HBsAg and HBV DNA from the serum, with or without anti-HBs seroconversion after a finite course of therapy, with the persistence of low amounts of intrahepatic covalently closed circular DNA (cccDNA) and HBV DNA integration. HBV cure is the ideal goal of antiviral treatment, but it is difficult to achieve with current therapies.[33,34] One of the main causes that promotes viral persistence is the lasting exposure to high antigen load, which is believed to play a critical role in immune impairment.[35,36] In particular, both T-and B-cell responses are defective in chronic HBV infection as well as the innate response, which results inefficient.[4,5,37]

The decrease in the antiviral efficiency of virus-specific T lymphocytes observed in patients chronically infected with HBV is believed to contribute to viral persistence.[38] Prolonged exposure to viral antigens leads to the progressive loss of effector functions in a phenomenon known as T lymphocyte "exhaustion." Functionally impaired CD8 T cells were first described in the late 1990s, in the mouse model of chronic lymphocytic choriomeningitis mammarenavirus (LCMV) infection, showing that virus-specific CD8 T cells were unable to efficiently process effector functions.[39] Subsequently, this dysfunctional response has also been characterized in various chronic infections, including CHB.[39,40]

Associated with the progressive loss of T-cell effector function and proliferative potential, several distinctive cellular and functional features of the exhausted phenotype have been recognized, including a distorted cell metabolism, an epigenetic program distinct from that of effector and memory T cells, the altered expression and use of transcription factors, and the high expression of multiple co-inhibitory receptors.[39,40]

In addition, as a further factor contributing to viral persistence, the liver displays an "immunosuppressive" environment, affecting the ability of the immune system to control HBV[41] (**Fig. 1**).

The Role of Antigen Burden and Persistence in T-Cell Exhaustion

Persistently elevated antigen expression levels are closely associated with T-cell dysfunction (see **Fig. 1**). In particular, the amount of antigen expressed by liver cells is believed to influence the fate of effector CD8 cells. A first clear evidence of the

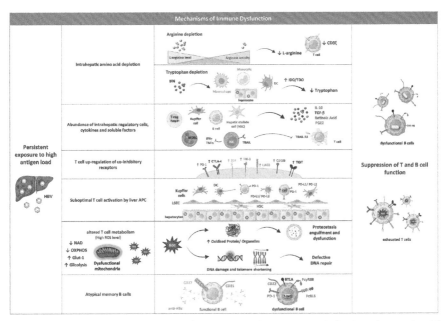

Fig. 1. Mechanisms of immune dysfunction in chronic HBV infection (created with BioRender.com).

role of antigen load within the liver was provided by using a recombinant adeno-associated viral vector system, in which a selective antigen expression was induced in mouse hepatocytes in vivo. In this model, only frequencies lower than 25% of antigen-expressing hepatocytes can induce long-term CD8 T-cell function, whereas in the presence of high percentage of transduced hepatocytes, virus-specific CD8 T cells become less responsive up to T-cell exhaustion and deletion.[42,43] Studies performed in chronic HBV patients have revealed a hierarchy of T-cell functional responsiveness in different clinical conditions of HBV infection and control linked to serum HBsAg concentrations, with maximal T-cell functionality in patients achieving HBsAg clearance following an acute self-limited hepatitis. At the opposite in patients with high levels of viremia and antigenemia T-cell responses are maximally dysfunctional. In addition, in long-term NUC-treated patients, an improved T-cell reactivity can be detected as a likely result of viral load drop and liver inflammation resolution, with better T-cell enhancement in patients who achieved sustained loss of serum HBsAg and anti-HBs seroconversion.[22]

Evidence that high antigenic load represents a barrier to HBV cure was further supported by experiments performed in a mouse model of persistent HBV infection, where in mice with high antigen level therapeutic vaccination was unable to induce envelope and core-specific CD8 T-cell responses in the spleen and in the liver, whereas expansion of antiviral T-cell responses and control of infection were obtained on vaccination in mice harboring low or intermediate antigen levels.[44]

Interestingly, HBV-specific T-cell functions were efficiently restored by therapeutic vaccination also in highly antigenemic mice but only after the decline of hepatic antigen expression by RNA interference. This evidence allowed proposing a sequential strategy based first on antigen decrease by antiviral treatment, followed by heterologous prime-boost vaccination, with protein priming to induce CD4- and B-cell-mediated responses followed by Modified vaccinia Ankara virus vector boosting to optimize CD8 induction.[45] However, recent studies performed in different mouse models of HBV infection have debated the evidence that high levels of antigen expression can impact on CD8 T-cell responses. Specifically, HBV core expression by 100% hepatocytes induced CD8 T-cell dysfunction, whereas a strong reduction in the levels of hepatocellular core Ag expression was per se not sufficient to elicit effector T-cell differentiation.[46] This study pointed to antigen presentation as a crucial factor inducing T-cell dysfunction rather than high antigen levels, because hepatocyte T cell priming promoted a dysfunctional T-cell differentiation program, whereas antigen presentation by Kupffer cells allowed T-cell differentiation into effector T cells.[47] These conclusions were further supported by another study where both mice with elevated serum HBsAg titers and animals that reached HBsAg clearance showed comparable levels of cluster of differentiation 8 (CD8) T-cell responses.[48] Finally, a recent study has shown that patients' age was inversely correlated with HBs-specific T-cell responses, suggesting that the duration of infection and HBsAg exposure, rather than the amount of antigen, may represent a critical factor inducing progressive decline of HBs-specific T cells in chronic HBV infection. These results highlighted the possibility that earlier treatments may be more beneficial for HBsAg loss.[20]

Upregulation of Co-Inhibitory Receptors

During acute infections, overexpressed inhibitory receptors play a role in containing the intensity of the immune response, thus preventing excessive tissue damage, and return to a lower expression level when the pathogen is eliminated. Instead, in chronic infection, many of these receptors, such as PD-1, T-cell immunoglobulin domain and Mucin domain 3 (TIM-3), cytotoxic T lymphocyte antigen 4 (CTLA4), 2B4, lymphocyte-activation gene 3 (LAG3), and CD160, have been found to be stably upregulated, thus contributing to peripheral tolerance establishment by inhibiting T lymphocytes proliferation and function.[39]

The first inhibitory receptor to be described is PD-1, which recognizes two ligands, programmed death ligand 1 (PD-L1) and PD-L2, expressed by immune and non-immune cells or only by dendritic cells (DCs), macrophages, and germinal center B cells, respectively.[49] On binding, tyrosine residues on the cytoplasmic domain of PD-1 become phosphorylated, resulting in the recruitment of the phosphatase SHP-2, which then reduces the activation of downstream signaling intermediates, leading to a reduction in both cytokine production and T lymphocyte proliferation.[50–53] PD-1 signaling imprints also a modification to T-cell metabolism, by inhibiting glycolysis and amino acid transport while enhancing fatty acid β-oxidation.[52] Moreover, in PD-1[high] tumor-infiltrating T cells, mitochondria result greatly dysfunctional, with lower mitochondrial membrane potential, higher mass, and abnormal morphology.[54,55]

In addition to PD-1, other inhibitory receptors that negatively regulate T-cell functions are also expressed.[56] One of these is CTLA-4, a member of the CD28 family, shown to inhibit T lymphocyte activation by competing with the costimulatory molecule CD28 for binding to B7 receptors and by inhibiting glycolysis.[57,58]

In general, co-expression of several inhibitory receptors on T cells indicates a deeper state of exhaustion. As an example, Tim-3 (T-cell immunoglobulin and mucin-domain containing-3) co-expression with PD-1 can identify virus-specific T cells less functional than those expressing PD-1 alone in chronic LCMV infection.[56,59]

As in other chronic infections, also in chronic HBV infection, co-inhibitory receptors have been found significantly upregulated and associated to functional impairment on CD8 and CD4 T cells,[60–67] with maximal overexpression in the intrahepatic compartment[61,62,68] (see **Fig. 1**). However, it is now well-known that the virus-specific T-cell population is not uniformly exhausted, as PD-1 expression by T cells to different HBV epitopes, such as to $core_{18-27}$ and $pol_{455-463}$, did not result proportional to the degree of their functional impairment, which has been detected to be higher in polymerase-specific cells.[16] Moreover, different expression levels of co-inhibitory receptors, together with differentiation markers and transcription factors, have been found associated to various degrees of T-cell dysfunction even within the same T-cell specificity.[18] Interestingly, the co-expression of PD-1 with other markers, such as CD127, TOX, CD39, and Bcl-2, allowed calculating the exhaustion level of HBV-core-specific CD8 T cells from different treatment naïve CHB patients, which inversely correlates with their cytokine production capacity. Of note, such "Exhaustion Score" turned out to be useful to predict the likelihood to respond in vitro to immune modulation.[14]

In chronic HBV infection, high expression of co-inhibitory receptors has been associated to functional impairment also in case of B cells,[9] particularly those specific for the viral envelope,[69] which resulted in an atypical differentiation stage, with altered signaling, homing, survival, and function.[8] Blocking the PD-1/PD-L1 inhibitory signaling could partially restore the B-cell function, as previously shown also for T cells.[6,9]

Intracellular Pathways Defects in Exhausted T Cells

Different studies have been performed to assess whether blockade of inhibitory receptors, such as PD-1, can allow restoring the T-cell function,[6] but the general conclusion is that in chronic HBV infection, this strategy can only allow a partial improvement of the T-cell function. To identify specific defects that could represent new molecular targets for correction of T-cell dysregulation, HBV-specific CD8 T cells isolated from patients with an active CHB were tested in a transcriptomic approach.[70] By gene set enrichment analysis of such data, general gene downregulation resulted to be the prevalent transcriptional phenotype of exhausted HBV-specific CD8 cells compared with functional HBV-specific cells from patients who spontaneously resolved an acute hepatitis B.[70]

The most significantly downregulated biological processes were related to the mitochondrial function, the proteasome, DNA repair, and transcription. In addition, a relevant set of negative transcriptional regulators, such as histone deacetylase 1 (HDAC1), for example, resulted upregulated, contributing to further amplification of gene silencing.[70]

Downregulated genes associated with mitochondria were related to metabolism, such as the Krebs cycle and fatty acid β-oxidation, transmembrane transporters, mitochondria fission, and fusion and to the electron transport chain, with oxidative phosphorylation (OXPHOS).[70] These findings confirmed previous results evidencing a metabolic unbalance in exhausted HBV-specific CD8 cells that were dependent by glucose metabolism, because poorly able to use OXPHOS for their energy needs.[71]

Moreover, a significantly higher percentage of lymphocytes with depolarized mitochondria were detected among virus-specific CD8 cells from chronic HBV patients than in controls, together with significantly higher mitochondrial reactive oxygen species (ROS) content.[70,71] As a further confirmation of the key role of ROS in the T-cell dysfunction, mitochondria-targeted antioxidant compounds led to a significant improvement of the T-cell antiviral function.[70] Interestingly, culturing HBV-specific T cells in the presence of such antioxidants allowed also to improve telomeres' length, which had been detected significantly shorter in HBV as compared with influenza (FLU)-specific control CD8 cells, witnessing a faster induction of senescence in exhausted T cells.[72] ROS overproduction is expected to induce damage to cellular components, including proteins and DNA. Indeed, when cellular proteostasis was studied, an accumulation of intracellular aggresomes was observed, as well as a defective upregulation of the autophagosome marker LC3 when cells were treated with chloroquine, suggesting a higher accumulation of intracellular aggregates and a less efficient proteostasis function[73] (see **Fig. 1**).

The induction of elevated DNA damage in conjunction with an altered function of some mediators of the DNA damage response was also detected, including a reduced poly-(ADP-ribose) polymerization (PARylation) by the poly-(adenosine diphosphate [ADP]-ribose) polymerases (PARPs).[72] The latter are DNA damage sensors activated by DNA lesions that catalyze PARylation using NAD molecules as donors of ADP-ribose monomers to recruit several DNA damage factors to the sites of the DNA lesions.[74] High DNA damage should stimulate a DNA repair response, which resulted instead defective, leading to persistent DNA repair activation with potential NAD depletion by PARP enzymes.[72] This would be further enhanced by the enzymatic activity of the upregulated CD38, the major cellular NAD consumer,[75] which expression indeed resulted inversely correlated with the T-cell antiviral function, as well as to PARylation levels.[72] Moreover, NAD decrease can potentially lead to diminished acetyl-CoA availability for the tricarboxylic acid cycle (TCA) cycle and then for energy production but also for histone acetylation, contributing to chromatin condensation and gene silencing.[76] Nicotinamide adenine dinucleotide (NAD) depletion would also affect sirtuins' activity, which intervene into mitochondrial regulation, and affect telomere length and DNA repair pathways,[77] potentially generating a vicious cycle which would maintain persistent DNA damage and NAD consumption.

Although methods currently used to measure intracellular NAD are not feasible due to the extremely low frequencies of HBV-specific CD8 cells in peripheral blood of patients with chronic HBV infection, NAD supplementation by administration of the NAD precursor in association with CD38 inhibition has been demonstrated to significantly improve altered intracellular pathways as well as T-cell antiviral activity.[72]

The Liver Microenvironment

The liver is an essential metabolic organ, where the direct contact between nutrients or pathogen-derived molecules from the gut and resident cells is favored by the slow blood flow in fenestrated liver sinusoids to the space of Dissè. Liver sinusoidal endothelial cells (LSECs), hepatic stellate cells (HSCs), intravascular liver-resident macrophages (Kupffer cells), and liver DCs line the liver capillary system to mediate the interaction between hepatocytes, circulating antigens, and extravasating leukocytes. As a consequence, many intrahepatic mechanisms are active to ensure protection from excessive immune responses against non-self-antigens. Some of these are represented by the unique features of the hepatic immune population, the production of regulatory cytokines, and of other soluble regulatory mediators.[78] Indeed, different intrahepatic cell populations, such as DCs, Kupffer cells, HSC, and LSECs, but also Tregs, greatly contribute to intrahepatic tolerance by secreting the immunoregulatory cytokines interleukine (IL)-10, transforming growth factor (TGF)-β, and by acting as suboptimal antigen-presenting cells expressing high levels of ligands for co-inhibitory receptors (eg, PD-L1, PD-L2) in response to interferon I(FN) production (see **Fig. 1**). Indeed, high PD-L1 levels represent one reason why intrahepatic antigen presentation results far less efficient than at peripheral level. In addition, the presence of low oxygen concentrations in the inflamed liver can further induce PD-L1 expression as well as recruitment and development of the regulatory population of myeloid-derived suppressor cells (MDSC).[79] CD8 T cells can also be primed by antigen presented on the hepatocytes, although resulting either in dysfunctional T cells[46] or in apoptosis mediated by the proapoptotic protein Bcl-2 Interacting Mediator of cell death (BIM)[80] or by Fas–FasL interaction.[81]

Among factors documented to constrain T cells, amino acid-degrading enzymes released by damaged cells can cause the depletion of available amino acids. The enzymes tryptophan-2,3-dioxygenase and indoleamine 2,3-dioxygenase 1 (IDO1),[82] respectively, expressed by hepatocytes or induced in liver-infiltrating immune cells by pro-inflammatory cytokines, can degrade tryptophan (Trp) with the formation of catabolic by-products, collectively called kynurenines (Kyn).[83,84] In case of immune cells, the role of the inducible IDO activity can represent an antimicrobial defense strategy by depleting Trp from the microenvironment but also a mechanism to control a potentially harmful unrestrained immune activation.[85] However, in the inflamed, persistently infected liver, high expression of Trp-degrading enzymes contribute to antiviral immune responses curtailing, and thus to viral persistence. Indeed, low Trp concentrations in conjunction with the presence of Kyn in the culture medium, was observed to induce the downregulation of the TCR ζ-chain, impairing both proliferation and cytokine secretion in CD8 T cells,[86] up to T-cell apoptosis[87] and to favor the emergence of IL-10 and TGF-β producing CD4 Treg cells.[86,88] Also NK cell proliferation resulted in vitro hindered by tryptophan catabolites derived from IDO1 activity.[89] These effects are, at least in part, mediated by Kyn activation of the aryl hydrocarbon receptor, a ligand-operated transcription factor, which is engaged in promoting IL-10 and TGF-β production by regulatory T cells T_R1 and Treg while reducing major histocompatibility complex (MHC) class II molecule expression and favoring anti-inflammatory T-cell polarization by DC.[90]

Also shortage of the essential amino acid L-arginine due to the presence of arginase I, derived from dying hepatocytes, MDSC and other liver-infiltrating cells, represents a crucial factor leading to T-cell cycle inhibition and CD3ζ chain downregulation and documented both in course of acute and chronic HBV infection as a mechanism devoted to limit immune cell-mediated liver damage.[91,92]

In addition, inflammatory stimuli lead to the production of prostaglandins (PG) by infiltrating myeloid cells, among which the best known PGE2 is acknowledged among soluble mediators of liver immune tolerance,[93] by binding to four subtypes of receptor (EP1, EP2, EP3, and EP4)[94] on most major immune cell subsets.[95] Although diverse and even opposite PGE2 immunoregulatory effects have been described, a large number of studies have documented PGE2-mediated dampening of the immune response during chronic inflammation, such as cancer and chronic viral infections.[96–98] These findings are in line with significantly elevated PGE2 serum levels in patients with chronic HBV infection.[99] Also, B cells have been shown an altered differentiation on PGE2 exposure, with immunoglobulin (Ig)-class switching, and enhanced development of IL-10 producing Breg,[100] as well as macrophages, which resulted polarized toward the M2 phenotype[101] and NK cells that were described as suppressed in their cytotoxicity and cytokine production potential.[102,103]

Another liver metabolism-derived molecule with immunoregulatory functions is retinoic acid (RA), which derives from HSCs. These cells, following liver damage-induced activation, release their lipid droplet content, where retinyl esters are stored.[104,105] In coculture experiments of HSCs and DCs in the presence of low concentrations of TGF-β, the RA-dependent CD4 T-cell differentiation into FoxP3 + Treg cells has been shown.[106] Moreover, in mouse HSC RA can stimulate the expression of the RA early inducible gene 1, which acts as a ligand for NK cells, sensitizing in this way early activated HSCs to NK cell killing.[107]

The Negative Regulatory Role of Natural Killer Cells

Regulation of adaptive immunity by NK cells has been widely demonstrated in animal and human models of viral infection.[7] NK cells are highly present within the liver, where they play direct and indirect antiviral activity by cytokine secretion and by promoting DC maturation, recruitment and antigen cross-presentation, ultimately resulting in T-cell response enhancement.[7] A negative regulatory role for NK cells has also been reported because they constrain effective antiviral adaptive immunity by deleting activated T cells through cytolytic granules or death receptor pathways mainly mediated by NKG2D- and TRAIL-dependent mechanisms[108–111] (see **Fig. 1**). Moreover, checkpoint inhibitory pathways were also described as direct mechanisms of T-cell restraint exploited by NK cells, including PD-1/PD-L1 and NK group 2 member A/Human Leukocyte Antigens E (NKG2A/HLA-E) signaling. In particular, NKG2A was shown to contribute to the inhibition of HIV-infected target cell clearance by NK cells[112] and is often co-expressed with PD-1 on activated CD8 T cells leading to dampening both T and NK antitumor responses.[113]

A critical role in this negative modulation of the T-cell response was also played by the NK cell activating receptor NCR1 (NKp46) in an LCMV infection, because inhibition of NCR1 ligand expression on T lymphocytes by type I IFNs can protect T cells against the NCR1-mediated NK cell attack.[114]

In patients with chronic HBV infection, NK cells seem to be impaired in their antiviral capacity showing a functional dichotomy, because in most of the reports, NK cell cytotoxicity seems to be preserved, whereas NK cell capacity to produce IFN-γ and TNF-α is defective, making NK cells more pathogenic than protective.[108,115] During chronic HBV infection, the immune suppressive cytokine milieu of the liver can impair IFN-γ production by NK cells, limiting their antiviral activity through the inhibitory effect of IL10 and TGF-β.[116] However, NK cells can upregulate the death ligand TRAIL which can not only engage the upregulated TRAIL receptor on liver cells, amplifying the liver damage, but also the R2 receptors expressed on HBV-specific T cells, deleting them.[108] Another mechanism involved in the regulatory activity of NK cells on HBV-specific T cells is mediated by NKG2D interaction with its specific ligand expressed on CD4 T cells. The upregulation of the NKG2D ligand MICA on HBV-specific CD4 T cells leads to NK-cell activation and cytotoxicity.[117] Importantly, NK cell depletion and blockade of TRAIL and NKG2D further improve the HBV-specific T-cell functions, confirming the negative regulatory role played by NK cells in chronic HBV patients.[108,115,117] Recently, this negative regulation was investigated in a mouse model of CHB, where NK cell depletion elicited an enhancement of antigen-specific T-cell responses to chimp adenoviral vector vaccination. Liver-resident NK cells served a crucial negative role constraining vaccine-induced antiviral HBV-specific CD8 T cells by their upregulation of PD-L1. However, PD-L1 blockade in combination with cytokine activation of NK cells provided help to boost vaccine-induced HBV-specific CD8 T cells.[118] This study was further confirmed in human CHB, highlighting the relevance of PD-L1-dependent regulation of T cells by cytokine-activated NK cells.[118]

Also overexpression of galectin-9 on NK cells has been reported to play an immunomodulatory role in CHB patients by promoting CD8 T-cell dysfunction through galectin-9 (Gal-9)/TIM-3 axis. Blocking Gal-9/TIM-3 pathway in vitro could partially restore HBV-specific CD8 T-cell responses, suggesting this checkpoint signaling as a potential therapeutic target for immunotherapy.[119]

FINAL REMARKS

Immune reconstitution strategies aimed at recovering functionally efficient T-cell responses can be crucial for a cure of chronic HBV infection. An efficient strategy should probably intervene at multiple levels, as many different pathogenetic mechanisms are believed to affect the immune response to the virus. Many levels of evidence, including the progressive T-cell impairment observed in association to increasing antigenemia levels in HBV-infected patients, suggest that antigen decline can represent a first step in this direction. In this regard, besides currently used NUCs, new and potentially more efficient antivirals could be used, once clinically available, in order to also reduce the number of infected hepatocytes. Then, different types of interventions to strengthen immune responses can be programmed. Among these, checkpoint blockade represents one strategy directed toward both innate and adaptive responses, provided that autoimmune reactions are excluded. In addition, several other immune reconstitution strategies to enhance adaptive cell functions directly, ranging from therapeutic vaccination to metabolic or epigenetic modulation, or indirectly through innate cells stimulation, are arising. Although it is not known to what extent a full functional immune recovery, after decades of chronic antigen stimulation, is still possible, several studies are currently under evaluation and hopefully will provide more data about safety and effectiveness of different approaches. Besides a well-balanced time for interventions add-on, another crucial aspect to be pursued is the development of reliable predictors of the individual response to a given strategy. Indeed, within the wide range of different clinical settings associated with chronic HBV infection, a great variability of patients' immunologic profiles is becoming more clearly evident. In this context, the presence of T cells with a variable degree of exhaustion, associated with a different individual representation of T-cell subsets with a different sensitivity to immune rejuvenation, could probably constitute one important aspect to evaluate, in order to identify patients that could take advantage more significantly from immune-modulatory strategies.

CLINICS CARE POINTS

- Understanding the mechanisms of the immunologic defects related to host immunity is essential to overcome cell-mediated immune dysfunction and to identify possible new immunomodulatory therapeutic strategies.
- Immune dysregulated pathways and cellular functions may represent new targets for novel therapies to be applied in a combination treatment approach.
- Identification of reliable biomarkers based on immunologic parameters could allow selecting patients with different capacity to respond to novel immunomodulatory therapy.

DISCLOSURE

The authors declare no conflict of interest.

REFERENCES

1. GBD 2019 Hepatitis B Collaborators. Global, regional, and national burden of hepatitis B, 1990–2019: a systematic analysis for the Global Burden of Disease Study 2019. Lancet Gastroenterol Hepatol, 2022; 7: 796–829.
2. World Health Organization. Global health sector strategy on viral hepatitis 2016-2021. Towards ending viral hepatitis. World Health Organization 2016;. https://apps.who.int/iris/handle/10665/246177.
3. Lampertico P, Agarwal K, Berg T, et al. EASL 2017 Clinical Practice Guidelines on the management of hepatitis B virus infection. J Hepatol 2017;67(2):370–98.

4. Bertoletti A, Ferrari C. Adaptive immunity in HBV infection. J Hepatol 2016;64(1): S71–83.

5. Maini MK, Gehring AJ. The role of innate immunity in the immunopathology and treatment of HBV infection. J Hepatol 2016;64(1):S60–70.

6. Fisicaro P, Barili V, Rossi M, et al. Pathogenetic mechanisms of T cell dysfunction in chronic HBV infection and related therapeutic approaches. Front Immunol 2020;11:849.

7. Fisicaro P, Rossi M, Vecchi A, et al. The good and the bad of natural killer cells in virus control: perspective for anti-HBV therapy. Int J Mol Sci 2019;20(20). https:// doi.org/10.3390/ijms20205080.

8. Burton AR, Pallett LJ, McCoy LE, et al. Circulating and intrahepatic antiviral B cells are defective in hepatitis B. J Clin Invest 2018;128(10):4588–603.

9. Salimzadeh L, Le Bert N, Dutertre C-A, et al. PD-1 blockade partially recovers dysfunctional virus–specific B cells in chronic hepatitis B infection. J Clin Invest 2018;128(10):4573–87.

10. Ferrari C. HBV and the immune response. Liver Int 2015;35(s1):121–8.

11. Penna A, Artini M, Cavalli A, et al. Long-lasting memory T cell responses following self-limited acute hepatitis B. J Clin Invest 1996;98(5):1185–94.

12. Rehermann B, Ferrari C, Pasquinelli C, et al. The hepatitis B virus persists for decades after patients' recovery from acute viral hepatitis despite active maintenance of a cytotoxic T-lymphocyte response. Nat Med 1996;2(10):1104–8.

13. Jeng W-J, Papatheodoridis GV, Lok ASF. Hepatitis B. Lancet 2023. https://doi. org/10.1016/S0140-6736(22)01468-4.

14. Rossi M, Vecchi A, Tiezzi C, et al. Phenotypic CD8 T cell profiling in chronic hepatitis B to predict HBV-specific CD8 T cell susceptibility to functional restoration in vitro. Gut 2023. https://doi.org/10.1136/gutjnl-2022-32720z. gutjnl-2022-327202.

15. Cheng Y, Zhu YO, Becht E, et al. Multifactorial heterogeneity of virus-specific T cells and association with the progression of human chronic hepatitis B infection. Sci Immunol 2019;4(32):eaau6905.

16. Schuch A, Salimi Alizei E, Heim K, et al. Phenotypic and functional differences of HBV core-specific versus HBV polymerase-specific CD8+ T cells in chronically HBV-infected patients with low viral load. Gut 2018;68(5):905–15.

17. Hoogeveen RC, Robidoux MP, Schwarz T, et al. Phenotype and function of HBV-specific T cells is determined by the targeted epitope in addition to the stage of infection. Gut 2019;68(5):893–904.

18. Heim K, Binder B, Sagar, et al. TOX defines the degree of CD8+ T cell dysfunction in distinct phases of chronic HBV infection. Gut 2021;70(8):1550–60.

19. Kennedy PTF, Sandalova E, Jo J, et al. Preserved T-cell function in children and young adults with immune-tolerant chronic hepatitis B. Gastroenterology 2012; 143(3):637–45.

20. Le Bert N, Gill US, Hong M, et al. Effects of hepatitis B surface antigen on virus-specific and global T cells in patients with chronic hepatitis B virus infection. Gastroenterology 2020;159(2):652–64.

21. Mason WS, Gill US, Litwin S, et al. HBV DNA integration and clonal hepatocyte expansion in chronic hepatitis B patients considered immune tolerant. Gastroenterology 2016;151(5):986–98.e4.

22. Boni C, Laccabue D, Lampertico P, et al. Restored function of HBV-specific T cells after long-term effective therapy with nucleos(t)ide analogues. Gastroenterology 2012;143(4):963–73.e9.

23. Bertoletti A. The challenges of adopting immunological biomarkers in the management of chronic HBV infection. J Hepatol 2022;77(2):299–301.
24. Tsukuda S, Watashi K. Hepatitis B virus biology and life cycle. Antiviral Res 2020;182:104925.
25. Karayiannis P. Hepatitis B virus: virology, molecular biology, life cycle and intrahepatic spread. Hepatol Int 2017;11(6):500–8.
26. Wong DK-H, Seto W-K, Cheung K-S, et al. Hepatitis B virus core-related antigen as a surrogate marker for covalently closed circular DNA. Liver Int 2017;37(7):995–1001.
27. Testoni B, Lebossé F, Scholtes C, et al. Serum hepatitis B core-related antigen (HBcrAg) correlates with covalently closed circular DNA transcriptional activity in chronic hepatitis B patients. J Hepatol 2019;70(4):615–25.
28. Kramvis A. Genotypes and genetic variability of hepatitis B virus. Intervirology 2014;57(3–4):141–50.
29. Buster EHCJ, Hansen BE, Lau GKK, et al. Factors that predict response of patients with hepatitis B e antigen-positive chronic hepatitis B to peginterferon-alfa. Gastroenterology 2009;137(6):2002–9.
30. Viganò M, Grossi G, Loglio A, et al. Treatment of hepatitis B: is there still a role for interferon? Liver Int 2018;38:79–83.
31. Sonneveld MJ, Chiu S-M, Park JY, et al. Probability of HBsAg loss after nucleo(s)tide analogue withdrawal depends on HBV genotype and viral antigen levels. J Hepatol 2022;76(5):1042–50.
32. Chan HL-Y, Hui AY, Wong ML, et al. Genotype C hepatitis B virus infection is associated with an increased risk of hepatocellular carcinoma. Gut 2004;53(10):1494–8.
33. Wong GLH, Gane E, Lok ASF. How to achieve functional cure of HBV: stopping NUCs, adding interferon or new drug development? J Hepatol 2022;76(6):1249–62.
34. Lim SG, Baumert TF, Boni C, et al. The scientific basis of combination therapy for chronic hepatitis B functional cure. Nat Rev Gastroenterol Hepatol 2023. https://doi.org/10.1038/s41575-022-00724-5.
35. Bertoletti A, Boni C. HBV antigens quantity: duration and effect on functional cure. Gut 2022;71(11):2149–51.
36. Montali I, Vecchi A, Rossi M, et al. Antigen load and T cell function: a challenging interaction in HBV infection. Biomedicines 2022;10(6):1224.
37. Burton AR, Maini MK. Human antiviral B cell responses: emerging lessons from hepatitis B and COVID-19. Immunol Rev 2021;299(1):108–17.
38. Bertoletti A, Le Bert N. Fine-tuning TLR-7-based therapy for functional HBV cure. Hepatol Commun 2019;3(10):1289–92.
39. McLane LM, Abdel-Hakeem MS, Wherry EJ. CD8 T cell exhaustion during chronic viral infection and cancer. Annu Rev Immunol 2019;37(1):457–95.
40. Barili V, Vecchi A, Rossi M, et al. Unraveling the multifaceted nature of CD8 T cell exhaustion provides the molecular basis for therapeutic T cell reconstitution in chronic hepatitis B and C. Cells 2021;10(10):2563.
41. Protzer U, Maini MK, Knolle PA. Living in the liver: hepatic infections. Nat Rev Immunol 2012;12(3):201–13.
42. Wong YC, Tay SS, McCaughan GW, et al. Immune outcomes in the liver: is CD8 T cell fate determined by the environment? J Hepatol 2015;63(4):1005–14.
43. Tay SS, Wong YC, McDonald DM, et al. Antigen expression level threshold tunes the fate of CD8 T cells during primary hepatic immune responses. Proc Natl Acad Sci U S A 2014;111(25):E2540–9.

44. Backes S, Jäger C, Dembek CJ, et al. Protein-prime/modified vaccinia virus Ankara vector-boost vaccination overcomes tolerance in high-antigenemic HBV-transgenic mice. Vaccine 2016;34(7):923–32.

45. Michler T, Kosinska AD, Festag J, et al. Knockdown of virus antigen expression Increases therapeutic vaccine efficacy in high-titer hepatitis B virus carrier mice. Gastroenterology 2020;158(6):1762–75.e9.

46. Bénéchet AP, De Simone G, Di Lucia P, et al. Dynamics and genomic landscape of CD8+ T cells undergoing hepatic priming. Nature 2019;574(7777):200–5.

47. Iannacone M, Guidotti LG. Immunobiology and pathogenesis of hepatitis B virus infection. Nat Rev Immunol 2022;22(1):19–32.

48. Fumagalli V, Di Lucia P, Venzin V, et al. Serum HBsAg clearance has minimal impact on CD8+ T cell responses in mouse models of HBV infection. J Exp Med 2020;217(11). https://doi.org/10.1084/jem.20200298.

49. Keir ME, Butte MJ, Freeman GJ, et al. PD-1 and its ligands in tolerance and immunity. Annu Rev Immunol 2008;26(1):677–704.

50. Riley JL. PD-1 signaling in primary T cells. Immunol Rev 2009;229(1):114–25.

51. Yokosuka T, Takamatsu M, Kobayashi-Imanishi W, et al. Programmed cell death 1 forms negative costimulatory microclusters that directly inhibit T cell receptor signaling by recruiting phosphatase SHP2. J Exp Med 2012;209(6):1201–17.

52. Boussiotis VA. Molecular and biochemical aspects of the PD-1 checkpoint pathway. N Engl J Med 2016;375(18):1767–78.

53. Hui E, Cheung J, Zhu J, et al. T cell costimulatory receptor CD28 is a primary target for PD-1–mediated inhibition. Science 2017;355(6332):1428–33.

54. Thommen DS, Koelzer VH, Herzig P, et al. A transcriptionally and functionally distinct PD-1(+) CD8(+) T cell pool with predictive potential in non-small-cell lung cancer treated with PD-1 blockade. Nat Med 2018;24(7):994–1004.

55. Ogando J, Sáez ME, Santos J, et al. PD-1 signaling affects cristae morphology and leads to mitochondrial dysfunction in human CD8+ T lymphocytes. J Immunother Cancer 2019;7(1):151.

56. Blackburn SD, Shin H, Haining WN, et al. Coregulation of CD8+ T cell exhaustion by multiple inhibitory receptors during chronic viral infection. Nat Immunol 2009;10(1):29–37.

57. Schildberg FA, Klein SR, Freeman GJ, et al. Coinhibitory pathways in the B7-CD28 ligand-receptor family. Immunity 2016;44(5):955–72.

58. Patsoukis N, Bardhan K, Chatterjee P, et al. PD-1 alters T-cell metabolic reprogramming by inhibiting glycolysis and promoting lipolysis and fatty acid oxidation. Nat Commun 2015;6(1):6692.

59. Jin H-T, Anderson AC, Tan WG, et al. Cooperation of Tim-3 and PD-1 in CD8 T-cell exhaustion during chronic viral infection. Proc Natl Acad Sci U S A 2010;107(33):14733–8.

60. Boni C, Fisicaro P, Valdatta C, et al. Characterization of hepatitis B virus (HBV)-Specific T-cell dysfunction in chronic HBV infection. J Virol 2007;81(8):4215–25.

61. Fisicaro P, Valdatta C, Massari M, et al. Combined blockade of programmed death-1 and activation of CD137 increase responses of human liver T cells against HBV, but not HCV. Gastroenterology 2012;143(6):1576–85.e4.

62. Bengsch B, Martin B, Thimme R. Restoration of HBV-specific CD8+ T cell function by PD-1 blockade in inactive carrier patients is linked to T cell differentiation. J Hepatol 2014;61(6):1212–9.

63. Raziorrouh B, Heeg M, Kurktschiev P, et al. Inhibitory phenotype of HBV-specific CD4+ T-cells is characterized by high PD-1 expression but absent coregulation of multiple inhibitory molecules. PLoS One 2014;9(8):e105703.

64. Dong Y, Li X, Zhang L, et al. CD4+ T cell exhaustion revealed by high PD-1 and LAG-3 expression and the loss of helper T cell function in chronic hepatitis B. BMC Immunol 2019;20(1):27.
65. Nebbia G, Peppa D, Schurich A, et al. Upregulation of the tim-3/galectin-9 pathway of T cell exhaustion in chronic hepatitis B virus infection. PLoS One 2012;7(10):e47648.
66. Schurich A, Khanna P, Lopes AR, et al. Role of the coinhibitory receptor cytotoxic T lymphocyte antigen-4 on apoptosis-Prone CD8 T cells in persistent hepatitis B virus infection. Hepatology 2011;53(5):1494–503.
67. Raziorrouh B, Schraut W, Gerlach T, et al. The immunoregulatory role of CD244 in chronic hepatitis B infection and its inhibitory potential on virus-specific CD8+ T-cell function. Hepatology 2010;52(6):1934–47.
68. Fisicaro P, Valdatta C, Massari M, et al. Antiviral intrahepatic T-cell responses can Be restored by blocking programmed death-1 pathway in chronic hepatitis B. Gastroenterology 2010;138(2):682–93.e4.
69. Le Bert N, Salimzadeh L, Gill US, et al. Comparative characterization of B cells specific for HBV nucleocapsid and envelope proteins in patients with chronic hepatitis B. J Hepatol 2020;72(1):34–44.
70. Fisicaro P, Barili V, Montanini B, et al. Targeting mitochondrial dysfunction can restore antiviral activity of exhausted HBV-specific CD8 T cells in chronic hepatitis B. Nat Med 2017;23(3):327–36.
71. Schurich A, Pallett LJ, Jajbhay D, et al. Distinct metabolic requirements of exhausted and functional virus-specific CD8 T cells in the same host. Cell Rep 2016;16(5):1243–52.
72. Montali I, Ceccatelli Berti C, Morselli M, et al. Deregulated intracellular pathways define novel molecular targets for HBV-specific CD8 T cell reconstitution in chronic hepatitis B. J.Hepatol 2023. https://doi.org/10.1016/j.jhep.2023.02.035.
73. Acerbi G, Montali I, Ferrigno GD, et al. Functional reconstitution of HBV-specific CD8 T cells by in vitro polyphenol treatment in chronic hepatitis B. J Hepatol 2021;74(4):783–93.
74. Covarrubias AJ, Perrone R, Grozio A, et al. NAD+ metabolism and its roles in cellular processes during ageing. Nat Rev Mol Cell Biol 2021;22(2):119–41.
75. Aksoy P, White TA, Thompson M, et al. Regulation of intracellular levels of NAD: a novel role for CD38. Biochem Biophys Res Commun 2006;345(4):1386–92.
76. Cantó C, Menzies KJ, Auwerx J. NAD(+) metabolism and the control of energy homeostasis: a balancing act between mitochondria and the nucleus. Cell Metab 2015;22(1):31–53.
77. Shahgaldi S, Kahmini FR. A comprehensive review of Sirtuins: with a major focus on redox homeostasis and metabolism. Life Sci 2021;282:119803.
78. Kubes P, Jenne C. Immune responses in the liver. Annu Rev Immunol 2018;36: 247–77.
79. Wen Q, Han T, Wang Z, et al. Role and mechanism of programmed death-ligand1 in hypoxia-induced liver cancer immune escape (Review). Oncol Lett 2020;19(4):2595–601.
80. Mehrfeld C, Zenner S, Kornek M, et al. The contribution of non-professional antigen-presenting cells to immunity and tolerance in the liver. Front Immunol 2018;9:635.
81. Horst AK, Neumann K, Diehl L, et al. Modulation of liver tolerance by conventional and nonconventional antigen-presenting cells and regulatory immune cells. Cell Mol Immunol 2016;13(3):277–92.

82. Terness P, Bauer TM, Röse L, et al. Inhibition of allogeneic T cell proliferation by indoleamine 2,3-dioxygenase-expressing dendritic cells: mediation of suppression by tryptophan metabolites. J Exp Med 2002;196(4):447–57.
83. Dai H, Dai Z. The role of tryptophan catabolism in acquisition and effector function of memory T cells. Curr Opin Organ Transplant 2008;13(1):31–5.
84. Badawy AA-B. Kynurenine pathway of tryptophan metabolism: regulatory and functional aspects. Int J Tryptophan Res 2017;10. 1178646917691938.
85. Cervenka I, Agudelo LZ, Ruas JL. Kynurenines: tryptophan's metabolites in exercise, inflammation, and mental health. Scienc 2017;357(6349). https://doi.org/10.1126/science.aaf9794.
86. Fallarino F, Grohmann U, You S, et al. The combined effects of tryptophan starvation and tryptophan catabolites down-regulate T cell receptor ζ-chain and induce a regulatory phenotype in naive T cells. J Immunol 2006;176(11):6752–61.
87. Fallarino F, Grohmann U, Vacca C, et al. T cell apoptosis by tryptophan catabolism. Cell Death Differ 2002;9(10):1069–77.
88. Hill M, Tanguy-Royer S, Royer P, et al. Ido expands human CD4+CD25high regulatory T cells by promoting maturation of LPS-treated dendritic cells. Eur J Immunol 2007;37(11):3054–62.
89. Frumento G, Rotondo R, Tonetti M, et al. Tryptophan-derived catabolites are responsible for inhibition of T and natural killer cell proliferation induced by indoleamine 2,3-dioxygenase. J Exp Med 2002;196(4):459–68.
90. Rothhammer V, Quintana FJ. The aryl hydrocarbon receptor: an environmental sensor integrating immune responses in health and disease. Nat Rev Immunol 2019;19(3):184–97.
91. Sandalova E, Laccabue D, Boni C, et al. Increased levels of arginase in patients with acute hepatitis B suppress antiviral T cells. Gastroenterology 2012;143(1):78–87.e3.
92. Das A, Hoare M, Davies N, et al. Functional skewing of the global CD8 T cell population in chronic hepatitis B virus infection. J Exp Med 2008;205(9):2111–24.
93. Crispe IN. Immune tolerance in liver disease. Hepatology 2014;60(6):2109–17.
94. Harris SG, Padilla J, Koumas L, et al. Prostaglandins as modulators of immunity. Trends Immunol 2002;23(3):144–50.
95. Hata AN, Breyer RM. Pharmacology and signaling of prostaglandin receptors: multiple roles in inflammation and immune modulation. Pharmacol Ther 2004;103(2):147–66.
96. Sreeramkumar V, Fresno M, Cuesta N. Prostaglandin E 2 and T cells: friends or foes? Immunol Cell Biol 2012;90(6):579–86.
97. Chen JH, Perry CJ, Tsui Y-C, et al. Prostaglandin E2 and programmed cell death 1 signaling coordinately impair CTL function and survival during chronic viral infection. Nat Med 2015;21(4):327–34.
98. Zelenay S, van der Veen AG, Böttcher JP, et al. Cyclooxygenase-dependent tumor growth through evasion of immunity. Cell 2015;162(6):1257–70.
99. Li X, Xie T, Gao L, et al. Prostaglandin E2 facilitates Hepatitis B virus replication by impairing CTL function. Mol Immunol 2018;103:243–50.
100. Chen R, Cao Y, Tian Y, et al. PGE2 ameliorated viral myocarditis development and promoted IL-10-producing regulatory B cell expansion via MAPKs/AKT-AP1 axis or AhR signaling. Cell Immunol 2020;347:104025.

101. Németh K, Leelahavanichkul A, Yuen PST, et al. Bone marrow stromal cells attenuate sepsis via prostaglandin E2–dependent reprogramming of host macrophages to increase their interleukin-10 production. Nat Med 2009;15(1):42–9.
102. Park A, Lee Y, Kim MS, et al. Prostaglandin E2 secreted by thyroid cancer cells contributes to immune escape through the suppression of natural killer (NK) cell cytotoxicity and NK cell differentiation. Front Immunol 2018;9:1859.
103. Kalinski P. Regulation of immune responses by prostaglandin E2. J Immunol 2012;188(1):21–8.
104. Friedman SL. Hepatic stellate cells: protean, multifunctional, and enigmatic cells of the liver. Physiol Rev 2008;88(1):125–72.
105. Haaker MW, Vaandrager AB, Helms JB. Retinoids in health and disease: a role for hepatic stellate cells in affecting retinoid levels. Biochim Biophys Acta - Mol Cell Biol Lipids 2020;1865(6):158674.
106. Dunham RM, Thapa M, Velazquez VM, et al. Hepatic stellate cells preferentially induce Foxp3+ regulatory T cells by production of retinoic acid. J Immunol 2013;190(5):2009–16.
107. Radaeva S, Wang L, Radaev S, et al. Retinoic acid signaling sensitizes hepatic stellate cells to NK cell killing via upregulation of NK cell activating ligand RAE1. Am J Physiol Liver Physiol 2007;293(4):G809–16.
108. Peppa D, Gill US, Reynolds G, et al. Up-regulation of a death receptor renders antiviral T cells susceptible to NK cell–mediated deletion. J Exp Med 2013; 210(1):99–114.
109. Lang PA, Lang KS, Xu HC, et al. Natural killer cell activation enhances immune pathology and promotes chronic infection by limiting CD8+ T-cell immunity. Proc Natl Acad Sci U S A 2012;109(4):1210–5.
110. Zingoni A, Ardolino M, Santoni A, et al. NKG2D and DNAM-1 activating receptors and their ligands in NK-T cell interactions: role in the NK cell-mediated negative regulation of T cell responses. Front Immunol 2012;3:408.
111. Cerboni C, Zingoni A, Cippitelli M, et al. Antigen-activated human T lymphocytes express cell-surface NKG2D ligands via an ATM/ATR-dependent mechanism and become susceptible to autologous NK- cell lysis. Blood 2007;110(2):606–15.
112. Ramsuran V, Naranbhai V, Horowitz A, et al. Elevated HLA-A expression impairs HIV control through inhibition of NKG2A-expressing cells. Science 2018; 359(6371):86–90.
113. André P, Denis C, Soulas C, et al. Anti-NKG2A mAb is a checkpoint inhibitor that promotes anti-tumor immunity by unleashing both T and NK cells. Cell 2018; 175(7):1731–43.e13.
114. Crouse J, Bedenikovic G, Wiesel M, et al. Type I interferons protect T cells against NK cell attack mediated by the activating receptor NCR1. Immunity 2014;40(6):961–73.
115. Boni C, Lampertico P, Talamona L, et al. Natural killer cell phenotype modulation and natural killer/T-cell interplay in nucleos(t)ide analogue-treated hepatitis e antigen-negative patients with chronic hepatitis B. Hepatology 2015;62(6):1697–709.
116. Peppa D, Micco L, Javaid A, et al. Blockade of immunosuppressive cytokines restores NK cell antiviral function in chronic hepatitis B virus infection. PLoS Pathog 2010;6(12):e1001227.
117. Huang W-C, Easom NJ, Tang X-Z, et al. T cells infiltrating diseased liver express ligands for the NKG2D stress surveillance system. J Immunol 2017;198(3):1172–82.

Novel Assays to Solve the Clinical and Scientific Challenges of Chronic Hepatitis B

Thomas Tu, PhD[a,b,*], Harout Ajoyan, BSc[a],
Jacob George, MBBS, FRACP, PhD, FAASLD[a]

KEYWORDS

- Hepatitis elimination • Point-of-care testing • Public health • Cure • Rapid test

KEY POINTS

- Clinical tests to guide diagnosis, monitoring, and treatment of chronic hepatitis B are right for the purpose in settings with strong testing infrastructure and high patient engagement.
- However, most cases of chronic Hepatitis B are in limited resource settings, in remote locales, or with low engagement in health care systems.
- Newly developed rapid diagnostic tests and point-of-care tests can overcome some of these barriers to optimal care for hepatitis B.
- Other novel assays can also support the development of curative therapies for chronic hepatitis B infection.

INTRODUCTION

Chronic Hepatitis B is the most common blood-borne virus infection, affecting 262 million people worldwide. It is a major cause of liver disease and is responsible for ~800,000 deaths each year from either liver cancer (hepatocellular carcinoma, HCC) or liver failure[1] resultant from immune-mediated chronic inflammation and persistence of the virus. Chronic hepatitis B is presently incurable as the forms of the virus that persist in the liver and are not targeted by current treatments. Instead, existing treatments suppress virus replication and limit inflammation, but most patients need to take these indefinitely given the high risk of viral reactivation if treatment is stopped.

HEPATITIS B INFECTION

Hepatitis B is caused by infection with the hepatitis B virus (HBV), an enveloped circular double-stranded DNA virus (**Fig. 1**). Upon exposure, HBV specifically infects the

[a] Storr Liver Centre, The Westmead Institute for Medical Research, The University of Sydney at Westmead Hospital, Westmead, New South Wales, Australia; [b] Centre for Infectious Diseases and Microbiology, Sydney Infectious Diseases Institute, The University of Sydney at Westmead Hospital, Westmead, New South Wales, Australia
* Corresponding author.
E-mail address: t.tu@sydney.edu.au

Clin Liver Dis 27 (2023) 837–855
https://doi.org/10.1016/j.cld.2023.05.002
1089-3261/23/© 2023 Elsevier Inc. All rights reserved.

liver.theclinics.com

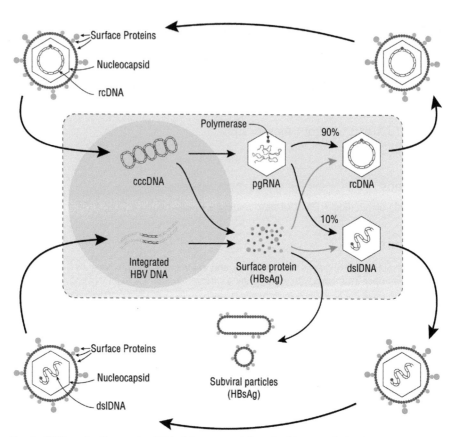

Fig. 1. HBV replication cycle. HBV virions containing double-stranded relaxed circular (rc) DNA (*top*) enter the hepatocytes through receptor-mediated endocytosis. The viral genome is transported to the nucleus, where it is converted into cccDNA, the template for all viral mRNAs and pregenomic (pg)RNA. pgRNA is encapsidated by viral capsid proteins (HBV core protein) along with the viral polymerase, which reverse-transcribes the pgRNA to generate rcDNA. The mature nucleocapsid is then enveloped in HBV surface antigen and secreted from the cell. In 5% to 10% of virions, double-stranded linear (dsl)DNA (*bottom*) is generated as a byproduct of reverse-transcription instead of rcDNA. Nucleocapsids containing this form also can be packaged into virus particles. Only dslDNA genomes can integrate into the host genome upon infection of new cells. Although integrated HBV DNA cannot produce new virus, both cccDNA and integrated HBV DNA can produce HBV surface protein.

hepatocytes. The virus is then transported to the nucleus, and its genome is converted to covalently closed circular DNA (cccDNA), the template for all viral RNA transcripts. These include pregenomic RNA, which is encapsidated by HBV core antigen (HBcAg) and then reverse-transcribed into double-stranded DNA. DNA-containing nucleocapsids are then enveloped by host membranes studded with the HBV surface antigen (HBsAg) and secreted from the cell as virions.

In some infection events, instead of forming cccDNA, the genomes of incoming viruses can integrate into the host genome.[2] HBV DNA integration occurs in all patients, early in an infection (within days),[3,4] and can even persist after viral clearance. Although these integrated forms are replication-deficient, they can encode full-length

HBsAg. HBsAg from integrated HBV and cccDNA forms can be secreted from the cell as immunomodulatory subviral particles, in excess of viral particles at a ratio of greater than 10,000:1.[5]

Chronic HBV infection is characterized by several phases. Initially, all hepatocytes are infected. As virus replication is noncytopathic, there is no liver damage. The virus can then evade the immune response for decades[6] until such time as the immune system is triggered (through unknown mechanisms) and attacks infected hepatocytes,[7] resulting in inflammation and fibrosis. The resultant inflammation kills infected hepatocytes, but this response is frequently self-limited (again through unknown mechanisms). Eventually, through interactions with the immune response, the liver settles at a new equilibrium with low levels of virus replication and a minority of infected cells that drive continual low-level immune-mediated liver injury. Thus, virus persistence is key to the chronic liver damage associated with HBV infection.

CURRENT METHODS FOR DIAGNOSIS AND CLINICAL MONITORING OF HEPATITIS B

In high-resource settings, laboratory diagnosis of hepatitis B is simple, widely available, robust, and economical. Laboratory-based assays for circulating HBsAg have been used for decades as a sensitive measure for infection with hepatitis B. Moreover, similar assays are available to determine previous exposure (anti-HBc antibodies), indicating exposure and presence of cccDNA; resolution of chronic infection or protection by vaccination (anti-HBs antibodies); and the raising of an antiviral immune response with HBV e antigen and antibodies against it.

Despite these long-established assays, only $\sim$10% of people with chronic hepatitis B are diagnosed and even fewer are in care or on appropriate treatment ($\sim$5%). Multiple factors (financial, sociologic, policy-associated, medical, and scientific) can contribute to these low rates (**Table 1**).[8] Existing systems have not significantly expanded the number of people diagnosed, in care, and appropriately treated to a level required to meet World Health Organization (WHO) targets for the global elimination of hepatitis B as a public health threat. Urgent changes are needed.

In this article, the authors review the potential of new assays to address these hurdles and improve the well-being of the millions living with chronic hepatitis B. The authors have broadly separated the unresolved issues into clinical (diagnosis, provision of care, and determining disease progression) and scientific (quantifying intrahepatic forms of the virus and antiviral responses to further cure research) problems.

UNRESOLVED CLINICAL ISSUES

Current tests are effective in providing accurate clinical information for hepatitis B management, particularly in high-resource settings, where patients are engaged in care and can afford repeated visits to the clinic and the associated tests. However, these tests face limitations in specific contexts in high-, middle-, and low-income countries. In recent years, novel assays (including point-of-care assays, rapid tests, dried blood spot assays, and those detecting new viral targets) have been developed to address the key unresolved issues and attempt to improve linkage to care (**Fig. 2**).

Increasing Diagnosis Rates

Most people ($\sim$90%) living with hepatitis B are undiagnosed. Timely access to testing for HBsAg (the marker of current HBV infection) remains limited in many cases for multiple reasons: awareness of HBV as a health threat, the stigma associated with HBV, lack of access to testing infrastructure, costs of the tests, requirements for cold

Table 1
Contributors to low rates of diagnosis, linkage to care, and treatment uptake that are addressed by novel tests

Theme	Issue	Affects	Improvement by New Assays
Financial	Direct costs of diagnostic tests, medications, and monitoring	Diagnosis, monitoring, treatment	Cheaper tests
	Indirect costs of testing and monitoring (travel, days off, and so forth)	Diagnosis, monitoring, treatment	Reduced time between testing and interpretation, reducing number of clinic visits
	Lack of adequate medical insurance coverage	Diagnosis, monitoring, treatment	Point-of-care assays decouple testing from centralized laboratory services
Policy	Complicated rules for hepatitis B treatment and management	Monitoring, treatment	Simplified outputs from novel tests
	Risk-based screening/diagnosis difficult to implement	Diagnosis	Increased accessibility of diagnostic tests to enable universal testing
Sociological	Test result anxiety	Diagnosis, monitoring, treatment	Reduced time between testing and interpretation
	Stigma and discrimination of having hepatitis B	Diagnosis, monitoring, treatment	Enables more accessible testing (eg, self-testing/self-monitoring)
	Poor availability of accessible information about hepatitis B	Diagnosis, monitoring, treatment	Improve linkage to care by reducing time between testing and interpretation, enabling better provision of information
	Current treatments are not curative	Diagnosis, monitoring, treatment	New tests can support curative research
Medical/scientific	Centralized laboratory diagnosis requires multiple clinic visits, presenting multiple opportunities for loss to follow-up	Diagnosis, monitoring, treatment	Reduced time between testing and interpretation, reducing number of clinic visits
	Laboratory infrastructure not universally available	Diagnosis, monitoring, treatment	Point-of-care assays have reduced dependence on laboratory infrastructure and trained staff
	Cold-chain or same-day delivery required for some tests	Diagnosis, monitoring, treatment	Use of dried blood spots as a sample, point-of-care assays do not require sample transport

Current approach

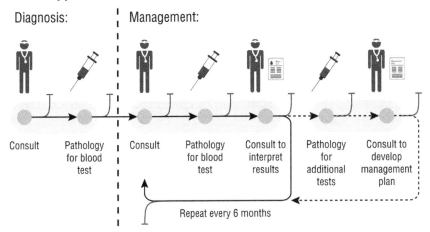

Potential approaches with novel tests

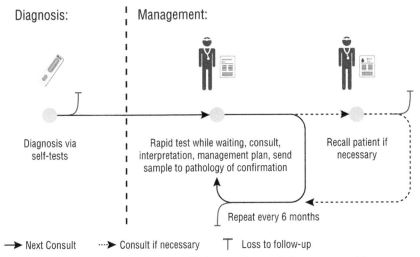

Fig. 2. Novel test assays could dramatically improve loss to follow-up rates. The current clinical diagnosis and management (*top*) involves multiple visits to various health care providers, with the potential for loss to follow-up (*red line*) at each point. Novel test assays enable a complete revolution in the model of care (*bottom*). Greater entry into care could be enabled by diagnosis using self-tests. Tests required for management and interpretation of the results can be carried out within the same consult using rapid tests, which would limit the risks to loss to follow-up. To ensure quality of diagnosis, rapid tests can be complemented by existing laboratory-based tests, recalling the patient only when necessary (eg, conflicting results).

delivery of blood samples to a pathology laboratory (difficult in remote settings), and the requirement for several clinical visits to receive and understand test results.

A novel approach to overcome some of these aspects is the use of point-of-care assays, particularly rapid test assays to detect HBsAg. Multiple rapid tests for HBsAg have been prequalified by the WHO and require only small volumes of blood, serum, or plasma either via fingerstick (<1–2 μL) or venipuncture (~5 mL). These rapid tests use lateral flow technology to return a visible and interpretable result within 15 minutes. This potentially leads to reduced loss to follow-up as only one clinic visit is required for testing, interpretation of the results, and (if necessary) provision of counseling, information, and follow-up procedures. Indeed, greater linkage to care has been linked to rapid tests compared with diagnosis by standard-of-care venipuncture.[10] Rapid tests are also likely to be cheaper given less reliance on laboratory infrastructure.

Following the uptake and ubiquity of rapid antigen tests for SARS-CoV-2, self-testing for HBsAg using rapid tests could conceivably be implemented and improve diagnosis rates. This would allow timely results (as they do not require making doctors' appointments), thereby limiting test/result anxiety. Self-testing at home may also circumvent exposure to community stigma.

In general, rapid tests have high specificity (pooled value of ~99% in meta-analyses[11]) but have lower sensitivity (pooled value of ~90%) compared with the greater than 95% sensitivity for laboratory-based chemiluminescence immunoassays (CLIA) and enzyme-linked immunosorbent assays (ELISA). Recent studies with the Bioline WD test have shown greater than 99% sensitivity,[12,13] but this high rate is not reflected in all regions (eg, high rates of false negatives were observed in a study in Pakistan,[14] potentially owing to HBsAg mutants). If performance can be broadened and improved, rapid tests could be useful even in high-resource countries to complement existing tests and improve linkage to care. Such tests would also simplify universal screening,[15,16] suggested as a strategy to dramatically increase HBV diagnosis rates given the ease of their distribution, use, and interpretation.

An alternative approach to expanding diagnosis is the use of blood spot tests in remote settings to overcome requirements for immediate shipping of blood samples. For this approach, drops of blood (produced by a lancet to the finger) are blotted to filter paper and sent to central laboratories for CLIA/ELISA tests to detect HBsAg (and HBV DNA, as described in later discussion). The ease of finger-prick tests and use of room-temperature delivery (or by regular mail) theoretically increases the access of testing in remote settings. Studies have shown comparable sensitivity and specificity to standard CLIA/ELISA diagnosis methods (92%–100% sensitivity and 100% specificity),[17,18] but some degradation occurs with medium-term (~1 month) storage at room temperature.[18]

Clinical Monitoring and Identifying Patients Eligible for Antiviral Treatment

Diagnosis is just the first step in preventing the health impacts of chronic HBV infection. Ongoing care requires the monitoring of several viral markers. A major clinical decision in chronic hepatitis B management is determining patient eligibility for antiviral treatment (the most effective therapeutic intervention to prevent liver disease progression). Measuring liver damage (described in later discussion) and HBV DNA levels is recommended before treating most patients under existing international guidelines[19–21] and in proposed simplified guidelines for treatment.[22,23] The current approach to measuring viral load relies on a laboratory-based quantitative polymerase chain reaction (qPCR) assay on DNA extracted from serum or whole blood. As with current approaches for HBV diagnosis, these have multiple drawbacks (see **Table 1**), some of which can be addressed with new assays.

The fully automated, continuous, random-access GeneXpert platform qPCR has been implemented with great success for rapid testing of HCV RNA in mobile clinics, leading to increased linkage to hepatitis C care and immediate patient access to antiviral treatment using a "test and cure" approach.[24] Kits for this platform have now been developed to quantify HBV DNA from 0.6 mL of plasma or serum, returning a result within an hour. Studies have shown excellent agreement of these rapid tests with standard laboratory-based assays.[25–28] Moreover, these assays have been tested on dried blood spots with good agreement with serum results (although with a higher lower limit of detection of ~ 1000 IU/mL),[27,28] adding flexibility for samples acquired in remote areas.

However, these new assays may require significant upfront equipment costs (eg, for staff training, assay cartridges, and the platform itself) that may not be feasible in low-resource settings. However, several PCR-free assays could significantly reduce this initial barrier to entry. Loop-mediated isothermal amplification assays amplify HBV DNA at a single temperature (rather than cycling through multiple temperatures), dispensing the need for a thermocycler. Moreover, these tests can detect clinically relevant HBV DNA levels using a visual (turbidimetric or fluorometric) output within 1 hour.[29–31] Isothermic DNA amplification has been combined with CRISPR-based detection assays as a more sensitive method to detect HBV DNA.[32,33] However, these remain difficult to translate into point-of-care assays in remote settings, given the requirement for temperature-sensitive enzymes to carry out amplification.

An alternative to directly measuring HBV DNA is using surrogate markers. HBV core-related antigen (HBcrAg, a composite of the secreted HBV e antigen, HBcAg, and a core-related protein called p22cr) has been shown to be well correlated with circulating HBV DNA levels in untreated patients. Thus, quantitative laboratory-based HBcrAg assays[34] and rapid HBcrAg point-of-care tests[35] have been suggested as potential methods to broaden access to guideline-centered treatment, particularly in areas lacking qPCR infrastructure.

Assessing Liver Disease Progression

Another important criterion for treatment eligibility is the presence of liver damage. The standard marker of liver damage is serum liver alanine aminotransferase (ALT) measured by ELISAs in pathology laboratories. Given the shortcomings of laboratory-based assays as outlined above, several groups have developed point-of-care assays for ALT with reasonably high sensitivity and specificity relative to laboratory-based assays.[36–39] This may help people with hepatitis B–related liver flares to access timely medication to prevent ongoing liver injury. However, it is also clear that one-off ALT testing can be an insensitive measure for intrahepatic inflammation, which is evident in 20% to 30% of patients with even persistently normal ALTs.[40,41] Thus, more sensitive measures for liver inflammation are required to ensure appropriate provision of care for people with hepatitis B.

Past liver injury and subsequent persistent liver fibrosis are also indicators for treatment eligibility. In high-resource settings, this is generally determined either by liver biopsy (and subsequent histopathologic interpretation) or by noninvasive methods (elastography-based or MRI-based technologies). Given the immediacy of point-of-care results, their noninvasive nature, and relative ease of use, elastography-based technologies have been widely used to assess the stage of liver fibrosis in chronic liver diseases, including hepatitis B. However, the platform (and training of users) is not universally available, particularly in primary care or low resource settings.

To overcome these barriers, various algorithms to predict liver fibrosis stage have been developed based on a combination of surrogate markers, including patient features (eg, age, sex, ethnicity, body mass index), comorbidities (eg, diabetes), and results of standard blood tests (eg, ALT, AST, GGT, and platelet count).[42] In the future, these may be determined with point-of-care tests: not only with liver function tests (described above) but also for platelet counts. Several portable cytometry-based assays requiring only a finger-prick's worth of blood have been developed and agree well with gold-standard laboratory-based blood count approaches.[43,44]

Most liver fibrosis algorithms have been developed for various chronic liver diseases, but disease cause significantly affects their predictive power. For example, the Fib-4 algorithm (which considers patient age, AST, ALT, and platelet counts) works well for patients with Metabolic-associated Fatty Liver Disease (MAFLD) alone, but accuracy was reduced for patients with both MAFLD and HBV.[45] Moreover, sensitivity at early stages of fibrosis remains relatively low. Thus, their main utility is excluding significant (F2 or more) or advanced (F3/F4) chronic liver disease, rather than detecting minor injury. Given the presence of these lower levels of liver injury can be considered grounds for treatment in some cases, greater research should be carried out to develop more sensitive measures.

Viral Sequencing

The viral DNA sequence can have significant ramifications on patient prognosis and disease progression, an understanding of epidemiologic events (eg, spreading clusters), and likely response to therapies.[46] For example, DNA mutations in the polymerase gene driven by prior treatment with (and subsequent resistance to) lamivudine is contraindicated for treatment with entecavir because of increased risk of viral resistance.[47,48] Mutations in the Pre-surface regions of the viral genome selected by the immune response have been associated with an increased risk of liver disease and cancer.[49,50]

Naturally circulating variations in the viral population can also be clinically relevant. Eight HBV genotypes have been described in detail to date with 10 total known HBV genotypes, each having a relatively well-defined geographic distribution. Moreover, each genotype has been reported to respond differently to treatments (eg, genotype A and D are more susceptible to interferon treatment compared with genotype B and C) and carries different risks of liver cancer (eg, people with genotype C HBV are more likely to progress to liver cancer compared with those infected with genotype B).[51]

However, viral DNA sequencing and genotyping are not carried out for routine clinical management, owing to high costs, dependence on specialized laboratories to carry out the assay and to interpret sequencing results, and the long turnaround times (generally weeks). Current assays include qPCR assays with genotype-specific probes or conventional PCR followed by capillary sequencing of the HBsAg and polymerase genes. Greater access to these tests could improve the provision of care for chronic patients with HBV. Astbury and colleagues[52] developed a mobile next-generation sequencing pipeline (based on Oxford Nanopore technology) using dried blood spots to genotype viruses and identify resistance mutations without the need for DNA extraction. Although this approach still requires PCR and specialized analysis of sequencing data, it may broaden the availability of next-generation sequencing to laboratory settings with PCR capacity and enhance the delivery of optimum care.

As an alternative approach, Song and colleagues[53] have developed a point-of-care lateral flow assay using antibodies specific for the surface antigens of the 4 most common viral genotypes (A to D) and a pan-genotypic antibody. Notably, given that this serotyping assay is based on the HBsAg and not HBV DNA, the assay can be used even with patients on antiviral treatment (unlike PCR-based assays).

Assessing Liver Cancer Risk

Chronic hepatitis B is the single greatest cause of HCC worldwide. Unlike other causes of HCC, HBV-associated HCC can occur in the presence or absence of cirrhosis. Thus, simply staging liver fibrosis is unable to accurately stratify patients into high and low liver cancer risk. Currently, patients with chronic HBV are monitored for HCC using abdominal ultrasound to detect liver masses or by measuring serum alpha-fetoprotein (AFP). These however are not sensitive for small or early-stage HCCs (eg, AFP is elevated in only ~50% of patients with HCC[54]). Additional host proteins (such as Lens culinaris agglutinin–reactive AFP, and des gamma-carboxy prothrombin) can improve sensitivity, particularly when combined with other clinical aspects (gender and age). The GALAD scoring algorithm based on these aspects have shown more sensitive performance compared with existing screening and surveillance measures in detecting early liver cancers in patients with chronic HBV[55–57] and fatty liver disease.[58] Further research continues to understand the power of the GALAD algorithm in larger and more diverse populations.

Despite many studies, serum levels of viral products do not appear to accurately predict cancer risk in all contexts.[59] One notable exception is the use of integrated HBV DNA to determine liver cancer recurrence. HBV-associated HCC often contains copies of the virus DNA integrated into unique positions in the host genome. Circulating DNA and urine are both known to contain fragments of liver-derived DNA, including integrated HBV DNA from hepatocytes and tumor tissue. Thus, tumor-specific fragments detected by specific PCR have been used to predict cancer recurrence after resection.[60,61] However, assays to detect these junctions are bespoke and require significant expertise to design and develop.

Other groups have developed liver cancer markers based on the methylation of circulating cellular DNA fragments. The genomes of liver cancers often display altered methylation patterns compared with normal hepatocytes, and these are maintained in circulating DNA fragments. Panels of methylated DNA sequences have been defined and quantified by several groups to differentiate unaffected patients and patients with liver cancer with promising results.[62,63] In particular, a group from Exact Sciences achieved a higher specificity and sensitivity for early-stage HCC compared with GALAD or AFP by combining with AFP and Lens culinaris agglutinin-reactive AFP and quantifying a panel of 3 methylated DNA sequences from 3 mL of plasma.[64] This approach appeared to perform equally well regardless of cause or gender, suggesting it could be of value when considering patients with multiple liver comorbidities.

Another context where HBV proteins may play a role in determining cancer risk is "occult" HBV infection (defined as having HBV DNA while being HBsAg-negative). Occult HBV is associated with increased HCC risk, although it is unclear whether this is due to a population with HBsAg below the limit of detection for standard HBsAg assays. Indeed, using an ultra-high-sensitivity HBsAg assay (100× more sensitive than standard HBsAg assays), Wong and colleagues[65] found that 36.8% of patients ostensibly negative for HBsAg by standard assays were HBsAg-positive (in some cases, >10 years after supposed seroconversion). These data are consistent with lower sensitivity assays (10× more sensitive than the standard HBsAg ELISA) with positive rates of 7% to 26%.[66,67] Such assays provide an approach for clinical research to determine if low-level HBsAg may contribute or be associated with increased cancer or disease progression risk.

Transmission Risk

Recent studies in blood recipients have suggested that the minimum infectious dose of HBV is as low as 15 IU.[68] The lower limit of detection of current HBV DNA PCR assays (10 IU/mL) is too low to completely rule out this level of virus in the context of blood and organ donation. Indeed, blood from patients on antiviral treatment (below the limit of quantification by qPCR) was sufficient for establishing infection in immuno-compromised mice with humanized livers.[69]

Although organs from donors previously exposed to HBV (anti-HBc Ab positive) are still considered for transplant with appropriate analysis of risk factors and patient consent,[70] blood donations from people previously exposed to HBV are excluded in some countries because of concerns about transmission.[71]

Increasing sensitivity of current tests for HBV could expand the pool of safe blood donors.[72] There may be little chance of directly detecting lower than current detection limits given the amount of DNA template available in the extracted samples. However, a high-sensitivity HBsAg test may be able to detect residual virions: 0.5 mIU/mL of HBsAg (10× lower than the lower limit of detection by standard HBsAg assays at 0.05 IU/mL) corresponds to 4 IU/mL of HBV DNA,[72] so could identify potentially infectious donors missed by PCR. As mentioned, this assay would also detect blood from donors with occult hepatitis B, which accounts for a large proportion of transfusion-related HBV infections.[73,74]

UNRESOLVED SCIENTIFIC ISSUES FOR CURE RESEARCH

New curative strategies are being developed to target the underlying levels of persistent viral forms (cccDNA and integrated HBV DNA), their transcriptional activity, and/or activation of an antiviral immune response. Monitoring these aspects is difficult with currently used assays, and so novel tests have been developed to assess the effectiveness of new treatment strategies more readily (**Fig. 3**).

Measuring Levels of Intrahepatic Hepatitis B Virus DNA

Many investigational therapies affect viral replication (or even expression) but not the underlying viral DNA templates responsible for viral persistence and rebound after treatment cessation. Hence, circulating HBV DNA or protein markers (ie, current tests for HBV) can present poor surrogates for intrahepatic levels of HBV. To directly quantify cccDNA and integrated HBV DNA, several molecular methods have been developed, although these require invasive needle biopsies to achieve sufficient cellular input for analysis and can have low specificity, sensitivity, and precision.[75–77] Given these significant drawbacks, most of these assays are only suitable for occasional monitoring. Ongoing efforts to develop new highly sensitive methods to quantify cccDNA and integrated DNA (eg, from fine needle aspirate [FNA] liver samples) are being pursued.

Measuring the Transcriptional Activity of Intrahepatic Hepatitis B Virus DNA

To overcome these barriers, both newly applied and newly developed surrogate measures for transcriptionally active HBV DNA have been developed.[78] Serum levels of HBV DNA significantly correlate with levels of cccDNA in untreated people with HBV but loses this strong association once patients are on antiviral therapy. Levels of HBsAg quantified using ELISAs in laboratory diagnostic settings provide a measure of viral transcriptional activity (even in people treated with reverse-transcriptase inhibitors) and are increasingly measured in patient management to decide on the cessation of antiviral therapy or clinical trials of novel HBV treatment strategies.

A shortcoming to this approach is that the source of HBsAg (either cccDNA or integrated HBV DNA) remains unclear. As cccDNA is responsible for posttreatment viral rebound, this is the key molecule to be targeted with new treatment strategies. To determine if investigational therapies are reducing transcriptionally active cccDNA, several new serum assays have been developed. Most widely used are assays measuring circulating HBV RNA (detected by reverse-transcription qPCR) or HBcrAg (ELISA), both only produced by cccDNA. However, ~30% of patients with HBV test

Approaches to measure

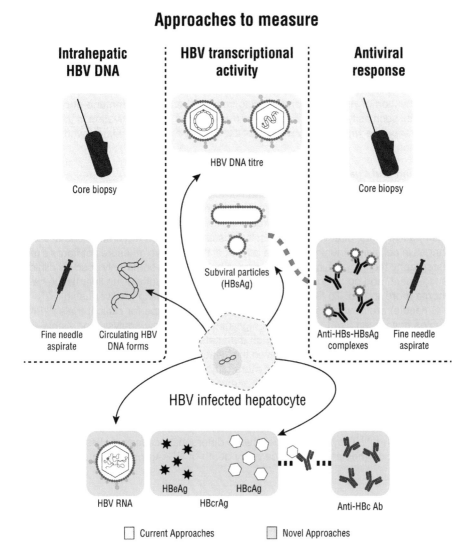

Fig. 3. Novel assays to support HBV cure research. Several aspects of HBV and patient response that are crucial for HBV cure research remain difficult to measure in clinical trial participants, including intrahepatic HBV DNA, HBV transcriptional activity, and the intrahepatic antiviral immune response. Quantification of intrahepatic HBV DNA quantification currently requires invasive core biopsies to achieve sufficient cellular input, which limits its use for serial monitoring. More sensitive PCR-based assays may use minimally invasive FNA samples instead. Circulating HBV DNA forms (eg, integrated HBV DNA) may also play a role in the future. Viral titer and quantitative HBsAg can be used as an indication of total viral transcriptional activity but cannot distinguish between cccDNA or integrated HBV DNA. Measuring HBV RNA, HBcrAg, and anti-HBc Abs may provide an indication of cccDNA-specific activity. Direct assessment of hepatic cells using invasive biopsies is required for the quantification of antiviral immunity changes; less-invasive FNAs as well as anti-HBs-HBsAg complex quantification are being considered an alternate novel approach.

negative for these markers using current assays.[79] Thus, higher-sensitivity assays are needed if these are to be used in the future for clinical trials.

In an alternate approach, Caviglia and colleagues[80] investigated the use of serum levels of anti-HBc as a surrogate marker for cccDNA, showing high correlation ($r = 0.785$) and detection even in occult hepatitis B (where cccDNA is at low concentrations, ~ 1 per 10,000 cells). Supporting this, anti-HBc titers have been used to predict reactivation of HBV infection following immunotherapy[81] or immune-suppressive conditions, such as lymphoma[82,83] or liver transplant.[84] This reactivation in the face of antiviral response may explain why anti-HBc has also been correlated with disease progression.[85]

Quantifying and Characterizing Antiviral Responses

Both direct-acting antivirals and immunotherapies are likely to cause changes in antiviral immunity. However, these have been technically difficult to measure in people with chronic hepatitis B. Given that circulating immune cells do not necessarily reflect intrahepatic events, direct accessing of liver tissues has been required to characterize changes in cellular immunity. With the advent of noninvasive measures of fibrosis (eg, elastography techniques), core biopsies have become less commonly used for clinical management, and so opportunities to study antiviral immunity using liver tissue have become more limited. To fill this void, FNAs (directly sampling the liver using a 23- to 25-G needle) are now considered an important sample type for clinical trials.[86] FNA samples have been used for in-depth high-dimensional flow analysis and single-cell transcriptomics to provide large and rich data sets on intrahepatic cell types and their expression profiles.[87–89] However, given the invasive nature of these tests, serial sampling to monitor changes over time is more difficult to carry out.

Some antiviral responses have been measured in the circulation. Immune complexes of anti-HBs-HBsAg may be one marker particularly important for the development of curative treatments.[90] Increased levels of these immune complexes may represent reinvigoration of humoral immunity and indeed have been found to precede a functional cure.[91] They may also be used to differentiate causes of HBsAg reduction (eg, via antibody-mediated clearance or by death of HBsAg-producing cells).[92]

SUMMARY

Most people living with HBV live in developing countries and have limited access to laboratory-based diagnosis or monitoring. To ensure that 2030 WHO elimination goals for hepatitis B are met (reducing incidence by 90% and mortality due to chronic hepatitis B by 65% relative to 2015 levels[93]), huge leaps in diagnosis and treatment rates are required (currently at $\sim 10\%$ and $\sim 5\%$ worldwide, respectively).[1] These aspects can be addressed on a policy level. Current screening and treatment guidelines could be expanded so that a greater proportion of the affected population are diagnosed and get appropriate care. Novel assays can help achieve this: for example, universal screening for HBV (as opposed to the current paradigm of risk-based screening) could become more cost-effective with cheaper tests.[94] Also, the impact of simplified treatment algorithms (eg, the 2022 Chinese treatment guidelines in which most HBV DNA-positive people with chronic hepatitis B are considered for antiviral treatment) can be multiplied significantly by the broader availability of tests for HBV DNA or appropriate surrogate markers. These results fit into suggested schemes to meet the 2030 WHO elimination goals for hepatitis B (eg, the 5-line guideline—test all adults, vaccinate all HBV-negative adults, test HBV-positive people for hepatitis delta virus, increase treatment, and monitor for liver disease).

Thus, a key part of the solution is developing and implementing assays to measure various aspects of HBV infection quickly, easily, cheaply, and preferably without dependence on centralized laboratory services. Although some approaches described in this have already been trialed and implemented in the field (eg, point-of-care assays for HBV antigens, antibodies, and HBV DNA), most still require substantial validation across laboratories and settings, as well as cost-benefit justification for their use. These novel assays do not address all issues that prevent successful linkage to care, but such developments can significantly broaden public health capabilities and accelerate cure research, both of which are crucial to the elimination of the impacts of chronic hepatitis B.

CLINICS CARE POINTS

- Global hepatitis B control requires knowing the hepatitis B status of every person (HBsAg, anti-HBs, anti-HBc) to vaccinate, monitor, and (if necessary) treat them.
- Upcoming assays potentially provide cheap and highly-sensitive measurements of these aspects that can feed into simple management and treatment algorithms.
- Point of care testing for surface antigen and HBV DNA are key to monitor control of viral replication, particularly in remote or resource limited settings.
- Loss-to-follow up could be reduced by the new assays by simplifying and speeding up testing thereby facilitating appropriate provision of care, and immediately informing patient management.

CONFLICT OF INTEREST

The authors have no relevant affiliations or financial involvement with any organization or entity with a financial interest in or financial conflict with the subject matter or materials discussed in the manuscript. This includes employment, consultancies, honoraria, stock ownership or options, expert testimony, grants or patents received or pending, or royalties.

FUNDING

Work on this manuscript was in part supported by Ideas grants 2002565 and 2021586 from the National Health and Medical Research Council (NHMRC) of Australia, and by the Robert W Storr bequest to the Sydney Medical Foundation, University of Sydney.

REFERENCES

1. Polaris Observatory C. Global prevalence, treatment, and prevention of hepatitis B virus infection in 2016: a modelling study. Lancet Gastroenterol Hepatol 2018; 3(6):383–403.
2. Tu T., Budzinska M.A., Shackel N.A., et al., HBV DNA integration: molecular mechanisms and clinical implications, *Viruses*, 9 (4), 2017,75.
3. Tu T., Budzinska M.A., Vondran F.W.R., et al., Hepatitis B virus DNA integration occurs early in the viral life cycle in an in vitro infection model via sodium taurocholate cotransporting polypeptide-dependent uptake of enveloped virus particles, *J Virol*, 92 (11), 2018, e02007-17.

4. Tu T., Zehnder B., Qu B., et al., *De novo* synthesis of hepatitis B virus nucleocapsids is dispensable for the maintenance and transcriptional regulation of cccDNA. JHEP Reports, 3(1), 2020, 100195.

5. Gerlich WH. Medical virology of hepatitis B: how it began and where we are now. Virol J 2013;10:239.

6. Mutz P., Metz P., Lempp F.A., et al., HBV bypasses the innate immune response and does not protect HCV from antiviral activity of interferon, *Gastroenterology*, 154 (6), 2018, 1791–1804 e22.

7. Chua C.G., Mehrotra A., Mazzulli T., et al., Optimized ex vivo stimulation identifies multi-functional HBV-specific T cells in a majority of chronic hepatitis B patients, *Sci Rep*, 10 (1), 2020, 11344.

8. Tu T., Block J.M., Wang S., et al., The lived experience of chronic hepatitis B: a broader view of its impacts and why we need a cure, *Viruses*, 12 (5), 2020, 515.

10. Ho E., Michielsen P., Van Damme P., et al., Point-of-care tests for hepatitis B are associated with a higher linkage to care and lower cost compared to venepuncture sampling during outreach screenings in an asian migrant population, *Ann Glob Health*, 86 (1), 2020, 81.

11. Amini A, Varsaneux O, Kelly H, et al. Diagnostic accuracy of tests to detect hepatitis B surface antigen: a systematic review of the literature and meta-analysis. BMC Infect Dis 2017;17(Suppl 1):698.

12. Dembele B, Affi-Aboli R, Kabran M, et al. Evaluation of four rapid tests for detection of hepatitis B surface antigen in ivory coast. J Immunol Res 2020;2020: 6315718.

13. Segeral O., Phirum W., Khan O., et al., In-field evaluation of SD Bioline HBsAg whole blood rapid test in pregnant women in Cambodia: the ANRS 12345 TA PROHM study, *Diagn Microbiol Infect Dis*, 101 (2), 2021, 115452.

14. Farooq A, Waheed U, Zaheer HA, et al. Detection of HBsAg mutants in the blood donor population of Pakistan. PLoS One 2017;12(11):e0188066.

15. Su S., Wong W.C., Zou Z., et al., Cost-effectiveness of universal screening for chronic hepatitis B virus infection in China: an economic evaluation, *Lancet Global Health*, 10 (2), 2022, e278–e287.

16. Allard N.L., MacLachlan J.H., Tran L., et al., Time for universal hepatitis B screening for Australian adults, *Med J Aust*, 215 (3), 2021, 103–105 e1.

17. Mohamed S., Raimondo A., Pénaranda G., et al., Dried blood spot sampling for hepatitis B virus serology and molecular testing, *PLoS One*, 8 (4), 2013, e61077.

18. Yamamoto C., Nagashima S., Isomura M., et al., Evaluation of the efficiency of dried blood spot-based measurement of hepatitis B and hepatitis C virus sero-markers, *Sci Rep*, 10 (1), 2020, 3857.

19. Terrault NA, Lok ASF, McMahon BJ, et al. Update on prevention, diagnosis, and treatment of chronic hepatitis B: AASLD 2018 hepatitis B guidance. Hepatology 2018;67(4):1560–99.

20. Sarin SK, Kumar M, Lau GK, et al. Asian-Pacific clinical practice guidelines on the management of hepatitis B: a 2015 update. Hepatol Int 2016;10(1):1–98.

21. European Association for the Study of the Liver. Electronic address, e.e.e. and L. European Association for the Study of the, EASL 2017 Clinical Practice Guidelines on the management of hepatitis B virus infection. J Hepatol 2017;67(2): 370–98.

22. Wong R.J., Kaufman H.W., Niles J.K., et al., Simplifying treatment criteria in chronic hepatitis B: reducing barriers to elimination, *Clin Infect Dis*, 76(3), 2022, e791-e800.

23. Dieterich D., Graham C., Wang S., et al., It is time for a simplified approach to hepatitis B elimination, *Gastro Hep Advances*, 2 (2), 2023, 209–218.

24. Trickey A., Fajardo E., Alemu D., et al., Impact of hepatitis C virus point-of-care RNA viral load testing compared with laboratory-based testing on uptake of RNA testing and treatment, and turnaround times: a systematic review and meta-analysis, *Lancet Gastroenterol Hepatol*, 8 (3), 2023, 253–270.

25. Auzin A.M., Slavenburg S., Peters C., et al., Rapid, random-access, and quantification of hepatitis B virus using the Cepheid Xpert HBV viral load assay, *J Med Virol*, 93 (6), 2021, 3999–4003.

26. Marcuccilli F., Chevaliez S., Muller T., et al., Multicenter evaluation of the cepheid xpert((R)) HBV viral load test, *Diagnostics*, 11 (2), 2021, 297.

27. Poiteau L, Wlassow M, Hézode C, et al. Evaluation of the xpert HBV viral load for hepatitis B virus molecular testing. J Clin Virol 2020;129:104481.

28. Jackson K., Tekoaua R., Li X., et al., Real-world application of the Xpert(R) HBV viral load assay on serum and dried blood spots, *J Med Virol*, 93 (6), 2021, 3707–3713.

29. Chen C.M., Ouyang S., Lin L.Y., et al., Diagnostic accuracy of LAMP assay for HBV infection, *J Clin Lab Anal*, 34 (7), 2020, e23281.

30. Quoc N.B., Phuong N.D.N., Chau N.N.B., et al., Closed tube loop-mediated isothermal amplification assay for rapid detection of hepatitis B virus in human blood, *Heliyon*, 4 (3), 2018, e00561.

31. Vanhomwegen J., Kwasiborski A., Diop A., et al., Development and clinical validation of loop-mediated isothermal amplification (LAMP) assay to diagnose high HBV DNA levels in resource-limited settings, *Clin Microbiol Infect*, 27 (12), 2021, 1858 e9-e1858 e15.

32. Chen X, Tan Y, Wang S, et al. A CRISPR-Cas12b-based platform for ultrasensitive, rapid, and highly specific detection of hepatitis B virus genotypes B and C in clinical application. Front Bioeng Biotechnol 2021;9:743322.

33. Ding R., Long J., Yuan M., et al., CRISPR/Cas12-based ultra-sensitive and specific point-of-care detection of HBV, *Int J Mol Sci*, 22 (9), 2021, 4842.

34. Maasoumy B., Wiegand S.B., Jaroszewicz J., et al., Hepatitis B core-related antigen (HBcrAg) levels in the natural history of hepatitis B virus infection in a large European cohort predominantly infected with genotypes A and D, *Clin Microbiol Infect*, 21 (6), 2015, 606 e1-e10.

35. Shimakawa Y, Ndow G, Kaneko A, et al. Rapid point-of-care test for hepatitis B core-related antigen to diagnose high viral load in resource-limited settings. Clin Gastroenterol Hepatol 2022;S1542-3565(22):00554-7.

36. Pollock N.R., Rolland J.P., Kumar S., et al., A paper-based multiplexed transaminase test for low-cost, point-of-care liver function testing, *Sci Transl Med*, 4 (152), 2012, 152ra129.

37. Pollock NR, Colby D, Rolland JP. A point-of-care paper-based fingerstick transaminase test: toward low-cost "lab-on-a-chip" technology for the developing world. Clin Gastroenterol Hepatol 2013;11(5):478–82.

38. Howell J., Van H., Pham M., et al., Validation of a novel point-of-care test for alanine aminotransferase measurement: a pilot cohort study, *Liver Int*, 43 (5), 2023, 989–999.

39. Resmi PE, Sachin Kumar S, Alageswari D, et al. Development of a paper-based analytical device for the colourimetric detection of alanine transaminase and the application of deep learning for image analysis. Anal Chim Acta 2021;1188: 339158.

40. Seto W.K., Lai C.L., Ip P.P., et al., A large population histology study showing the lack of association between ALT elevation and significant fibrosis in chronic hepatitis B, *PLoS One*, 7 (2), 2012, e32622.
41. Kumar M, Sarin SK, Hissar S, et al. Virologic and histologic features of chronic hepatitis B virus-infected asymptomatic patients with persistently normal ALT. Gastroenterology 2008;134(5):1376–84.
42. Joseph J. Serum marker panels for predicting liver fibrosis - an update. Clin Biochem Rev 2020;41(2):67–73.
43. Dickerson W.M., Yu R., Westergren H.U., et al., Point-of-care microvolume cytometer measures platelet counts with high accuracy from capillary blood, *PLoS One*, 16 (8), 2021, e0256423.
44. Larsson A, Smekal D, Lipcsey M. Rapid testing of red blood cells, white blood cells and platelets in intensive care patients using the HemoScreen point-of-care analyzer. Platelets 2019;30(8):1013–6.
45. Wang Q., Xie W., Liu L., et al., Serum markers for predicting advanced fibrosis in patients with chronic hepatitis B and nonalcoholic fatty liver disease, *Medicine (Baltim)*, 100 (18), 2021, e25327.
46. Revill P.A., Tu T., Netter H.J., et al., The evolution and clinical impact of hepatitis B virus genome diversity, *Nat Rev Gastroenterol Hepatol*, 17 (10), 2020, 618–634.
47. Levine S, Hernandez D, Yamanaka G, et al. Efficacies of entecavir against lamivudine-resistant hepatitis B virus replication and recombinant polymerases in vitro. Antimicrobial Agents Chemother 2002;46(8):2525–32.
48. Reijnders JG, Deterding K, Petersen J, et al. Antiviral effect of entecavir in chronic hepatitis B: influence of prior exposure to nucleos(t)ide analogues. J Hepatol 2010;52(4):493–500.
49. Yeung P., Wong D.K., Lai C.L., et al., Association of hepatitis B virus pre-S deletions with the development of hepatocellular carcinoma in chronic hepatitis B, *J Infect Dis*, 203 (5), 2011, 646–654.
50. Su IJ, Wang HC, Wu HC, et al. Ground glass hepatocytes contain pre-S mutants and represent preneoplastic lesions in chronic hepatitis B virus infection. J Gastroenterol Hepatol 2008;23(8 Pt 1):1169–74.
51. Kao JH, Chen PJ, Lai MY, et al. Hepatitis B genotypes correlate with clinical outcomes in patients with chronic hepatitis B. Gastroenterology 2000;118(3):554–9.
52. Astbury S, Costa Nunes Soares MM, Peprah E, et al. Nanopore sequencing from extraction-free direct PCR of dried serum spots for portable hepatitis B virus drug-resistance typing. J Clin Virol 2020;129:104483.
53. Song LW, Wang YB, Fang LL, et al. Rapid fluorescent lateral-flow immunoassay for hepatitis B virus genotyping. Anal Chem 2015;87(10):5173–80.
54. Luo CL, Rong Y, Chen H, et al. A logistic regression model for noninvasive prediction of AFP-negative hepatocellular carcinoma. Technol Cancer Res Treat 2019;18:1533033819846632.
55. Yang J.D., Addissie B.D., Mara K.C., et al., GALAD score for hepatocellular carcinoma detection in comparison with liver ultrasound and proposal of GALADUS score, *Cancer Epidemiol Biomarkers Prev*, 28 (3), 2019, 531–538.
56. Li L, et al. Validation of the GALAD model and establishment of a new model for HCC detection in Chinese patients. Front Oncol 2022;12:1037742.
57. Schotten C.,Ostertag B., Sowa J.P., et al., GALAD score detects early-stage hepatocellular carcinoma in a European cohort of chronic hepatitis B and C patients, *Pharmaceuticals*, 14 (8), 2021, 735.

58. Best J., Bechmann L.P., Sowa J.P., et al., GALAD score detects early hepatocellular carcinoma in an international cohort of patients with nonalcoholic steatohepatitis, *Clin Gastroenterol Hepatol*, 18 (3), 2020, 728–735 e4.
59. Liu Y, Veeraraghavan V, Pinkerton M, et al. Viral biomarkers for hepatitis B virus-related hepatocellular carcinoma occurrence and recurrence. Front Microbiol 2021;12:665201.
60. Li C.L., Ho M.C., Lin Y.Y., et al., Cell-free virus-host chimera DNA from hepatitis B virus integration sites as a circulating biomarker of hepatocellular cancer, *Hepatology*, 72 (6), 2020, 2063–2076.
61. Li W, Cui X, Huo Q, et al. Profile of HBV integration in the plasma DNA of hepatocellular carcinoma patients. Curr Genomics 2019;20(1):61–8.
62. Kisiel J.B., Dukek B.A., V S R Kanipakam R., et al., Hepatocellular carcinoma detection by plasma methylated DNA: discovery, phase I pilot, and phase II clinical validation, *Hepatology*, 69 (3), 2019, 1180–1192.
63. Goncalves E, et al. DNA methylation fingerprint of hepatocellular carcinoma from tissue and liquid biopsies. Sci Rep 2022;12(1):11512.
64. Chalasani N.P., Ramasubramanian T.S., Bhattacharya A., et al., A novel blood-based panel of methylated DNA and protein markers for detection of early-stage hepatocellular carcinoma, *Clin Gastroenterol Hepatol*, 19 (12), 2021, 2597–2605 e4.
65. Wong DK, Inoue T, Mak LY, et al. A longitudinal study to detect hepatitis B surface and core-related antigens in chronic hepatitis B patients with hepatitis B surface antigen seroclearance using highly sensitive assays. J Clin Virol 2022;160:105375.
66. Seto W.K., Tanaka Y., Wong D.K., et al., Evidence of serologic activity in chronic hepatitis B after surface antigen (HBsAg) seroclearance documented by conventional HBsAg assay, *Hepatol Int*, 7 (1), 2012, 98–105.
67. Wong DK, Chen C, Mak LY, et al. Detection of the hepatitis B surface antigen in patients with occult hepatitis B by use of an assay with enhanced sensitivity. J Clin Microbiol 2022;60(2):e0220421.
68. Candotti D., Assennato S.M., Laperche S., et al., Multiple HBV transfusion transmissions from undetected occult infections: revising the minimal infectious dose, *Gut*, 68 (2), 2019, 313–321.
69. Burdette D.L., Lazerwith S., Yang J., et al., Ongoing viral replication and production of infectious virus in patients with chronic hepatitis B virus suppressed below the limit of quantitation on long-term nucleos(t)ide therapy, *PLoS One*, 17 (4), 2022, e0262516.
70. Huprikar S, Danziger-Isakov L, Ahn J, et al. Solid organ transplantation from hepatitis B virus-positive donors: consensus guidelines for recipient management. Am J Transplant 2015;15(5):1162–72.
71. Committee, J.U.K.U.B.T.a.T.T.S.P.A. Hepatitis B. 2023 cited 2023 09/02/2023; Available at: https://www.transfusionguidelines.org/dsg/wb/guidelines/he016-hepatitis-b.
72. Gerlich WH, Glebe D, Schüttler CG. Hepatitis B viral safety of blood donations: new gaps identified. Annals of Blood 2018;3(38).
73. Allain JP, Mihaljevic I, Gonzalez-Fraile MI, et al. Infectivity of blood products from donors with occult hepatitis B virus infection. Transfusion 2013;53(7):1405–15.
74. Harvala H., Reynolds C., Gibney Z., et al., Hepatitis B infections among blood donors in England between 2009 and 2018: is an occult hepatitis B infection a risk for blood safety?, *Transfusion*, 61 (8), 2021, 2402–2413.

75. Zhang H, Tu T. Approaches to quantifying hepatitis B virus covalently closed circular DNA. Clin Mol Hepatol 2022;28(2):135–49.
76. Allweiss L., Testoni B., Yu M., et al., Quantification of the hepatitis B virus cccDNA: evidence-based guidelines for monitoring the key obstacle of HBV cure, *Gut*, 72 (5), 2023, 972–983.
77. Tu T, Zhang H, Urban S. Hepatitis B virus DNA integration: in vitro models for investigating viral pathogenesis and persistence. Viruses 2021;13(2):180.
78. Tu T, Bommel FV, Berg T. Surrogate markers for hepatitis B virus covalently closed circular DNA. Semin Liver Dis 2022;42(3):327–40.
79. Ghany M.G., King W.C., Lisker-Melman M., et al., Comparison of HBV RNA and hepatitis B core related antigen with conventional HBV markers among untreated adults with chronic hepatitis B in north America, *Hepatology*, 74 (5), 2021, 2395–2409.
80. Caviglia G.P., Olivero A., Ciancio A., et al., Analytical and clinical evaluation of a novel assay for anti-HBc IgG measurement in serum of subjects with overt and occult HBV infection, *Diagn Microbiol Infect Dis*, 96 (4), 2020, 114985.
81. Wu Y., Wang X., Lin X., et al., Quantitative of serum hepatitis B core antibody is a potential predictor of recurrence after interferon-induced hepatitis B surface antigen clearance, *J Microbiol Immunol Infect*, 54 (2), 2021, 238–244.
82. Cerva C, Salpini R, Alkhatib M, et al. Highly sensitive HBsAg, anti-HBc and anti HBsAg titres in early diagnosis of HBV reactivation in anti-HBc-positive onco-haematological patients. Biomedicines 2022;10(2).
83. Matsubara T, Nishida T, Shimoda A, et al. The combination of anti-HBc and anti-HBs levels is a useful predictor of the development of chemotherapy-induced reactivation in lymphoma patients with resolved HBV infection. Oncol Lett 2017; 14(6):6543–52.
84. Cholongitas E, Papatheodoridis GV, Burroughs AK. Liver grafts from anti-hepatitis B core positive donors: a systematic review. J Hepatol 2010;52(2):272–9.
85. Yuan Q, Song LW, Cavallone D, et al. Total hepatitis B core antigen antibody, a quantitative non-invasive marker of hepatitis B virus induced liver disease. PLoS One 2015;10(6):e0130209.
86. Gehring A.J., Mendez P., Richter K., et al., Immunological biomarker discovery in cure regimens for chronic hepatitis B virus infection, *J Hepatol*, 77 (2), 2022, 525–538.
87. Gill U.S., Pallett L.J., Thomas N., et al., Fine needle aspirates comprehensively sample intrahepatic immunity, *Gut*, 68 (8), 2019, 1493–1503.
88. Sprengers D., van der Molen R.G., Kusters J.G., et al., Flow cytometry of fine-needle-aspiration biopsies: a new method to monitor the intrahepatic immunological environment in chronic viral hepatitis, *J Viral Hepat*, 12 (5), 2005, 507–512.
89. Nkongolo S, Mahamed D, Kuipery A, et al. Longitudinal liver sampling in patients with chronic hepatitis B starting antiviral therapy reveals hepatotoxic CD8+ T cells. J Clin Invest 2023;133(1).
90. Corti D, Benigni F, Shouval D. Viral envelope-specific antibodies in chronic hepatitis B virus infection. Curr Opin Virol 2018;30:48–57.
91. Xu H., Locarnini S., Wong D., et al., Role of anti-HBs in functional cure of HBeAg+ chronic hepatitis B patients infected with HBV genotype A, *J Hepatol*, 76 (1), 2022, 34–45.

92. Bazinet M., Anderson M., Pântea V., et al., Analysis of HBsAg immunocomplexes and cccDNA activity during and persisting after NAP-based therapy, *Hepatol Commun*, 5 (11), 2021, 1873–1887.
93. World Health O. Global health sector strategy on viral hepatitis 2016-2021. Towards ending viral hepatitis. Geneva: World Health Organization; 2016.
94. Xiao Y., Hellard M.E., Thompson A.J., et al., The cost-effectiveness of universal hepatitis B screening for reaching WHO diagnosis targets in Australia by 2030, *Med J Aust*, 218 (4), 2023, 168–173.

Overview of New Targets for Hepatitis B Virus

Immune Modulators, Interferons, Bifunctional Peptides, Therapeutic Vaccines and Beyond

James Lok, MA, MBBS, MRCP, Maria Fernanda Guerra Veloz, MD, PhD, Kosh Agarwal, B Med Sci (Hons), MBBS, MRCP, MD*

KEYWORDS

- Hepatitis B virus • Treatment • Immune modulators • Vaccination

KEY POINTS

- Chronic hepatitis B virus (HBV) infection is characterized by exhaustion of the adaptive immune response, with a reduction in their proliferative and cytotoxic capacity.
- Immunomodulatory agents have been developed including Toll-like receptor agonists, therapeutic vaccines, and checkpoint inhibitors.
- Given the pleotropic nature of HBV persistence, it is likely that a combination of immunomodulators and direct acting antivirals will be required to achieve the highest rates of functional cure.
- The heterogeneity of clinical outcomes demands a personalized approach to pharmacotherapy and predictive biomarkers.

INTRODUCTION

Hepatitis B virus (HBV) is a global health problem with 262 million people affected worldwide. Chronic infection may be established within the liver, especially if exposure occurs early in life, and this predisposes to serious complications such as cirrhosis, hepatic decompensation, and hepatocellular carcinoma. Elimination of the virus is challenging due to integration of its genetic material into host DNA and formation of a transcriptional template (covalently closed circular DNA, cccDNA) that is resistant to endonuclease enzymes. In addition, there is exhaustion of the HBV-specific immune response with a reduction in cytotoxic and proliferative capability. For many years, nucleos(t)ide analogs (NA) have been the cornerstone of treatment given their high barrier to resistance and favorable side-effect profile; however, functional cure (defined as serum HBsAg $\leq$ 0.05 IU/mL) is rarely achieved and prolonged courses

Institute of Liver Studies, King's College Hospital, London, SE5 9RS, UK
* Corresponding author.
E-mail address: kosh.agarwal@kcl.ac.uk

Clin Liver Dis 27 (2023) 857–876
https://doi.org/10.1016/j.cld.2023.05.003
1089-3261/23/© 2023 Elsevier Inc. All rights reserved.

liver.theclinics.com

are required to achieve clinical benefit. The World Health Organization has targeted a 90% reduction in the incidence of viral hepatitis by the year 2030. Achieving this ambitious goal will require the expansion of screening programs, improved linkage to care, and a broader repertoire of therapeutic options.

VIRAL LIFE CYCLE

HBV is a member of the Hepadnaviridae family of viruses and has a relaxed circular, partially double-stranded DNA genome (rcDNA). Its life cycle and therapeutic targets are summarized in **Fig. 1**. In summary, 42 nm Dane particles bind to sodium taurocholate co-transporting peptide (NTCP) on the basolateral surface of hepatocytes, triggering clathrin-mediated endocytosis and internalization to the endosomal compartment.[1,2] Following disassembly of its nucleocapsid, rcDNA is transported to the nucleus and converted into cccDNA by a series of host enzymes[3]; this episomal structure is inherently stable and forms the template for pre-genomic (pgRNA, 3.5kb) and sub-genomic RNA expression (2.4 kb, 2.1 kb, 0.7 kb).[4] Transcriptional activity fluctuates during the course of infection and is influenced by viral proteins (core, HBx), host transcriptional factors (Smc5/6), and epigenetic modifiers (eg, histone acetylation).[5,6]

The multifunctional HBV polymerase is responsible for the encapsidation of pgRNA, synthesis of the minus and positive DNA strands, and degradation of the RNA template. Early in the viral life cycle, nucleocapsids containing newly synthesized rcDNA are transported back to the nucleus and amplify the cccDNA reservoir. In later stages, nucleocapsids are encapsulated by surface proteins and released into the bloodstream by exocytosis.[7] During reverse transcription of rcDNA into cccDNA, primer

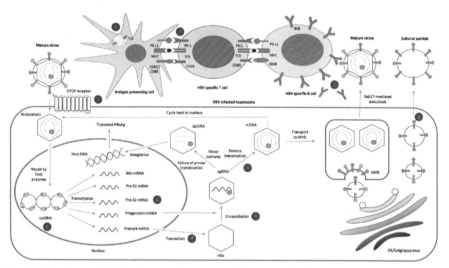

Fig. 1. Overview of HBV therapeutic targets: (a) entry inhibitors, (b) cccDNA targeting agents (CRISPR/Cas system, zinc finger nucleases, transcription activator-like endonucleases, base editors), (c) RNA destabilizers (PAPD5/7 inhibitors), (d) translation inhibitors (small interfering RNAs, antisense oligonucleotides), (e) capsid assembly modulators, (f) inhibitors of HBV polymerase (chain terminating nucleos(t)ide analogs, active site polymerase inhibitor nucleotides, (g) HBsAg secretion inhibitors (nucleic acid polymers, STOPS), (h) pattern recognition receptor agonists (Toll-like receptors, RIG-I, NOD-2), (i) checkpoint inhibitors (eg, PD-1/PD-L1 pathway), (j) monoclonal antibodies.

translocation may fail to occur and this leads to the formation of double-stranded linear DNA; the structure integrates into the host genome at the site of DNA breaks and is an additional source of subgenomic RNA transcripts.[8] Integration is purported to drive cellular transformation through *cis*-mediated mutagenesis and contribute to the exhaustion of HBV-specific immune responses.[9]

Limitations of Current Treatment

Chain terminating NAs, such as tenofovir disoproxil fumarate (TDF), tenofovir alafenamide (TAF), and entecavir (ETV), have been the mainstay of HBV treatment for over a decade.[10,11] Following intracellular activation, they are incorporated into the elongating viral genome and cause chain termination through a combination of steric hindrance and/or absence of a 3'-OH group. ETV also competes with endogenous deoxyguanosine nucleotides and inhibits protein priming. TAF is a phosphonamidate prodrug that delivers the active metabolite (tenofovir diphosphate) more efficiently to target cells. The subsequent reduction in systemic exposure reduces the risk of off-target effects, including renal impairment and bone demineralization.[12] All 3 agents are orally administered, well tolerated, and reduce the risk of liver-related complications; however, they have no direct effect on cccDNA transcriptional activity and so functional cure is seldom achieved.[13] Virological relapse is common after treatment withdrawal, occurring in up to 60% of patients at 12 months, and may precipitate hepatic decompensation.[14,15]

Interferons stimulate an array of IFN-stimulated gene (ISG) products and these have broad suppressive effects on HBV activity. Interferon-α (IFN-α) increases cytidine deaminase activity (APOBEC3) and triggers G-to-A hypermutation throughout the viral genome.[16] In addition, it promotes the degradation of pgRNA, impedes HBV RNA nuclear export, and recruits transcriptional co-repressors to cccDNA.[17,18] Pegylated IFN-α is administered subcutaneously on a weekly basis and offers the advantages of finite treatment duration; however, side effects are often prohibitive (including blood dyscrasias, psychiatric disturbances) and durable response to monotherapy is suboptimal. In the 48-week registrational study, 4.0% of HBeAg-negative patients treated with PEG IFN-α achieved HBsAg loss within 6 months of treatment completion.[19] Given its pleotropic antiviral effects, there has been renewed interest in combining PEG IFN-α with other therapeutic classes, as described below.

ANTIVIRAL STRATEGIES
Capsid Assembly Modulation

HBV core proteins are expressed from the precore/core open reading frame (ORF) and play a key role in the viral life cycle, including capsid formation, encapsidation of pgRNA-viral polymerase complex, and amplification of the cccDNA reservoir. In addition, they upregulate HBV transcriptional activity by interacting with CpG islands and disrupting nucleosome packaging.[20,21] Structurally, these proteins comprise 3 domains (alpha-helical rich N-terminal domain, linker region, arginine rich C-terminal domain) and dimerize with T = 4 (or occasionally T = 3) icosahedral symmetry.[22] Capsid assembly modulators (CAMs) are a broadly divided into 2 subgroups: type 1 CAMs trigger the formation of aberrant capsid structures, whereas type 2 CAMs result in morphologically "normal" capsids that are devoid of pgRNA polymerase. CAMs achieve rapid suppression of HBV DNA (up to 4 $\log_{10}$ IU/mL) and RNA (up to 3 $\log_{10}$ IU/mL) within 28 days of treatment initiation, an effect that may be synergized by NAs. For example, in a phase IIa study (NCT03577171) comprising HBeAg-positive patients with baseline HBV DNA $\geq 2 \times 10^5$ IU/mL, 24-week treatment with entecavir + vebicorvir (class II CAM) resulted in a more profound reduction in HBV DNA (-5.33 $\log_{10}$ IU/mL vs -4.20 $\log_{10}$ IU/mL) compared with entecavir alone. In the combination group, 92% achieved a normal alanine aminotransferase (ALT) by week 24 versus 42% in the entecavir monotherapy cohort.[23] On a cautionary note, HBsAg seroconversion is rarely achieved with early generation CAMs and resistant mutants frequently emerge. In the JADE study (NCT03361956), virological break-through (defined as >1 $\log_{10}$ IU/mL increase in HBV DNA from nadir) occurred in 5/28 patients receiving JNJ-6379 75 mg monotherapy (class II CAM) between weeks 16 and 20. T33N variants were detectable in these subjects and resulted in an 85-fold change in EC_{50}.[24]

For CAMs to have a prominent role in HBV cure programs, it is imperative that they contribute to HBsAg loss through their secondary mechanism (ie, disrupting the pool of cccDNA). ALG-000184 (prodrug of ALG-001075) is a next generation class II CAM with excellent antiviral potency in preclinical studies. It has pangenotypic activity, including against most NA/CAM-resistant HBV strains, and is projected to achieve concentrations required to engage this secondary mode of action (EC_{50} 70.0 mM). Preliminary data from a phase I clinical trial (NCT04536337) have shown that a pro-found reduction in HBV DNA can be achieved with this compound after 28 days of treatment (mean decline 4.2 $\log_{10}$ IU/mL at 100 mg dose, 4.0 $\log_{10}$ IU/mL at 300 mg dose). In parallel, there was a modest HBsAg reduction in 3 out of 7 subjects (range of 0.23–0.78 $\log_{10}$ IU/mL).[25]

Active site polymerase inhibitor nucleotides

In contrast with chain terminating NAs, active site polymerase inhibitor nucleotides (ASPINs) distort the HBV polymerase active site and impede all its enzyme functions (ie, protein priming, primer elongation, DNA synthesis). ATI-2173 is the phosphorami-date prodrug of clevudine and remains the only ASPIN in clinical development.[26] In the phase II study (NCT04847440), treatment naïve subjects received a combination of TDF + ATI-2173 (25 mg or 50 mg OD) or TDF + placebo for 90 days.[27] Across the 3 cohorts, a similar reduction in HBV DNA levels was demonstrated at the end of treat-ment (-3.53 $\log_{10}$ IU/mL TDF + placebo, -3.72 $\log_{10}$ IU/mL TDF + 25 mg ATI-2173, -3.54 $\log_{10}$ IU/mL TDF + 50 mg ATI-2173). However, the combination of ATI-2173 + TDF achieved more sustained off-treatment virological suppression; at follow-up week 12, the mean HBV DNA reduction was -0.66 $\log_{10}$ IU/mL with TDF monotherapy, compared to -3.20 $\log_{10}$ IU/mL and -3.50 $\log_{10}$ IU/mL in the TDF/ATI-2173 combination arms.[27] Research into this prodrug has been halted as one participant developed bradycardia and hypotension, shortly after receiving triple com-bination therapy (ATI-2173, TDF, and vebicorvir). They had been fasting for 20 hours and were taking a thiazide-like diuretic (indapamide), but the FDA was sufficiently con-cerned to request an independent cardiology assessment. A separate trial exploring the combination of ATI-2173 and AB-279 (GalNAc conjugated siRNA) has been terminated.

Translation inhibitors: small interfering RNAs and antisense oligonucleotides

Oligonucleotides have the potential to treat a wide range of diseases and are broadly divided into 2 types. Small interfering RNAs (siRNA) have a characteristic duplex struc-ture, comprising an antisense (23 nucleotide) and passenger (21 nucleotide) strand. They interact with an RNA-induced silencing complex (RISC) and direct the cleavage of complementary RNA transcripts by Argonaute 2 (AGO2). In contrast, antisense ol-igonucleotides (ASOs) are single-stranded nucleic acid polymers that promote the degradation of target molecules by RNaseH.[28] Both have the potential to stimulate the innate immune response by interacting with pattern recognition receptors (PRRs), such as Toll-like receptors (TLRs) and retinoic acid inducible gene 1 (RIG-I). Double-stranded RNA molecules (siRNA) interact with TLR3 or RIG-I, single-stranded RNA (siRNA) with TLR7 or TLR8, and single-stranded DNA with TLR9.

Effective delivery of these oligonucleotides to the liver is challenging and must overcome their inherent biochemical (large, hydrophilic, polyanionic) properties and the abundance of nucleases in the extracellular space. Plasma stability may be enhanced through chemical alterations of the nucleotide backbone, including 2'-ribose substitutions (2'-OMe, 2'-MOE), replacement of phosphodiester linkages, and the addition of linked nucleic acids.[28] Conjugation with triennial N-acetylgalactosamine (GalNAc) residues further enhances hepatocyte delivery; this naturally occurring glycoprotein binds to high capacity asialoglycoprotein receptors (ASGPR) on the hepatocyte surface (up to 500,000 receptor copies per cell) and rapidly dissociates from oligonucleotides following endocytosis.[29]

Currently, there are 4 siRNA molecules in clinical development (JNJ-3989, AB-729, RG-6346, and VIR-2218). VIR-2218 is a GalNAc-conjugated siRNA that incorporates ESC+ (Enhanced Stabilization Chemistry Plus) technologies; in a phase II study exploring different dosing strategies, the 6-dose regimen (200 mg every 4 weeks) was associated with a more pronounced (-1.96 vs -1.61 $\log_{10}$ IU/mL at nadir) and sustained (1.76 vs -0.87 $\log_{10}$ IU/mL at week 44) reduction in HBsAg, compared with the 2-dose regimen. No treatment associated serious adverse event (SAEs) were reported.[30] Meanwhile, preliminary data suggest an additive effect between VIR-2218, PEG IFN-α, and VIR-3434 (Fc engineered monoclonal antibody against HBsAg). In an ongoing phase II study (NCT04412863), anti-HBs seroconversion was achieved in 30.8% of patients who received a combination of VIR-2218 (up to 13 doses) plus PEG IFN-α (up to 44 weeks). At week 48, a greater reduction in HBsAg (2.9 ± 1.36 $\log_{10}$ IU/mL) was observed in this cohort, compared with recipients of VIR-2218 monotherapy.[31] Similarly, in the VIR-2218-1006 study (NCT04856085), the combination of VIR-2218 and VIR-3434 achieved a mean reduction in HBsAg >2.5 $\log_{10}$ IU/mL across all cohorts, with most patients achieving HBsAg levels <10 IU/mL at the end of treatment.[32] Additional data from these combination studies are eagerly awaited.

JNJ-3989 is a 2:1 mixture of 2 GalNAc-conjugated siRNA molecules (JNJ-3976, JNJ-3924), and data are emerging from the REEF platform studies. In the phase IIb REEF-1 trial (NCT03982186), participants were randomized to receive (i) NA monotherapy (ii) NA + JNJ-3989 (40, 100, or 200 mg/4 weeks) or (iii) NA + JNJ-3989 (100 mg/4 weeks) + JNJ-6369 (capsid assembly modulator) for 48 weeks. The primary endpoint was the proportion of patients who met NA stopping criteria at week 48, as defined by ALT <3 x ULN, HBV DNA <LLOQ, HBeAg negative, and HBsAg <10 IU/mL. A dose-dependent reduction in HBsAg was observed in response to JNJ-3989, with a mean reduction of -1.5 $\log_{10}$ IU/mL (40 mg), -2.1 $\log_{10}$ IU/mL (100 mg), and -2.6 $\log_{10}$ IU/mL (200 mg), respectively. Despite a gradual re-bound in HBsAg levels during follow-up, 19.1% of patients receiving the highest 200 mg dose met the primary endpoint. Unexpectedly, there was antagonism between JNJ-3989 and JNJ-6379 (mean HBsAg reduction of -1.8 $\log_{10}$ IU/mL at week 48).[33]

In the REEF-2 study (NCT04129554), 130 HBeAg-negative virologically suppressed chronic hepatitis B (CHB) patients were randomized to receive NA + JNJ-3989 (200 mg every 4 weeks) + JNJ-6379 (250 mg daily) or NA + placebo for 48 weeks, at which point all study intervention was stopped (including NA). The primary endpoint was HBsAg seroclearance at week 72. Although no participants achieved this primary endpoint, the mean change in HBsAg level at week 48 was -1.89 $\log_{10}$ IU/mL in the

JNJ-3989 + JNJ-6379 combination arm. 57.9% had declining (17.1%) or stable (40.8%) HBsAg levels off treatment through follow-up week 24.[34] Studies are ongoing to explore the combination of JNJ-3989 with JNJ-0535 (HBV DNA vaccine, NCT05123599) and nivolumab (PD-1 inhibitor, NCT05275023). Unfortunately, Johnson & Johnson has recently deprioritized their HBV program and the future of these assets is unknown.

To date, 4 different ASOs have entered clinical trials for the treatment of CHB infection, namely Bepirovirsen (GSK), GSK3389404 (GSK), RO7062931 (Roche), and ALG-020572 (Aligos). Bepirovirsen is an unconjugated ASO comprising a central portion of deoxynucleotides flanked by 2′-MOE modified ribonucleotides.[35] In the phase IIb B-CLEAR study (NCT04449029), 457 participants (227 receiving NA therapy, 230 not receiving NA therapy) were randomized in a 3:3:3:1 ratio into 4 different treatment arms: Cohort 1 (300 mg bepirovirsen once weekly for 24 weeks), Cohort 2 (bepirovirsen 300 mg for 12 weeks followed by 150 mg for 12 weeks), Cohort 3 (300 mg bepirovirsen for 12 weeks followed by placebo), and Cohort 4 (placebo for 12 weeks followed by 300 mg bepirovirsen for 12 weeks). The primary endpoint was HBsAg <LLOD (0.05 IU/mL) and HBV DNA <LLOQ (20 IU/mL), sustained for 24 weeks after the planned end of bepirovirsen treatment. In the cohort receiving bepirovirsen 300 mg for 24 weeks, persistent HBsAg and HBV DNA loss was achieved in 9% (NA treated) or 10% (NA untreated) of participants and was more common in those with lower baseline HBsAg titres (<1000 IU/mL).[35] Although these results are relatively modest, GSK has started enrolling participants into phase III studies (B-Well 1, NCT05630807; B-Well 2, NCT05630820) which will explore 24 weeks of bepirovirsen in the NA-suppressed HBeAg-negative population. Other studies have shown that bepirovirsen has additional immunomodulatory properties and activates non-parenchymal TLR signaling pathways[36]; this may explain its superior efficacy over GalNAc conjugated ASOs such as GSK3389404.[37]

Hepatitis B virus RNA destabilization

The stability of HBV RNAs is enhanced by the polyadenylation and guanylation of its poly(A) tail. This is carried out by host poly(A) polymerases (PAPD5/7) that interact with highly conserved stem loop sequences (SLα) on the surface of HBV RNA molecules.[38] AB-161 is a next-generation PAPD5/7 inhibitor that achieves antiviral effects at nanomolar EC_{50} values, and promising results are emerging from animal studies. However, adverse events have previously been reported with this drug class (AB-452, GS-8873, EDP-721) and so the safety profile of this compound must be carefully explored. An alternative target is the monocyte chemoattractant protein-induced protein-1 (MCPIP-1); this structure possesses RNase (as well as deubiquitinase) properties and plays a physiological role in resolving inflammation. MCPIP-1 accelerates HBV RNA degradation in hepatoma cell lines and suppresses proinflammatory cytokine production (including IL-1β, TNFα, and IL-6).[39]

Inhibition of HBsAg secretion

Nucleic acid polymers (NAPs) are single-stranded phosphorothioate oligonucleotides that interfere with the release of subviral particles, through their interactions with chaperone proteins (eg, DNAJB12).[40] NAPs selectively target the degradation of subviral particles, without affecting the production of HBV RNA, HBc/HBeAg, or Dane particles. In the REP 401 study (NCT02565719), triple combination therapy (TDF + PEG IFNα + REP 2139/2165) achieved high rates of HBsAg loss (60%) and most participants achieved HBsAg reduction >1 $\log_{10}$ IU/mL by the end of treatment (87.5%). Transaminase flares were common and correlated with the decline in HBsAg.[41] Efforts have been made to develop LNA-modified NAPs (STOPS, S-Antigen Transport-Inhibiting Oligonucleotide Polymers), but these compounds (ALG-020572) ultimately lacked efficacy in human studies.[42] It has been suggested that LNA modifications impart excessive structural rigidity and suppress functionality.[43]

Direct targeting of covalently closed circular DNA

Achieving sterilizing cure requires the silencing and/or elimination of the cccDNA transcriptional template; however, this is challenging due to its supercoiled structure and resistance to host endonucleases. In recent years, there has been growing interest in genome editing techniques, including zinc-finger nucleases (ZFNs), transcription activator-like endonucleases (TALENs), and the clustered regularly interspaced short palindromic repeats (CRISPR/Cas) system.[44] In the latter, Cas9 proteins are directed to target sequences by guide RNA molecules, triggering double-stranded DNA breaks and the insertion of mutagenic indels by recombination (NHEJ) mechanism.[45] This process requires a protospacer-adjacent motif within target DNA sites that is typically 2 to 6 nucleotides in length. *In vitro* studies have been promising, suggesting that engineered CRISPR/Cas systems can cause a dramatic reduction in cccDNA levels[46]; however, concerns remain about the optimal delivery systems, fate of mutated cccDNA variants, and potential for genome wide off-target effects. Other approaches to silencing cccDNA activity include base editing, epigenetic modifications and interference with transcriptional co-factors/co-repressors (eg, HBx, FXR-α). Direct acting antiviral therapies are summarized in **Table 1**.

IMMUNOMODULATORY STRATEGIES
Stimulation of Pattern Recognition Receptors

TLRs are expressed on plasma membranes (TLR1-2, TLR4-6) or within endosomal compartments (TLR3, TLR7-9), and represent a key component of the innate immune response. HBV subjugates this process by downregulating receptor expression, disrupting its interactions with adaptor proteins and preventing the ubiquitination of transcription factors.[47–49] TLR agonists are an attractive therapeutic class and several agents have entered clinical trials, including vesatolimod, RO7020531, and JNJ-4964 (TLR7 agonists), GS-9688 (TLR8 agonist), and AIC649 (TLR9 agonist).

TLR7 is predominantly expressed by plasmacytoid dendritic cells (pDCs) and B lymphocytes; upon ligand engagement, there is enhanced secretion of type I interferons (IFNα and β), proinflammatory cytokines (TNFα), and chemokines (IP-10, CXCL10). In addition, there is upregulation of antigen presentation, cross-priming of cytotoxic T cells, and plasma cell differentiation.[50] In the woodchuck model, vesatolimod achieved a sustained reduction in viral load and loss of surface antigen in almost one-third of cases.[51] However, in phase II studies comprising treatment naïve (NCT02579382) and NA-suppressed patients (NCT02166047), there was no significant decline in HBsAg at doses up to 4 mg per week. The failure to meet the primary endpoint may be reflective of the study dose; indeed, weekly doses of vesatolimod were capped to preferentially activate gut-associated lymphoid tissue and intrahepatic pDCs, whilst minimizing the systemic production of proinflammatory cytokines.[52,53] To improve the therapeutic window of TLR7 agonists, a liver targeted compound (APR002) has been developed that is internalized through OATP1B1/OATP1B3 receptors. In animal models, APR002 exhibits a higher liver-to-serum ratio (5.6) compared to vesatolimod, as well as lower volume of distribution and improved pharmacokinetics. Although both compounds achieved comparable levels of IFN-driven endpoints (ISG15 expression, serum IP-10), APR002 elicited lower levels of

Table 1
Summary of direct acting antivirals against HBV

Drug Class	MECHANISM OF ACTION	Examples	Clinical Development	Observations
Capsid assembly modulators (CAM)	Class I: induces aberrant capsid structures. Class II: induces morphologically "normal" capsids that are devoid of pgRNA-polymerase.	ABI-H0731 (Vebicorvir) JNJ-6379 ABI-H0731 EDP-514 ALG-000184	Phase I/II	First-generation CAMs have minimal effect on cccDNA pool and HBsAg levels. Virological breakthrough is common with monotherapy. Grade 2–4 ALT elevations are often observed.
Active site polymerase inhibitor nucleotides (ASPIN)	Inhibits all enzyme functions of HBV polymerase (ie, protein priming, primer elongation, DNA synthesis).	ATI-2173	Phase II	Sustained off-treatment virological suppression has been observed with the combination of ATI-2173 and tenofovir.
Translation inhibitor Small-interfering RNA	Directs cleavage of RNA transcripts by Argonaute 2.	JNJ-3989 AB-729 RG-6346 VIR-2218	Phase II	Dose-dependent reduction in HBsAg is achieved but the durability of these responses is unclear. HBsAg reduction alone is unlikely to fully reconstitute HBV specific immunity.
Antisense oligonucleotide	Promotes RNase H mediated degradation of target molecules.	Bepirovirsen GSK3389404 RO7062931	Phase I-III	Greatest antiviral potency has been demonstrated with bepirovirsen (non GalNAc conjugated ASO).
mRNA destabilizer	Inhibits host poly(A) polymerases (PAPD5/7).	ALG-020572 AB-161	Phase I	Limited efficacy and safety data in human subjects.
HBsAg secretion inhibitor Nucleic acid polymers (NAPs)	Inhibits release of subviral particles by interacting with HSP chaperones.	REP2139 REP2165	Phase II	Rates of HBsAg reduction are greater than other antiviral treatments. Transaminase flares are common and correlate with the decline in HBsAg. LNA-modified NAPs (STOPS) had no efficacy in a phase I trial.

IL-6 and TNFα.[54] Given these promising results, a phase I study of APR002 has been initiated (NCT05268198).

TLR8 recognizes ssRNA and is predominantly expressed by monocytes, myeloid dendritic cells, and CD4$^+$ regulatory T cells. GS-9688 (selgantolimod) is a highly selective TLR8 agonist that stimulates cytokine production (IL-12p40, IL-6, TNFα, IFN-γ), enhances NK cell function, and suppresses myeloid-derived suppressor cells (MDSCs). In addition, it increases the frequency of HBV-specific CD8$^+$ T cells, at least in those with HBsAg <2000 IU/mL.[55] Despite broad immunological effects, the impact of GS-9688 on HBV activity has been relatively modest in human subjects; for example, in a phase II clinical trial (NCT03491553) enrolling virally suppressed patients, the combination of GS-9688 (1.5 or 3 mg once weekly) + NA achieved HBsAg decline > 0.1 $\log_{10}$ IU/mL in 18% of participants by week 24. Side effects were relatively common, including nausea (46%), vomiting (23%), and headache (21%).[56] Similar results have been demonstrated in viraemic subjects.[57] Peripheral blood mononuclear cell (PBMC) studies have demonstrated increased expression of programmed death-ligand 1 (PD-L1) and galectin-9 on the surface of MDSCs after GS-9688 exposure[55]; this suggests that checkpoint inhibition may have a synergistic antiviral effect and a phase II study (GS-US-465–4439, NCT04891770) combining TAF + VIR-2218 + GS-9688 + nivolumab (PD-1 inhibitor) is exploring this further.

Inarigivir activates 2 cystolic PRRs (RIG-I, NOD-2) and interferes with the interaction between HBV polymerase and pgRNA.[58] In a phase II study (NCT02751996), treatment naïve participants were randomized 4:1 to receive inarigivir once daily for 12 weeks (at daily doses of 25, 50, 100, or 200 mg) or placebo, followed by TDF for an additional 3 months. Lead-in with inarigivir achieved modest reductions in HBV DNA (-0.58 $\log_{10}$ IU/mL at 25 mg dose, -1.54 $\log_{10}$ IU/mL at 200 mg dose) and HBsAg (10.9% achieved decrease >0.5 $\log_{10}$ IU/mL). After switching to TDF, a greater reduction in HBV DNA was observed in those who had received inarigivir (-5.70 $\log_{10}$ IU/mL at 200 mg dose), compared to those who had received placebo (-4.40 $\log_{10}$ IU/mL).[59] The clinical development of inarigivir has subsequently been terminated after serious idiosyncratic hepatoxicity was observed in a parallel phase II study comprising virally suppressed patients (CATALYST 206). Approximately 17% of subjects receiving the higher 400 mg daily dose of inarigivir developed hepatocellular injury at a mean duration of 16 weeks (range 13–21), including one fatality.[60] Despite the toxicity observed with higher doses of inarigivir, activation of cystolic PRRs remains a viable therapeutic option and other compounds should be explored. For example, activation of STING (Stimulation of IFN genes) receptors by 2'3'-cyclic GMP-AMP (cGAMP) or non-nucleotide agonists can efficiently inhibit cccDNA transcription in cell lines and animal models.[61,62] Next generation STING agonists are currently undergoing preclinical development.

Checkpoint Inhibition

Chronic infection is characterized by exhaustion of the HBV-specific T-cell response, with a reduction of their cytotoxic capabilities, increased levels of oxidative stress, and mitochondrial dysfunction.[63] The factors driving this process are diverse and include persistent viral antigenemia, contact-mediated apoptosis (via NKGD2-and TRAIL-pathways), and a suppressive cytokine milieu (IL-10, TGF-β).[64,65] In addition, there is depletion of key nutrients (arginine, tryptophan) and overexpression of co-inhibitory ligands (PD-1, galectin-9).[66,67] Given these observations, checkpoint inhibitory pathways are emerging as an important drug target and several agents are under investigation, including nivolumab (IgG4 PD-1 inhibitor), RO7191863 (GalNAc conjugated LNA oligonucleotide targeting PD-L1 mRNA), and envafolimab (single-domain

PD-L1 antibody). In a phase I study enrolling NA-suppressed patients (NP40479), 5 doses of RO7191863 3 mg/kg achieved a mean maximal decline in HBsAg of 0.3 ± 0.2 $\log_{10}$ IU/mL, and the most significant response was observed in those with baseline titres <2.5 $\log_{10}$ IU/mL.[68] Meanwhile, in a pilot study of patients on long-term NA therapy, a single dose of nivolumab (0.3 mg/kg) achieved a mean decline in HBsAg of -0.30 $\log_{10}$ IU/mL at week 12.[69] Envafolimab is another checkpoint inhibitor that has demonstrated potency in human populations; in a recent phase IIb study (NCT04465890) conducted in China, a total of 149 NA-suppressed patients (HBeAg negative, baseline HBsAg <10,000 IU/mL, and HBV DNA <20 IU/mL) were randomized to receive additional envafolimab (1 or 2.5 mg/kg every 2 weeks) or placebo for 24 weeks. Seven patients achieved HBsAg reduction >0.5 $\log_{10}$ IU/mL (all of whom had baseline HBsAg <500 IU/mL) and 3 achieved functional cure. ALT flares were observed in 15% of participants who received envafolimab but there was no significant change in bilirubin levels.[70]

Overall, these studies suggest that inhibition of the PD-1/PD-L1 pathway alone, or in combination with NA, has a modest effect on HBsAg (especially in those with high baseline titers). This highlights the pleotropic nature of T-cell exhaustion and the redundancy of these pathways. Phase I/II studies are ongoing to explore the combination of PD-1/PD-L1 inhibitors with siRNA (NCT05275023, NCT04225715), therapeutic vaccines (NCT05343481), and siRNA + TLR8 agonist (NCT04891770). From a safety perspective, nivolumab is commonly prescribed for oncological indications and there is a recognized risk of immune-mediated toxicities, including endocrinopathies, colitis, and skin disorders. Based on real-world cancer studies, it is estimated that up to 10% of patients treated with PD-1/PD-L1 inhibitors may develop $\geq$ grade 3 immune-related adverse event (AEs)[71]; however, higher doses of nivolumab are prescribed in this setting (240 mg every 2 weeks) and they are generally treating an older, more comorbid population. Further studies are needed to assess the risk of immune-mediated toxicities in chronic HBV infection and determine the risk–benefit profile of this approach.

Therapeutic Vaccination

Therapeutic vaccination describes the process of inoculating viral antigens to prime HBV-specific T-cell responses and re-invigorate existing immunity. Although promising results have been shown in mouse models, most therapeutic vaccines have failed to demonstrate efficacy in human populations. The reasons for this include limited epitope immunogenicity (and HLA restriction), suboptimal choice of vectors, and the tolerogenic liver milieu. In recent years, several modifications have been made to improve the efficacy of this approach. For example, JNJ-0535 is a DNA plasmid vaccine that encodes 2 HBV proteins (core, polymerase) and expresses epitopes that are highly conserved across HBV genotypes.[72] The vaccine is administered into skeletal tissue via electroporation-mediated intramuscular injection; this is designed to increase local inflammation within skeletal tissue, maximize the recruitment of antigen presenting cells, and enhance the priming of HBV-specific T-cell responses. However, in common with other vaccines, JNJ-0535 induces a stronger T-cell response in healthy controls versus HBV-infected individuals.[72] This may be due to the suppressive effect of high viral antigenemia and the synergistic effects of antigen reduction has been demonstrated in mouse models. For example, in a recent study by Michler and colleagues,[73] the lowering of antigen levels in HBV-transgenic mice followed by therapeutic vaccination achieved a more prominent CD8+ T-cell response compared with controls. A reduction in viral antigen alone or in combination with non-HBV vaccine components, failed to elicit significant HBV-specific T-cell responses. In human subjects, there is an ongoing phase Ib study (OSPREY, NCT05123599) to explore the combination of JNJ-0535 and JNJ-3989 in the NA-suppressed population (siRNA lead-in of 14.5 weeks).

TG1050 is a nonreplicative, adenoviral vaccine that encodes truncated HBV core, modified polymerase enzyme, and 2 surface domains. In mouse models, a single dose of the vaccine-induced HBV-specific T cells against all TG1050-encoded immunogens and core-specific T cells were detectable for up to 400 days post-infection.[74] In a phase Ib study (NCT02428400), multiple doses of TG1050 (10^9, 10^{10}, or 10^{11} virus particles) were well tolerated and induced a broad HBV-specific T-cell response. However, the priming of HBsAg-specific T cells was subdued and the reduction in serum HBsAg levels was relatively minor (<0.2 log_{10} IU/mL in most cases).[75]

The sequential delivery of adenoviral vectors and attenuated poxvirus may further enhance the T-cell response, as has been demonstrated against malaria, tuberculosis, and SARS-CoV-2. The HBV vaccine VTP-300 uses this heterologous prime-boost platform (ChAdOx1-MVA) and encodes 3 HBV proteins (polymerase, core, and surface antigen). Encouraging results are emerging from a phase Ib/IIa study (NCT04778904) in which NA-suppressed patients (n = 55) with a baseline HBsAg <4000 IU/mL were randomized into 4 cohorts: *Group 1* (n = 10) received MVA-HBV d0 and d28; *Group 2* (n = 18) received ChAdOx1-HBV d0 and MVA-HBV d28; *Group 3* (n = 18) received the same treatment as group 2 + nivolumab (0.3 mg/kg) at d28; *Group 4* (n = 9) revealed the same treatment as group 2 + nivolumab (0.3 mg/kg) at d0 and 28. The most pronounced antiviral affect was achieved in group 3, with a mean log_{10} reduction in HBsAg of −0.64 (3 months), −0.72 (6 months), and −0.99 (9 months), respectively. There were no vaccine-related SAEs and mild transaminase flares were limited to 2 patients.[76] These results suggest that the addition of low-dose nivolumab at the time of booster vaccination may enhance immunogenicity without increasing toxicity.

Monoclonal antibodies

VIR-3434 is a humanized monoclonal antibody that targets HBsAg and effectively opsonizes viral particles. In addition, its Fc region has been engineered to increase interaction with activating Fcγ (RIIa/RIIIa) receptors and suppress binding to FcγRIIb. This promotes antibody-dependent cellular cytotoxicity (ADCC), antibody-dependent cellular phagocytosis (ADCP), and HBV-specific T-cell responses (ie, vaccinal effect).[77] In a phase I study of HBeAg-negative NA-suppressed patients, a single dose of VIR-3434 (6 mg, 18 mg, 75 mg, or 300 mg) achieved rapid reduction in HBsAg. Most participants achieved >1 log_{10} IU/mL decrease within 1 to 3 days of dosing, an effect that was most durable in the 300 mg cohort.[78] As described above, interim data from an ongoing phase II study (VIR-2218–1006, NCT04856085) suggest an additive effect of VIR-3434 + VIR-2218 (siRNA) combination therapy.

Bifunctional Peptides

IMC-I109V eliminates HBV-infected hepatocytes through the recruitment of cytotoxic T cells, irrespective of their specificity. Structurally, it consists of an affinity-enhanced HBV-specific T-cell receptor (TCR) fused to a humanized anti-CD3 single-chain variable fragment; upon recognition of HLA-A*02:01-HBsAg, the effector domain binds to CD3 on the surface of neighboring T cells and directs them to the complex.[79] In an open-label phase I/II study (IMC-I109V-101) enrolling NA-suppressed HBeAg-negative patients, a single dose of IMC-I109V 0.8 mcg (at its minimum anticipated biological effect level) was well tolerated and cytokine release syndrome was not observed. Serum HBsAg levels transiently decreased by 11% to 15% during days 3

Table 2
Summary of immunomodulatory agents against HBV

Drug class	Mechanism of action	Examples	Clinical development	Observations
Activation of pattern recognition receptors				
TLR 7 agonists	Induces type I interferon (IFNα, β) production and plasma cell differentiation	Vesatolimod RO7020531 JNJ-4964	Phase I/II	Vesatolimod achieved no significant HBsAg decline in human studies (despite dose dependent induction of ISGs) Side effects relatively common, especially gastrointestinal disturbances.
TLR8 agonists	Stimulates cytokine production (IL-12p40, IL-6, TNFα, IFN-γ) and CD8+ T-cell responses. Inhibits myeloid-derived suppressor cells.	Selgantolimod	Phase II	Modest effects on HBsAg levels. Clinical development was terminated due to hepatocellular injury at 400 mg daily dose, including one fatality
RIG-I/NOD agonists	Induces type III interferon production (IFN-λ)	Inarigivir	Phase II	
Checkpoint inhibition PD-1/PD-L1 pathway	Blocks the interaction between PD-1 and PD-L1 Suppresses the dephosphorylation of the co-stimulatory CD28 receptor and other TCR-associated components	Nivolumab Zimberelimab RO7191863 Envafolimab	Phase I/II	The risk of immune-mediated toxicity is unclear
Therapeutic vaccination	Primes HBV specific T-cell responses and re-invigorates existing immunity	JNJ-0535 TG1050 VTP-300 GS-4774 BRII-179	Phase I/II	Most vaccines have demonstrated limited efficacy in human populations Efficacy may be enhanced by improving epitope immunogenicity, delivery systems, and co-administration with antigen reducing and/or checkpoint inhibitory agents
Monoclonal antibodies	Opsonization of viral particles Promotes ADCC, ADCP, and HBV specific T-cell responses	VIR-3434	Phase II	Potential to select immune escape variants

| Bifunctional peptides | TCR fused to anti-CD3 single-chain variable fragment. Recruits T cells to HBV-infected hepatocytes, regardless of antigen specificity | IMV-I109V | Phase I | Limited experience in human subjects Careful titration of dose is needed to prevent excess cytolysis and cytokine storm Currently restricted to HLA-A*02:01 positive individuals |

to 15 after the infusion, before returning to baseline within 3 weeks.[80] Moving forwards, the dose must be carefully titrated to prevent the overproduction of inflammatory cytokines and excessive cytolysis of infected hepatocytes. Given the variable frequency of HLA-A*02:01 among HBV-positive individuals, HLA nonrestrictive approaches will be required to maximize the potential of this approach.

Metabolic modulation

In chronic HBV infection, antigen-specific T cells display profound metabolic derangements including depolarization of mitochondria, repression of transcriptional activity, and dysregulation of proteostasis.[81] Acyl-CoA: cholesterol acyltransferase (ACAT) is an intracellular enzyme that esterifies cholesterol into neutral lipid droplets. Inhibition of this process diverts excess cholesterol to the plasma membrane, stabilizes TCR clusters, and enhances their response to ligand engagement; in addition, it improves the bioenergetic capacity of immune cells by restoring glycolysis and oxidative phosphorylation pathways.[82] In lieu of these findings, it will be interesting to explore the potency of ACAT suppression in human populations, especially as these compounds have previously been developed for the management of atherosclerotic disease.

Cellular inhibitor of apoptosis proteins (cIAP-1, cIAP-2) are restriction factors that prevent TNF-mediated elimination of HBV-infected hepatocytes.[83] Structurally, they contain baculovirus inhibitory repeat domains and are negatively regulated by second mitochondrial-derived activator of caspases.[84] APG-1387 is a highly selective IAP antagonist and results from a phase Ib study (NCT03585322) have recently been presented. In this study, treatment naïve participants (n = 49) received weekly doses of APG-1387 (7, 12, 20, or 30 mg) for 4 weeks, followed by a 12-week observation period. At the end of APG-1387 treatment, there was a significant decline in HBV DNA, HBsAg and HBeAg in the 12 and 30 mg cohorts. On a cautionary note, adverse events were relatively frequent, including Bell's palsy (14.3%), and this is a recognized off-target effect of this drug class.[85] Novel immunomodulatory strategies are summarized in **Table 2**.

SUMMARY

The World Health Organization has targeted the elimination of HBV as a global health problem by the year 2030. To achieve this goal, a range of new treatments have been developed, including translation inhibitors (siRNA, antisense oligonucleotides), immunomodulators (therapeutic vaccines, checkpoint inhibitors, pattern recognition receptor agonists), and monoclonal antibodies (eg, VIR-3434). Promising results are emerging from clinical trials and bepirovirsen has entered phase III development; however, the optimal strategy remains unclear and long-term safety data are lacking. Chronic HBV infection results in a heterogeneous clinical phenotype and our standards of care are well tolerated with a favorable side-effect profile; as we strive to achieve higher rates of functional cure, it is imperative that we minimize toxicity, adopt a personalized approach to pharmacotherapy, and use predictive biomarkers.

CLINICS CARE POINTS

- Nucleos(t)ide analogues are effective at suppressing HBV reverse transcription and reducing the risk of hepato-oncogenesis. However, functional cure is rarely achieved.
- New therapeutic classes have been developed including translation inhibitors, immunomodulators and monoclonal antibodies.

- Promising results are emerging from clinical trials but the optimal treatment combination remains unclear.

CONFLICT OF INTEREST STATEMENT

K. Agarwal is an advisor/speaker for Aligos, Arbutus, Assembly, Abbvie, Biotest, GLG, Gilead, Immunocore, Merck, Springbank, Shinoigi, Sobi and Vir. K. Agarwal has also received research grants from Gilead, Roche, Switzerland, and MSD. J. Lok and M.F. Guerra Veloz have no conflicts of interest to declare.

REFERENCES

1. Dane DS, Cameron CH, Briggs M. Virus-like particles in serum of patients with Australia-antigen-associated hepatitis. Lancet 1970;1(7649):695–8.
2. Yan H, Zhong G, Xu G, et al. Sodium taurocholate cotransporting polypeptide is a functional receptor for human hepatitis B and D virus. Elife 2012;1:e00049.
3. Wei L, Ploss A. Hepatitis B virus cccDNA is formed through distinct repair processes of each strand. Nat Commun 2021;12(1):1591.
4. Nassal M. HBV cccDNA: viral persistence reservoir and key obstacle for a cure of chronic hepatitis B. Gut 2015;64(12):1972–84.
5. Decorsière A, Mueller H, van Breugel PC, et al. Hepatitis B virus X protein identifies the Smc5/6 complex as a host restriction factor. Nature 2016;531(7594): 386–9.
6. Tropberger P, Mercier A, Robinson M, et al. Mapping of histone modifications in episomal HBV cccDNA uncovers an unusual chromatin organization amenable to epigenetic manipulation. Proc Natl Acad Sci U S A 2015;112(42):E5715–24.
7. Karayiannis P. Hepatitis B virus: virology, molecular biology, life cycle and intrahepatic spread. Hepatol Int 2017;11(6):500–8.
8. Meier MA, Calabrese D, Suslov A, et al. Ubiquitous expression of HBsAg from integrated HBV DNA in patients with low viral load. J Hepatol 2021;75(4):840–7.
9. Sze KM, Ho DW, Chiu YT, et al. Hepatitis B virus-telomerase reverse transcriptase promoter integration harnesses Host ELF4, Resulting in telomerase reverse transcriptase gene transcription in hepatocellular carcinoma. Hepatology 2021;73(1): 23–40.
10. European Association for the Study of the Liver. EASL 2017 clinical Practice Guidelines on the management of hepatitis B virus infection. J Hepatol 2017; 67(2):370–98.
11. Terrault NA, Lok ASF, McMahon BJ, et al. Update on prevention, diagnosis, and treatment of chronic hepatitis B: AASLD 2018 hepatitis B guidance. Hepatology 2018;67(4):1560–99.
12. Agarwal K, Brunetto M, Seto WK, et al. 96 weeks treatment of tenofovir alafenamide vs. tenofovir disoproxil fumarate for hepatitis B virus infection. J Hepatol 2018;68(4):672–81.
13. Buti M, Tsai N, Petersen J, et al. Seven-year efficacy and safety of treatment with tenofovir disoproxil fumarate for chronic hepatitis B virus infection. Dig Dis Sci 2015;60(5):1457–64.
14. Hall SAL, Vogrin S, Wawryk O, et al. Discontinuation of nucleot(s)ide analogue therapy in HBeAg-negative chronic hepatitis B: a meta-analysis. Gut 2022; 71(8):1629–41.

15. Agarwal K, Lok J, Carey I, et al. A case of HBV-induced liver failure in the REEF-2 phase II trial: implications for finite treatment strategies in HBV 'cure'. J Hepatol 2022;77(1):245–8.

16. Bonvin M, Achermann F, Greeve I, et al. Interferon-inducible expression of APO-BEC3 editing enzymes in human hepatocytes and inhibition of hepatitis B virus replication. Hepatology 2006;43(6):1364–74.

17. Liu Y, Nie H, Mao R, et al. Interferon-inducible ribonuclease ISG20 inhibits hepatitis B virus replication through directly binding to the epsilon stem-loop structure of viral RNA. PLoS Pathog 2017;13(4):e1006296.

18. Gao B, Duan Z, Xu W, et al. Tripartite motif-containing 22 inhibits the activity of hepatitis B virus core promoter, which is dependent on nuclear-located RING domain. Hepatology 2009;50(2):424–33.

19. Marcellin P, Lau GK, Bonino F, et al. Peginterferon alfa-2a alone, lamivudine alone, and the two in combination in patients with HBeAg-negative chronic hepatitis B. N Engl J Med 2004;351(12):1206–17.

20. Guo YH, Li YN, Zhao JR, et al. HBc binds to the CpG islands of HBV cccDNA and promotes an epigenetic permissive state. Epigenetics 2011;6(6):720–6.

21. Bock CT, Schwinn S, Locarnini S, et al. Structural organization of the hepatitis B virus minichromosome. J Mol Biol 2001;307(1):183–96.

22. Crowther RA, Kiselev NA, Böttcher B, et al. Three-dimensional structure of hepatitis B virus core particles determined by electron cryomicroscopy. Cell 1994;77(6):943–50.

23. Sulkowski MS, Agarwal K, Ma X, et al. Safety and efficacy of vebicorvir administered with entecavir in treatment-naïve patients with chronic hepatitis B virus infection. J Hepatol 2022;77(5):1265–75.

24. Janssen HLA, Hou J, Asselah T, et al. Randomised phase 2 study (JADE) of the HBV capsid assembly modulator JNJ-56136379 with or without a nucleos(t)ide analogue in patients with chronic hepatitis B infection. Gut 2023;72(7):1385–98.

25. Hou JL, Niu J, Ding Y, et al. Safety, pharmacokinetics (PK) and antiviral activity of the Capsid Assembly Modulator (CAM) ALG-000184 in subjects with HBeAg positive chronic hepatitis B (CHB). Presented at AASLD annual conference 2022, Abstract Number 33693.

26. Squires KE, Mayers DL, Bluemling GR, et al. ATI-2173, a novel liver-targeted non-chain-terminating nucleotide for hepatitis B virus cure regimens. Antimicrobial Agents Chemother 2020;64(9). 008366-20.

27. Tomas M, Jucov A, Anastasiy I, et al. Sustained 12 week off treatment antiviral efficacy of ATI-2173, a novel active site polymerase inhibitor nucleotide, combined with tenofovir disoproxil fumarate in chronic hepatitis B patients, a phase 2a clinical trial. J Hepatol 2022;77:S73.

28. Roberts TC, Langer R, Wood MJA. Advances in oligonucleotide drug delivery. Nat Rev Drug Discov 2020;19(10):673–94.

29. Prakash TP, Graham MJ, Yu J, et al. Targeted delivery of antisense oligonucleotides to hepatocytes using triantennary N-acetyl galactosamine improves potency 10-fold in mice. Nucleic Acids Res 2014;42(13):8796–807.

30. Lim YS, Yuen MF, Cloutier D, et al. Longer treatment duration of monthly VIR-2218 results in deeper and more sustained reductions in hepatitis B surface antigen in participants with chronic hepatitis B infection. J Hepatol 2022;77:S69–70.

31. Yuen MF, Lim YS, Cloutier D, et al. Preliminary 48-week safety and efficacy data of VIR-2218 alone and in combination with pegylated interferon alfa in participants with chronic HBV infection. Hepatology 2022;76:S19–20.

32. Gane E, Jucov A, Dobryanska M, et al. Safety, tolerability, and antiviral activity of the siRNA VIR-2218 in combination with the investigational neutralizing monoclonal antibody VIR-3434 for the treatment of chronic hepatitis B virus infection: preliminary results from the phase 2 MARCH trial. Hepatology 2022;76:S18–9.

33. Yuen MF, Asselah T, Jacobson I, et al. Effects of the siRNA JNJ-3989 and/or the capsid assembly modulator (CAM-N) JNJ-6379 on viral markers of chronic hepatitis B (CHB): results from the REEF-1 study. J Hepatol 2022;77:S864–5.

34. Agarwal K, Buti M, van Bommel F, et al. Efficacy and safety of finite 48-week treatment with the siRNA JNJ-3989 and the capsid assembly modulator (CAM-N) JNJ-6379 in HBeAg negative virologically suppressed (VS) chronic hepatitis B (CHB) patients: results from the REEF-2 study. J Hepatol 2022;77:S8.

35. Yuen MF, Lim SG, Plesniak R, et al. Efficacy and safety of bepirovirsen in chronic hepatitis B infection. N Engl J Med 2022;387(21):1957–68.

36. You S, Delahaye J, Ermler M, et al. Bepirovirsen, antisense oligonucleotide (ASO) against hepatitis B virus (HBV), harbors intrinsic immunostimulatory activity via Toll-like receptor 8 (TLR8) preclinically, correlating with clinical efficacy from the Phase 2a study. J Hepatol 2022;77:S873–4.

37. Yuen MF, Heo J, Kumada H, et al. Phase IIa, randomised, double-blind study of GSK3389404 in patients with chronic hepatitis B on stable nucleos(t)ide therapy. J Hepatol 2022;77(4):967–77.

38. Kim D, Lee YS, Jung SJ, et al. Viral hijacking of the TENT4-ZCCHC14 complex protects viral RNAs via mixed tailing. Nat Struct Mol Biol 2020;27(6):581–8.

39. Li M, Yang J, Zhao Y, et al. MCPIP1 inhibits Hepatitis B virus replication by destabilizing viral RNA and negatively regulates the virus-induced innate inflammatory responses. Antiviral Res 2020;174:104705.

40. Boulon R, Angelo L, Tetreault Y, et al. Ph-dependent interaction of NAPs with the HSP40 chaperone DNAJB12. Hepatology 2021;74:S512A.

41. Bazinet M, Pântea V, Placinta G, et al. Safety and efficacy of 48 Weeks REP 2139 or REP 2165, tenofovir disoproxil, and pegylated interferon alfa-2a in patients with chronic HBV infection naïve to nucleos(t)ide therapy. Gastroenterology 2020;158(8):2180–94.

42. Aligos Therapeutics. Aligos halting further development of STOPSTM drug candidate, ALG-010133. Press release. 6th January 2022. Available at: https://investor.aligos.com/news-releases/news-release-details/aligos-halting-further-development-stopstm-drug-candidate-alg. Accessed February 1, 2023.

43. Vaillant A. Editorial: in vitromechanistic evaluation of nucleic acid polymers: a cautionary tale. Mol Ther Nucleic Acids 2022;28:168–74.

44. Martinez MG, Smekalova E, Combe E, et al. Gene editing technologies to target HBV cccDNA. Viruses 2022;14(12):2654.

45. Ran FA, Hsu PD, Wright J, et al. Genome engineering using the CRISPR-Cas9 system. Nat Protoc 2013;8(11):2281–308.

46. Ramanan V, Shlomai A, Cox DB, et al. CRISPR/Cas9 cleavage of viral DNA efficiently suppresses hepatitis B virus. Sci Rep 2015;5:10833.

47. Wu J, Meng Z, Jiang M, et al. Hepatitis B virus suppresses toll-like receptor-mediated innate immune responses in murine parenchymal and nonparenchymal liver cells. Hepatology 2009;49(4):1132–40.

48. Wang H, Ryu WS. Hepatitis B virus polymerase blocks pattern recognition receptor signaling via interaction with DDX3: implications for immune evasion. PLoS Pathog 2010;6(7):e1000986.

49. Liu Y, Li J, Chen J, et al. Hepatitis B virus polymerase disrupts K63-linked ubiquitination of STING to block innate cytosolic DNA-sensing pathways. J Virol 2015; 89(4):2287–300.
50. Miyake K, Shibata T, Ohto U, et al. Emerging roles of the processing of nucleic acids and Toll-like receptors in innate immune responses to nucleic acids. J Leukoc Biol 2017;101(1):135–42.
51. Menne S, Tumas DB, Liu KH, et al. Sustained efficacy and seroconversion with the Toll-like receptor 7 agonist GS-9620 in the Woodchuck model of chronic hepatitis B. J Hepatol 2015;62(6):1237–45.
52. Agarwal K, Ahn SH, Elkhashab M, et al. Safety and efficacy of vesatolimod (GS-9620) in patients with chronic hepatitis B who are not currently on antiviral treatment. J Viral Hepat 2018;25(11):1331–40.
53. Janssen HLA, Brunetto MR, Kim YJ, et al. Safety, efficacy and pharmacodynamics of vesatolimod (GS-9620) in virally suppressed patients with chronic hepatitis B. J Hepatol 2018;68(3):431–40.
54. Korolowizc KE, Li B, Huang X, et al. Liver-targeted toll-like receptor 7 agonist combined with entecavir promotes a functional cure in the woodchuck model of hepatitis B virus. Hepatol Commun 2019;3(10):1296–310.
55. Amin OE, Colbeck EJ, Daffis S, et al. Therapeutic potential of TLR8 agonist GS-9688 (Selgantolimod) in chronic hepatitis B: remodeling of antiviral and regulatory mediators. Hepatology 2021;74(1):55–71.
56. Gane E, Dunbar P, Brooks A, et al. Safety and efficacy of the oral TLR8 agonist selgantolimod in individuals with chronic hepatitis B under viral suppression. J Hepatol 2023;78:513–23.
57. Janssen H, Lim YS, Kim HJ, et al. Safety and efficacy of oral TLR8 agonist, selgantolimod, in viremic adult patients with chronic hepatitis B. J Hepatol 2021; 75(2):S757–8.
58. Sato S, Li K, Kameyama T, et al. The RNA sensor RIG-I dually functions as an innate sensor and direct antiviral factor for hepatitis B virus. Immunity 2015; 42(1):123–32.
59. Yuen MF, Chen CY, Liu CJ, et al. A phase 2, open-label, randomized, multiple-dose study evaluating Inarigivir in treatment-naïve patients with chronic hepatitis B. Liver Int 2023;43(1):77–89.
60. Agarwal K, Afdhal N, Coffin C, et al. Liver toxicity in the Phase 2 Catalyst 206 trial of Inarigivir 400mg daily added to a nucleoside in HBV EAg negative patients. J Hepatol 2020;73:S125.
61. Guo F, Han Y, Zhao X, et al. STING agonists induce an innate antiviral immune response against hepatitis B virus. Antimicrobial Agents Chemother 2015;59(2): 1273–81.
62. Li Y, He M, Wang Z, et al. STING signaling activation inhibits HBV replication and attenuates the severity of liver injury and HBV-induced fibrosis. Cell Mol Immunol 2022;19(1):92–107.
63. Fisicaro P, Barili V, Montanini B, et al. Targeting mitochondrial dysfunction can restore antiviral activity of exhausted HBV-specific CD8 T cells in chronic hepatitis B. Nat Med 2017;23(3):327–36.
64. Kim JH, Ghosh A, Ayithan N, et al. Circulating serum HBsAg level is a biomarker for HBV-specific T and B cell responses in chronic hepatitis B patients. Sci Rep 2020;10(1):1835.
65. Aliabadi E, Urbanek-Quaing M, Maasoumy B, et al. Impact of HBsAg and HBcrAg levels on phenotype and function of HBV-specific T cells in patients with chronic hepatitis B virus infection. Gut 2022;71(11):2300–12.

66. Pallett LJ, Gill US, Quaglia A, et al. Metabolic regulation of hepatitis B immunopathology by myeloid-derived suppressor cells. Nat Med 2015;21(6):591–600.
67. Nebbia G, Peppa D, Schurich A, et al. Upregulation of the Tim-3/galectin-9 pathway of T cell exhaustion in chronic hepatitis B virus infection. PLoS One 2012;7(10):e47648.
68. Bishop H, Gane E, Lacombe K, et al. Liver-directed targeting of PD-L1 with RO7191863, a locked nucleic acid, in chronic hepatitis B: first report of phase 1 tolerability, pharmacokinetics, and pharmacodynamics. Hepatology 2021;74(6):1409A–10A.
69. Gane E, Verdon DJ, Brooks AE, et al. Anti-PD-1 blockade with nivolumab with and without therapeutic vaccination for virally suppressed chronic hepatitis B: a pilot study. J Hepatol 2019;71(5):900–7.
70. Wang G, Ciu Y, Xie Y, et al. ALT flares were linked to HBsAg reduction, seroclearance and seroconversion: interim results from a phase IIb study in chronic hepatitis B patients with 24-week treatment of subcutaneous PD-L1 Ab ASC22 (Envafolimab) plus nucleos(t)ide analogs. J Hepatol 2022;77:S70.
71. Johnson DB, Nebhan CA, Moslehi JJ, et al. Immune-checkpoint inhibitors: long-term implications of toxicity. Nat Rev Clin Oncol 2022;19(4):254–67.
72. De Creus A, Slaets L, Fevery B, et al. Therapeutic vaccine JNJ-0535 induces a strong HBV-specific T-cell response in healthy adults and a modest response in chronic HBV-infected patients. J Hepatol 2022;77:S72–3.
73. Michler T, Kosinska AD, Festag J, et al. Knockdown of virus antigen expression increases therapeutic vaccine efficacy in high-titer hepatitis B virus carrier mice. Gastroenterology 2020;158(6):1762–75.e9.
74. Martin P, Dubois C, Jacquier E, et al. TG1050, an immunotherapeutic to treat chronic hepatitis B, induces robust T cells and exerts an antiviral effect in HBV-persistent mice. Gut 2015;64(12):1961–71.
75. Zoulim F, Fournier C, Habersetzer F, et al. Safety and immunogenicity of the therapeutic vaccine TG1050 in chronic hepatitis B patients: a phase 1b placebo-controlled trial. Hum Vaccin Immunother 2020;16(2):388–99.
76. Lim YS, Evans T, Barnes E, et al. Phase 1b/2a study of heterologous ChAdOx1-HBV/MVA-HBV therapeutic vaccination (VTP-300) combined with low-dose nivolumab (LDN) in virally-suppressed patients with CHB on nucleos(t)ide analogues. Late breaker abstract AASLD annual conference 2022.
77. Lempp F, Vincenzetti L, Volz T, et al. Preclinical characterization of VIR-3434, a monoclonal antibody neutralizing hepatitis B virus that facilitates FcγR-mediated elimination of HBsAg. Hepatology 2021;74:513A–4A.
78. Agarwal K, Yuen MF, Wedemeyer H, et al. Dose-dependent durability of hepatitis B surface antigen reductions following administration of a single dose of VIR-3434, a novel neutralizing vaccinal monoclonal antibody. J Hepatol 2022;77:S831–2.
79. Fergusson JR, Wallace Z, Connolly MM, et al. Immune-mobilizing monoclonal T cell receptors mediate specific and rapid elimination of hepatitis B-infected cells. Hepatology 2020;72(5):1528–40.
80. Bourgeois S, Lim YS, Gane E, et al. IMC-I109V, a novel T cell receptor (TCR) bispecific (ENVxCD3) designed to eliminate HBV-infected hepatocytes in chronic HBV patients: interim data from a first-in-human study. J Hepatol 2022;77:S872–3.
81. Barili V, Vecchi A, Rossi M, et al. Unraveling the multifaceted nature of CD8 T cell exhaustion provides the molecular basis for therapeutic T cell reconstitution in chronic hepatitis B and C. Cells 2021;10(10):2563.

82. Schmidt NM, Wing PAC, Diniz MO, et al. Targeting human Acyl-CoA:cholesterol acyltransferase as a dual viral and T cell metabolic checkpoint. Nat Commun 2021;12(1):2814.

83. Ebert G, Preston S, Allison C, et al. Cellular inhibitor of apoptosis proteins prevent clearance of hepatitis B virus. Proc Natl Acad Sci U S A 2015;112(18):5797–802.

84. Bertrand MJ, Milutinovic S, Dickson KM, et al. cIAP1 and cIAP2 facilitate cancer cell survival by functioning as E3 ligases that promote RIP1 ubiquitination. Mol Cell 2008;30(6):689–700.

85. Zhang X, Xu X, Guan Y, et al. First-in-human study of APG-1387, targeting inhibitor of apoptosis proteins, for the treatment of patients with chronic hepatitis B. Hepatology 2022;76:S30–1.

Novel Drug Development in Chronic Hepatitis B Infection: Capsid Assembly Modulators and Nucleic Acid Polymers

Lung-Yi Mak, MD[a,b,1], Rex Wan-Hin Hui, MBBS[a,1],
Wai-Kay Seto, MD[a,b], Man-Fung Yuen, DSc, MD, PhD[a,b],*

KEYWORDS

- Functional cure • Subviral particles • Nucleocapsids

KEY POINTS

- Current therapy is insufficient to induce functional cure, defined as hepatitis B surface antigen seroclearance, among patients with chronic hepatitis B (CHB) infection.
- Nucleic acid polymers (NAPs) and capsid assembly modulators (CAMs) are 2 types of virus-directing therapies, among many others, that are being evaluated in clinical trials aiming to enhance functional cure in subjects with CHB infection.
- NAPs act by inhibiting the release of HBsAg from hepatocytes followed by lysosomal degradation. CAMs act by the formation of aberrant capsids or empty capsids, thereby prohibiting encapsidation of pregenomic RNA.
- NAPs (intravenous administration) in combination with nucleoside analogue and pegylated interferon were able to induce functional cure in around half of the subjects.
- CAMs (oral administration) are potent in suppressing viral nucleic acids but demonstrated minimal effects on HBsAg levels.

OVERVIEW

Chronic hepatitis B (CHB) infection affects 262 million of the global population and accounts for significant liver-related complications including liver failure, cirrhosis, hepatocellular carcinoma (HCC), liver transplant, and death.[1] The currently approved therapies with either pegylated interferon alpha (PEG-IFN) or nucleos(t)ide analogues

[a] Department of Medicine, School of Clinical Medicine, Queen Mary Hospital, Pokfulam Road 102, Hong Kong, China; [b] State Key Laboratory of Liver Research, 7/F, HK Jockey Club Building of Interdisciplinary Research, 5 Sassoon Road, Pokfulam, Hong Kong, China
[1] Authors contributed equally.
* Corresponding author. Department of Medicine, The University of Hong Kong, Pokfulam Road 102, Hong Kong, China.
E-mail address: mfyuen@hku.hk

Clin Liver Dis 27 (2023) 877–893
https://doi.org/10.1016/j.cld.2023.05.004
1089-3261/23/© 2023 Elsevier Inc. All rights reserved.
liver.theclinics.com

(NUCs) are imperfect drugs because of multiple issues including suboptimal efficacy for functional cure, need for long-term treatment for NUCs, and poor tolerability for PEG-IFN. In the past decade, potential new drug candidates for CHB are being increasingly identified and tested in clinical trials. These drugs can be broadly classified into virus-directing therapy, host targets, or immunomodulatory therapy. Many compounds from the last group have already been reviewed in the last chapter (Kosh Agarwal, "Overview of new targets for HBV: immune modulators, interferons, bifunctional peptides, therapeutic vaccines and beyond'). This article focuses on 2 virus-directing therapies: nucleic acid polymers (NAPs)/S-antigen transport-inhibiting oligonucleotide polymers (STOPS) and capsid assembly modulators (CAMs).

HEPATITIS B SURFACE ANTIGEN RELEASE INHIBITOR: NUCLEIC ACID polymers/ S-ANTIGEN TRANSPORT-INHIBITING OLIGONUCLEOTIDE POLYMERS
Origin of Hepatitis B Surface Antigen: Dane Particles and Subviral Particles

Hepatitis B virus (HBV) is a DNA virus (3.2 kb) that belongs to the Hepadnaviridae family. The DNA genome exists in the form of relaxed circular (rcDNA) or less ubiquitously double-stranded linear DNA (dslDNA). The rcDNA is composed of 4 open reading frames, one of which includes the gene for hepatitis B surface antigen (HBsAg) transcription. In the host nucleus, the rcDNA is repaired by host cell machinery to form the covalently closed circular DNA (cccDNA), where mRNA transcripts for small HBsAg (HBsAg-S), middle HBsAg, and large HBsAg (HBsAg-L) are transcribed from the S region, preS2 + S region, and preS1 + preS2+ S region, respectively (**Fig. 1**). These mRNA transcripts (2.1–2.4 kb) are transported to the cytoplasm, and translation of the HBsAg proteins occurs in the endoplasmic reticulum (ER). Here, all 3 HBsAg proteins are synthesized as multispanning transmembrane proteins to form the viral envelope following N-linked glycosylation at the asparagine residue (N146). These proteins then coat the genome-containing capsids in multivesicular bodies, with membrane remodeling through endosomal sorting complexes required for transport machinery and virion budding as infectious mature virions, also known as Dane particles. Subviral particles (SVPs) comprising only HBsAg, without infectious potential, are also synthesized in the ER, without glycosylation, which self-assemble in the ER-Golgi intermediate compartment and are exported from hepatocytes in the systemic circulation. SVPs are at 100,000-fold in excess to Dane particles.[2] Filamentous SVPs consists of all 3 HBsAg proteins, whereas spherical SVPs are made up of mainly HBsAg-S.[3] The composition of serum HBsAg showed specific patterns according to the disease phase.[4] HBsAg-S is the major component of the envelope and is the main bulk of envelope scaffolding. Some of the mature virions contain dslDNA, which is replication deficient, and the linear DNA is capable of host genome integration, forming another site for S mRNA transcription. Therefore, HBsAg is also produced from the integrated DNA and becomes the predominant source of HBsAg in hepatitis B e antigen (HBeAg)-negative phase.[5] However, for HBsAg originated from integrated DNA, their form of existence in the blood remains unknown (see **Fig. 1**).

Role and Implications of Hepatitis B Surface Antigen in Chronic Hepatitis B Infection

Viral entry and morphogenesis
The HBsAg proteins forming the HBV envelope allow attachment of the virion to hepatocytes. The low-affinity attachment of the highly conformational determinant region (a) of the HBsAg glycoprotein to heparan sulfate proteoglycans on hepatocytes allows the interaction of the pre-S1 domain of HBsAg-L with the entry receptor sodium

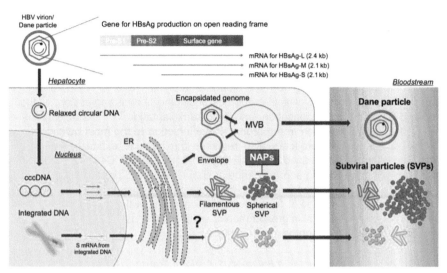

Fig. 1. HBsAg: production in the viral life cycle and proposed site of action for NAPs. Note: only parts relevant to HBsAg are illustrated. Following envelope-mediated viral entry, the relaxed circular DNA enters the host cell nucleus where covalently closed circular DNA is formed by host cell machinery. The mRNA transcripts for HBsAg-S, middle HBsAg (HBsAg-M), and HBsAg-L are transcribed from the S region, preS2 + S region, and preS1 + preS2+ S region, respectively. Without the coating of envelope proteins in the multivesicular bodies, genome-containing nucelocapsids cannot be released from cells as mature virions, that is, Dane particles. A large amount of subviral particles consisting of various compositions of HBsAg is also secreted. The question mark highlights that the form of existence for HBsAg originated from integrated DNA remains unknown. NAPs inhibit the secretion and promote intracellular degradation of subviral particles (SVPs), with minor or no effect on Dane particle secretion. ER, endoplasmic reticulum; MVB, multivesicular bodies. cccDNA, covalently-closed circular DNA; ER, endoplasmic reticulum; HBsAg, hepatitis B surface antigen; HBV, hepatitis B virus; MVB, multi-vesicular bodies; NAPs, nucleic acid polymers; SVPs, subviral particles.

taurocholate cotransporting polypeptide.[6] In addition, without the coating of envelope proteins, genome-containing nucleocapsids cannot be released from cells as mature virions (see **Fig. 1**).[7]

Immunopathogenesis

Among many viral antigens produced by HBV, HBsAg is believed to be the most contributory to the immunopathology in CHB infection.[8] SVPs can suppress the innate immune system through inhibition of inflammatory cytokines and enhanced production of immunosuppressive cytokines, resulting from abrogated interferon-stimulated gene transcription normally upregulated by Toll-like receptor signaling.[9,10] It has been shown that persistent exposure to viral antigens promotes a state of T-cell anergy and exhaustion,[11] in a time-dependent manner.[12] Excessive quantities of SVPs also act as a decoy for antibody against HBsAg (anti-HBs), which is the only neutralizing antibody produced by the host immune system with HBV specificity, further contributing to immune tolerance of HBV.[13]

Role in hepatocarcinogenesis

Apart from the deleterious effects on the immune system, HBsAg also plays a role in hepatocarcinogenesis. As discussed, HBsAg is produced from both the cccDNA and integrated DNA; the latter can potentially lead to the production of mutated HBsAg that is associated with ER stress as well as impaired DNA repair systems that contributes to HCC formation.[14–16]

Seroclearance of hepatitis B surface antigen as a clinical end point

The seroclearance of HBsAg from the blood of chronically HBV-infected subjects is associated with improved clinical outcomes, including fibrosis regression, reduced risk of HCC, liver decompensation, and liver transplantation.[17–19] Seroclearance of HBsAg marks the transition from chronic active infection to the most quiescent and low-risk phase and theoretically also reverses the immune exhaustion if HBsAg expression can be suppressed. The existing therapies with NUCs and PEG-IFN are only able to induce HBsAg seroclearance in about 1% to 2% patients and less than 4% patients annually, respectively.[20–26] HBsAg seroclearance is therefore recommended as the primary end point for phase 3 clinical trials, with a generally accepted threshold of achieving such in greater than or equal to 30% patients in addition to undetectable HBV DNA 6 months posttreatment.[27]

Mode of Action for Nucleic Acid Polymers/S-Antigen Transport-Inhibiting Oligonucleotide Polymers in Chronic Hepatitis B

NAPs belong to the antiviral polymer family of compounds that exert their antiviral effects governed by polymer length and hydrophobicity. NAPs are also classified as single-stranded phosphorothioate oligonucleotides (PS-ONs) that function based on their properties as amphipathic polymers which is sequence-independent, nor with antisense or immunomodulatory effects. In CHB, NAPs work by inhibiting the secretion of HBsAg out of hepatocytes. In vitro models using human HepG2.2.15 cells confirmed that REP 2139, one of the NAPs for CHB (see later), inhibits the secretion of SVPs, with minor or no effect on Dane particle secretion (see **Fig. 1**).[28] The host target of NAPs was proposed to be DNAJB12, a heat shock protein family (Hsp40) chaperone that is involved in the assembly of spherical SVPs.[29]

The first NAP with evidence of clinical activity in subjects with CHB was REP 2055 [sequence: $(dAdC)_{20}$], which was modified from REP 2031 (a 40-mer polycytidine homopolymer with no CpG motifs) by adding adenosine at every other position of the polypyrimidine sequence. REP 2055 lost its amphipathicity at acidic pH and failed to undergo tetramerization. However, in human studies (REP 101 study), REP 2055 was poorly tolerated due to proinflammatory cytokine induction (leading to fever, shivering, or headache),[30] leading to additional oligonucleotide modifications to block Toll-like receptor recognition of oligonucleotides and block degradation by endonucleases. REP 2139 is a PS-ON with the same length and sequence as REP 2055 but additionally includes an O-linked methyl group at the ribose 2′ position and methyl group at each cytidine base 5′ position, thereby being optimized for tolerability and activity in human subjects with or without hepatitis delta virus coinfection. REP 2165 is also a 40-mer PS-ON with a similar sequence to REP 2139, with substitution of 2′-O Me adenosine with 2′-OH adenosine at 3-ribose position, which increases susceptibility to nuclease attack. Additional formulation as a calcium chelate complex (REP 2139-Ca or REP 2165-Ca) or magnesium chelate complex (REP 2139-Mg or REP 2165-Mg) is intended to block chelation effects during administration of the compound, which is a common phenomenon for PS-ONs.[31]

STOPS are another class of PS-ONs containing novel chemistries to reduce HBsAg production by HBV-infected cells.[32] The prototype compound, ALG-10000, consists of 20 repeats of adenosine and 5-methylcytosine locked nucleic acid nucleotides connected by phosphorothioate linkages. ALG-10000 has been shown in cultured cell models to reduce extracellular HBsAg expression, with effective concentration for reduction of 50% HBsAg concentration (EC_{50}) being 4 nM and cellular cytotoxicity at 50% (CC_{50}) being greater than 1 μM. STOPS are shown to be potent in reducing extracellular HBsAg in in vitro models. In addition, STOPS do not lead to HBsAg accumulation and intracellular HBsAg was also reduced; this suggests that ALG-10000 acts on a process that precedes transport and trafficking of the HBsAg into the extracellular space. One key step is involvement of host factors such as glucose-regulated protein 78 (GRP78), which is a chaperone for membrane-associated protein and regulates unfolded protein response. STOPS treatment led to reduced amount of GRP78 and resulted in increased amounts of misfolded HBsAg, which are then subjected to degradation by cellular mechanisms.[32]

The first STOPS with clinical activity in subjects with CHB is ALG-010133. In the phase 1 study, ALG-010133 was in general well tolerated without serious adverse events, whereas the most common treatment-emergent adverse event was injection site reaction.[33] However, dosing of ALG-010133 in patients with CHB with up to 400 mg (estimated to achieve hepatic exposures >3 times EC_{90} for HBsAg inhibition) did not result in meaningful HBsAg reductions. In addition, higher dose levels up to 600 mg were deemed unlikely to reach the predefined 1 log HBsAg reduction. Therefore, the compound development was terminated by the pharmaceutical company.

Clinical Evidence on Nucleic Acid Polymers

Efficacy of nucleic acid polymers

In the REP 101 study, an open-label nonrandomized study, 8 HBeAg-positive subjects with CHB were given REP 2055 monotherapy at escalating doses, from 100 to 1200 mg for 2 subjects and 400 mg at least weekly for the other 6 subjects, for a maximum duration of 40 weeks. Regarding treatment efficacy, 7 of 8 subjects experienced on-treatment maximum reductions in serum HBsAg from 2.03 to 7.2 log and 3 subjects achieved HBsAg seroclearance. Transient detection of serum anti-HBs was associated with HBsAg reduction. Although serum HBV DNA generally correlated with serum HBsAg reduction, serum HBV DNA was still detectable at greater than or equal to 10^5 copies per mL in 3 subjects with significant HBsAg reduction. Long-term virological control (HBV DNA <2000 IU/mL, normal alanine aminotransferase [ALT] level) was observed only in 3 of 8 subjects.[30]

In the REP 102 study, REP 2139-Ca was given as a weekly 500 mg intravenous infusion for at least 20 weeks in 12 HBeAg-positive subjects with CHB. Patients who achieved greater than 2 log reduction in HBsAg levels and HBV DNA were then allowed to add on immunotherapy—either PEG-IFN or thymosin alpha 1—for an additional 12 weeks. Of the 12 subjects on monotherapy 9 experienced maximum on-treatment reduction in HBsAg of 2.79 to 7.10 log. Three subjects achieved HBsAg seroclearance, and the number increased to 8 following additional immunotherapy. Similar to REP 2055, anti-HBs was induced with HBsAg reduction, and the effect was relatively more sustainable and enhanced following addition of immunotherapy.[30]

REP 301 and REP 301-LTF involved subjects with HBV/HDV coinfection who were given combination REP 2139 with PEG-IFN.[34] Because this review focuses on CHB infection, the details of these 2 studies are not discussed in this article.

In the REP 401 study, which is a phase 2 open-label randomized study, 40 noncirrhotic previously treatment-naive HBeAg-negative subjects with CHB were given tenofovir disoproxil fumarate (TDF) for 24 weeks and then randomized to either the experimental arm with triple therapy consisting of weekly intravenous infusion of REP 2139-Mg/REP 2165-Mg + TDF + PEG-IFN for 48 weeks or the control arm with TDF + PEG-IFN for 24 weeks followed by additional REP 2139-Mg/REP

2165-Mg for an additional 48 weeks. During TDF monotherapy, no significant decline in HBsAg or detectable anti-HBs was observed. After adding REP 2139-Mg or REP 2165-Mg + PEG-IFN for the experimental arm, immediate and rapid decline of serum HBsAg in the magnitude of 4 to 6 log occurred in 15 of 20 subjects as early as 10 weeks of triple therapy. At week 48, HBsAg less than 1 IU/mL was observed in 14 of 20, HBsAg seroclearance (ie, HBsAg less than lower limit of detection of 0.05 IU/mL) was observed in 10 of 20 subjects, and detectable anti-HBs (≥10 mIU/mL) was seen in 11 of 20 participants. In contrast, for patients randomized to the control arm, HBsAg decline was modest, with only 3 of 20 subjects who had HBsAg decline of greater than 1 log without any HBsAg seroclearance or seroconversion. In part B of the same study that evaluated 48 weeks of NAPs (REP 2139-Mg vs REP 2165-Mg) with TDF + PEG-IFN, greater than 1 log HBsAg reduction from baseline was found in 27 of 36 subjects completing 24 to 48 weeks of follow-up, with 15 of 36 having sustained HBsAg seroclearance and 19 of 36 having sustained anti-HBs detectability. No significant differences in efficacy were observed between REP 2139-Mg and REP 2165-Mg.

Safety and tolerability of nucleic acid polymers

Asymptomatic and self-limiting elevations in serum ALT and aspartate aminotransferase (AST) levels were observed following HBsAg and HBV DNA reduction induced by NAPs.[30] Increase in ALT and AST levels were more frequent and severe in the experimental arm receiving NAPs, which correlated with the initial decrease in HBsAg, and were resolved during dosing and/or follow-up.[35] The mechanism of ALT flare was unknown. There are ongoing debates regarding the potential of liver toxicity with NAPs due to the possibility of accumulating HBsAg within hepatocytes, which has been reported in transgenic mice. Recent evidence may provide some insights into the fate of intracellular HBsAg on NAP treatment, suggesting that instead of being accumulated inside the hepatocytes, SVPs are readily degraded by intracellular pathways. This finding was elucidated by an in vitro cell culture model in which intracellular HBsAg is degraded by both proteosomal and lysosomal pathways, the latter being induced by the presence of NAPs, leading to dose-dependent reduction of intracellular HBsAg levels on REP 2139 treatment alongside 80% reduction in the extracellular HBsAg levels.[28]

Of note, REP 2055 and REP 2139-Ca infusion needs to be accompanied by mineral supplementation (calcium, magnesium, and vitamin D3). REP 2139-Ca monotherapy was better tolerated than REP 2055 among HBeAg-positive subjects with CHB as shown in the REP 102 study.[30] Unexpectedly, adverse effects of hair loss, dysphagia, and dysgeusia were observed in this trial, which were thought to be related to the heavy metal liberation by the compound—a common effect for PS-ONs that increases urinary mineral elimination[31]—in the trial subjects who belong to an area that is endemic for heavy metal exposure and probably predisposed to increased liberation of bodily stores of heavy metal during NAPs. Subsequent trials involving European sites excluded subjects with prior heavy metal exposure, and the adverse effects were not observed following dosing of REP 2139-Ca. Subsequent improvement in PS-ON stability as demonstrated by recent clinical studies may potentially call for abandoning the heavy metal exclusion requirement in future studies. Moreover, in REP 401 study, there were no significant differences in terms of adverse events between REP 2139-Mg and REP 2165-Mg. Common side effects, for example, thrombocytopenia, neutropenia, fever, and fatigue, were more attributable to the coadministered PEG-IFN.[35] Otherwise, no severe adverse events were reported in patients dosed with NAPs.

The Future of Nucleic Acid Polymers/S-Antigen Transport-Inhibiting Oligonucleotide Polymers

Despite impressive efficacy data of NAPs from the REP 401 study, it has been criticized for the small-scale, complicated dosing regimen and lack of NUC + NAPs arm (in the absence of PEG-IFN).[36] In addition, the nature of ALT flares was unknown, be it immune-mediated or drug-related toxicity. There was 1 case of viral rebound after 12 weeks of follow-up, which was accompanied by hepatic decompensation that improved on supportive care. No further data on subsequent condition of the subject were available because of withdrawal of consent.[35] More data are expected with respect to the mode of action of NAPs monotherapy with or without NUCs. Patients with various disease states, for example, high versus low baseline HBsAg, treatment naive versus treatment experienced, and those with cirrhosis, should be carefully evaluated. Speaking of usage of NAPs in cirrhotic patients, pilot data have demonstrated the safety and efficacy of subcutaneous injection of REP 2139-Mg with TDF in 2 subjects with chronic HBV/HDV coinfection with decompensated cirrhosis.[37] It is hoped that the subcutaneous use of REP 2139-Mg can be evaluated in patients with CHB monoinfection, with and without cirrhosis. For STOPS, an oral small molecule HBsAg inhibitor, called BJT-754, is currently in the preclinical phase of evaluation. Last, none of the studies discussed earlier have evaluated immunologic markers following dosing of NAPs or STOPS. It remains unanswered whether the observed reduction in circulating HBsAg can reinvigorate the polyfunctional T-cell response and lead to sustained control of viral infection. In addition, immunologic correlations will provide invaluable insights to elucidate the mechanisms of ALT flares following dosing. This should be an area to be explored for future trials involving NAPs or STOPS.

CAPSID ASSEMBLY MODULATORS
Core Protein and Nucleocapsids

The hepatitis B core antigen (HBcAg) is a 183-residue protein chain that is transcribed from the HBV core gene.[38]

The HBcAg has 3 domains, namely, the alpha-helix-rich N-terminal (required for nucleocapsid assembly), the linker region, and the arginine-rich C-terminal (required for viral replication).[39] The HBcAg self-assembles to form the 120-dimer icosahedral HBV nucleocapsid.[40,41] After formation, the nucleocapsid encapsidates the HBV pregenomic RNA (pgRNA) and HBV polymerase[42] and also acts as the site for reverse transcription of pgRNA to rcDNA.[43] As discussed earlier, nucleocapsids containing rcDNA can mature and be enveloped by HBsAg to form HBV virions or they can be disassembled and recycled to augment the cccDNA pool.[44] Aside from its contribution to HBV replication, the HBcAg also regulates HBV transcription through epigenetic mechanisms and modulates hepatic immune and apoptosis pathways.[45]

Mode of Action of Capsid Assembly Modulators

Given its important role in the HBV lifecycle, disruption of the HBcAg can directly inhibit HBV genetic replication and virion assembly. CAMs are a class of oral virus-directing agents that target the HBcAg and nucleocapsids. CAMs can be subdivided into 2 classes, including CAM-As, which induce formation of aberrant nucleocapsids, and CAM-Es, which induce formation of empty nucleocapsids (**Fig. 2**).[45]

The use of CAMs to induce aberrant nucleocapsid formation (ie, CAM-A action) was first reported in 2002, whereby the fluorescent dye 4,4'-dianilino-1,1'-binaphthyl-5,5'-disulfonic acid (bis-ANS) was demonstrated to bind to core proteins and mechanically interfere with nucleocapsid formation.[46] However, the evidence on bis-ANS was

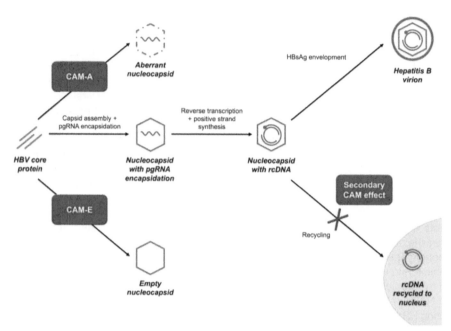

Fig. 2. Hepatitis B nucleocapsids and the effects of capsid assembly modulators.

limited to in vitro studies and has not been further developed.[45] Heteroaryldihydropyrimidine (HAP) is another compound with CAM-A properties. HAP activates nucleocapsid formation, but differentially strengthens protein bonding and misdirects formation of noncapsid polymers.[47] HAP and its derivatives have been developed, with agents including GLS4 and RO7049389 entering clinical trials. Recently, non-HAP CAM-A molecules have been identified as well, although data on these new molecules remain preliminary.[48]

CAM-E molecules stabilize dimer bonding to accelerate nucleocapsid assembly, inducing the formation of empty nucleocapsids without incorporation of pgRNA or HBV polymerase.[49] CAM-E molecules are more structurally diverse when compared with CAM-A, with main compounds including sulfamoylbenzamides and phenylpropenamides.[50,51] CAM-Es are more common in the currently developmental landscape and multiple agents have entered clinical trials.

With its primary action on nucleocapsid formation, CAMs can potently inhibit HBV replication to reduce circulating HBV DNA.[45] CAMs also have secondary effects on inducing mistimed uncoating of nucleocapsids, in turn interfering with cccDNA recycling.[52,53] It is hypothesized that the secondary effect of CAMs on cccDNA only occurs at higher drug concentrations, because more drug molecules are required to act on multiple binding sites to destabilize functioning HBV nucleocapsids. Reduction of the cccDNA pool can in turn limit pgRNA transcription and cccDNA-dependent viral protein production.[52,53]

Clinical Evidence on Capsid Assembly Modulator-As

GLS4 is the first-in-class CAM-A, and it requires pairing with ritonavir as a pharmacokinetic enhancer. GLS4 120 mg daily/ritonavir for 28 days in HBeAg-positive treatment-naive patients with HBV led to HBV DNA, pgRNA, and HBsAg reduction by

1.42 log, 0.75 log, and 0.06 log, respectively.[54] In a phase 2 trial, GLS4 120 mg/ritonavir combined with entecavir was compared against entecavir monotherapy and led to greater reduction of HBV DNA (5.02 vs 3.84 log), pgRNA (2.63 vs 0.27 log), and HBsAg (0.43 vs 0.21 log) at week 12. In the GLS4/ritonavir + entecavir group, 14.3% of patients had HBsAg decline greater than 1.5 log IU/mL, whereas no patients in the entecavir monotherapy group achieved this end point.[55]

RO7049389 is a newer CAM-A. After 28 days of treatment, RO7049389 induced HBV DNA reduction by 2.44 to 3.33 log and HBV RNA reduction by 2.09 to 2.77 log, whereas no apparent reduction in HBsAg, HBeAg, and hepatitis B core-related antigen (HBcrAg) levels was shown. Of note, all patients had rebound of HBV DNA and RNA within 28 days after end of treatment.[56] A phase 2 trial studied prolonged administration of RO7049389 ± pegylated interferon (Peg-IFN) for 48 weeks. Among NUC-treated patients, no HBsAg decline was observed during the study, whereas for treatment-naive patients, the RO7049389 + NUCs for 48 weeks led to maximal HBsAg decline by 0.40 to 0.45 log in 2 of 10 patients only, and the HBsAg reduction only occurred after grade 3 ALT flares. Finally, among treatment-naive patients started on the combination of RO7049389 + NUCs + Peg-IFN, mean HBsAg decline by 1.39 log was achieved after 48 weeks, and this effect was more prominent in HBeAg-positive patients (HBsAg decline by 1.64 log) and in patients with baseline HBsAg level greater than 4 log (HBsAg decline by 1.72 log).[57]

Clinical Evidence on Capsid Assembly Modulator-Es

NVR3-778 is the first oral CAM-E that was developed. NVR3-778 at 600 mg twice daily for 28 days in HBeAg-positive treatment-naive patients led to HBV DNA reduction by 1.43 log, although no significant changes in HBsAg, HBeAg, and HBcrAg levels were noted.[58] The combination of NVR3-778 (CAM) with Peg-IFN alpha has also been studied in a phase 1 study. After 28 days of treatment, the combination treatment led to HBV DNA and RNA reduction by 1.97 log and 2.10 log, respectively, which was higher than the reduction in NVR3-778 monotherapy (DNA reduction 1.43 log, RNA reduction 1.42 log) and Peg-IFN alpha monotherapy (DNA reduction 1.06 log, RNA reduction 0.89 log). The synergistic effect of CAM with Peg-IFN alpha was not demonstrable for HBsAg reduction.[58,59]

EDP-514, another CAM-E, has been studied in phase 1 studies. After 28 days of treatment, EDP-514 reduced HBV RNA by 2.00 to 2.88 log and 1.67 to 2.03 log in treatment-naive and NUC-treated patients, respectively. Nonetheless, EDP-514 did not induce any significant changes to HBsAg, HBcrAg, and HBeAg.[60,61]

CAM-Es have been further studied for longer treatment durations. After 24 weeks of treatment by vebicorvir (ABI-H0731) in treatment-naive patients, vebicorvir combined with entecavir led to greater HBV DNA and pgRNA reduction than entecavir alone (HBV DNA decrease by 5.33 vs 4.20 log, pgRNA decrease by 2.33 vs 0.63 log, respectively).[62] In a similar trial on NUC-treated patients, addition of vebicorvir to NUCs led to more patients achieving undetectable HBV DNA on a high-sensitivity HBV DNA assay (7% to 83% in HBeAg-positive patients, 63% to 94% in HBeAg-negative patients) and also led to significant pgRNA decline in HBeAg-positive patients by 1.68 log.[63] In both treatment-naive and on-treatment patients, the use of vebicorvir for 24 weeks did not enhance HBsAg or HBeAg decline.[62,63] However, in an extension trial in which vebicorvir was administered for an average of 76 weeks, more than 0.5 log reduction of HBsAg, HBeAg, and HBcrAg was achieved in 40%, 52%, and 88% of HBeAg-positive patients, respectively.[64,65] This HBsAg reduction effect was not observable in HBeAg-negative patients. The development of vebicorvir has now been halted due to resource reallocation.[66]

JNJ-6379 is another CAM-E that has been studied for extended treatment beyond 24 weeks. Among treatment-naive HBeAg-positive patients, JNJ-6379 250 mg daily with NUCs led to declines of HBV DNA (5.88 log), HBV RNA (3.15 log), and HBsAg (0.41 log).[67] Nonetheless, the effects of JNJ-6379 on HBsAg could not be repeated in treatment-naive HBeAg-negative patients or in on-treatment patients. Rebound in HBV RNA was noted with continued NUC treatment after withdrawal of JNJ-6379, confirming the direct effect of JNJ-6379 on HBV RNA.[67]

In recent years, newer-generation high-potency CAMs have been studied. ALG-000184 is one of the next-generation CAM-Es. After 4 weeks of treatment, ALG-000184 induced HBV DNA reduction of 3.8 log and 4.2 log in HBeAg-negative and -positive patients, respectively.[68] These reductions are higher than that observed in NVR3-778 (1.4 log reduction)[58] or ABI-H0731 (2.7 log reduction)[69] at 4 weeks. Among HBeAg-positive patients, 3 patients who received 4-week ALG-000184 at 300 mg daily achieved HBsAg decline of 0.23, 0.35, and 0.78 log, respectively, whereas 1 patient who received ALG-000184 at 100 mg daily achieved HBsAg decline of 0.52 log.[70]

A range of next-generation CAM-Es are currently in development. GLP26[71] and ABI-4334[72] are CAMs that are currently in preclinical development, whereas agents including ABI-H3733 (NCT04271592), ZM-H1505 R (NCT5484466), and QL-007 (NCT04157257) are further down the developmental pipeline and are in phase 2 trials (Table 1).[64]

CAMs are generally well-tolerated oral drugs, with the most common treatment-emergent adverse events being mild transient liver derangement, coryzal symptoms, and skin rash.[45] Nonetheless, incidences of grade 3/4 drug-induced hepatotoxicity have been reported in the phase 2 trials of ABI-H2158 and AB-506, both of which are CAM-Es. The development of these 2 agents has hence been discontinued.[66,73]

Combination of Novel Antivirals with Capsid Assembly Modulators

Combination regimens with novel HBV antivirals are currently studied, with an aim to generate synergistic antiviral effects to induce functional cure.[74] RNA interference by small interfering RNA (siRNA) or antisense oligonucleotides is one of the most promising novel therapeutic technique for HBV, and it has been studied in combination with CAMs.[59] The combination of JNJ-6379 (CAM) and JNJ-3989 (siRNA) has been studied in a phase 2 trial. Overall, the combination of JNJ-6379 and JNJ-3989 was well tolerated, and combination therapy did not enhance HBsAg, HBeAg, and HBcrAg

Table 1
Core protein allosteric modulators in clinical development

Class	Agent	Clinical Trial Registration
CAM-A	GLS4	NCT04147208
	RO7049389	NCT02952924
CAM-E	NVR3-778	NCT02112799 and NCT02401737
	EDP-514	NCT04470388
	ABI-H0731 (Vebicorvir)	NCT03576066 and NCT03577171
	JNJ-6379	NCT03361956
	ALG-000184	NCT04536337
	ABI-H3733	NCT04271592
	ZM-H1505R	NCT5484466
	QL-007	NCT04157257
	ABI-H2158	Development terminated
	AB-506	Development terminated

reduction when compared with the siRNA monotherapy groups. In contrast, the HBV RNA reduction in the combination group was 2.6 log, which was higher than the 1.9 log reduction in the siRNA monotherapy groups, highlighting the direct effects of CAMs on viral replication and RNA release.[75]

Vebicorvir has been studied in combination with AB-729 (siRNA) in HBeAg-negative patients. After 24 weeks of treatment, the percentage of patients in the AB-729 mono-therapy group achieving HBsAg less than 100 IU/mL and HBsAg less than 10 IU/mL was 69% and 0%, respectively. In comparison, the patients reaching HBsAg less than 100 IU/mL and less than 10 IU/mL were 58% and 29% in the combination therapy group, respectively. No patients in the vebicorvir monotherapy group achieved HBsAg less than 100 IU/mL. This combination study is ongoing and will further assess treatment responses at 48 weeks and off-treatment responses.[76] Another ongoing trial will study the combination of RO7049389 (CAM) + RG-6346 (siRNA) + RO7020531 (Toll-like receptor 7 agonist) + Peg-IFN alpha (NCT04225715).[74]

The Future for Capsid Assembly Modulators

Overall, CAMs are well-tolerated oral drugs that are effective in suppressing viral replication. Nonetheless, the suppressive effects of CAMs on HBV DNA and RNA are not sustainable in the long term, and most patients experience virological rebound after end of treatment.[45] Mechanistically, the effect of CAMs on viral proteins, most importantly HBsAg, is predicted to be minimal. Even with prolonged treatment beyond 24 weeks, the HBsAg reduction in CAM monotherapy has remained suboptimal, with most patients having HBsAg reduction by less than 0.5 log.[64,65,67] Longer duration treatment with more potent CAMs is likely required to achieve its secondary effect of reducing cccDNA recycling to in turn suppress viral proteins.[52,53] Newer-generation CAMs such as ALG-000184 seem to have higher in vivo potency than older agents,[70] yet there is no head-to-head comparison between these agents and the data for new-generation CAMs remain preliminary.

CAMs may require pairing with other agents to enhance HBsAg suppression. The pairing of RO7049389 + Peg-IFN did show mean HBsAg decline of 1.39 log after 48 weeks of treatment, although this effect was only observable in treatment-naive patients.[57] CAMs are also being studied in combination with other novel antivirals, particularly with emerging data on siRNA + CAM. Although CAMs do not seem to enhance HBsAg suppression on top of siRNA, the addition of CAMs may yield deeper HBV DNA and RNA suppression and the impact of this effect on functional cure remains to be determined.

As of now, the future role of CAMs in our expanding armamentarium against HBV remains undetermined. With companies reprioritizing their developmental pipelines to different agents or diseases, the developmental landscape of CAMs is anticipated to shift. The evidence on the newer-generation CAMs and on CAM-containing combination regimens is keenly anticipated, and upcoming data will influence the developmental direction for CAMs.

SUMMARY

NAPs and CAMs are 2 types of virus-directing therapies, among many others, that have shown efficacy and safety data in the quest of curing CHB. NAPs, given intravenously in combination with NUCs and PEG-IFN, were able to induce functional cure in around half of the subjects. CAMs are given orally and are potent in suppressing viral nucleic acids, but they only have modest or minimal effects on HBsAg suppression. It is unlikely that either compound will be able to be a stand-alone treatment to achieve functional cure. The available data call for the need for further evaluation of both compounds in various CHB populations.

CLINICS CARE POINTS

- Currently approved treatment for patients with chronic hepatitis B infection is insufficient to achieve functional cure (overall annual incidence 1%), which is defined as hepatitis B surface antigen seroclearance.

- Numerous new compounds are identified, and among many, capsid assembly modulators (CAMs) and nucleic acid polymers (NAPs) are two classes of virus-directing agents in clinical development.

- HBsAg has pleiotropic roles in CHB, including viral entry and morphogenesis, immunopathogenesis and hepatocarcinogenesis. NAPS are designed to knockdown HBsAg concentration by inhibiting release of HBsAg from hepatocytes followed by lysosomal degradation.

- NAPs (intravenous administration) in combination with nucleoside analogue and pegylated interferon were able to induce functional cure in around half of the subjects; however further confirmatory studies are needed.

- CAMs act by formation of aberrant capsids or empty capsids, thereby prohibiting encapsidation of pre-genomic RNA.

- CAMs (oral administration) are potent in suppressing viral nucleic acids but demonstrated minimal effects on HBsAg levels.

- The evidence on the newer-generation CAMs and on CAM-containing combination regimes is keenly anticipated, and upcoming data will influence the developmental direction for CAMs.

DISCLOSURE

L.-Y. Mak is an advisory board member for Gilead Sciences. W.-K. Seto received speaker's fees from AstraZeneca and Mylan, is an advisory board member of CSL Behring, is an advisory board member and received speaker's fees from AbbVie, and is an advisory board member and received speaker's fees and researching funding from Gilead Sciences. M.-F. Yuen serves as advisor/consultant for AbbVie, Assembly Biosciences, Aligos Therapeutics, Arbutus Biopharma, Bristol Myer Squibb, Clear B Therapeutics, Dicerna Pharmaceuticals, Finch Therapeutics, GlaxoSmithKline, Gilead Sciences, Immunocore, Janssen, Merck Sharp and Dohme, Hoffmann-La Roche and Springbank Pharmaceuticals, and Vir Biotechnology and receives grant/research support from Assembly Biosciences, Aligos Therapeutics, Arrowhead Pharmaceuticals, United States, Bristol Myer Squibb, Fujirebio Incorporation, Gilead Sciences, United States, Immunocore, Merck Sharp and Dohme, United States, Hoffman-La Roche, United States, Springbank Pharmaceuticals, and Sysmex Corporation, United States. R.W.-H. Hui has no conflict of interests.

REFERENCES

1. The Polaris Observatory Collaborators. CDA Foundation dashboard. Available at: https://cdafound.org/premium-dashboard/. Accessed April 1, 2023.
2. Blumberg BS. Australia antigen and the biology of hepatitis B. Science 1977; 197(4298):17–25.

3. Inoue J, Sato K, Ninomiya M, et al. Envelope proteins of hepatitis B virus: molecular biology and involvement in carcinogenesis. Viruses 2021;13(6). https://doi.org/10.3390/v13061124.

4. Pfefferkorn M, Bohm S, Schott T, et al. Quantification of large and middle proteins of hepatitis B virus surface antigen (HBsAg) as a novel tool for the identification of inactive HBV carriers. Gut 2018;67(11):2045–53.

5. Wooddell CI, Yuen MF, Chan HL, et al. RNAi-based treatment of chronically infected patients and chimpanzees reveals that integrated hepatitis B virus DNA is a source of HBsAg. Sci Transl Med 2017;9(409). https://doi.org/10.1126/scitranslmed.aan0241.

6. Ni Y, Lempp FA, Mehrle S, et al. Hepatitis B and D viruses exploit sodium taurocholate co-transporting polypeptide for species-specific entry into hepatocytes. Gastroenterology 2014;146(4):1070–83.

7. Bruss V, Ganem D. The role of envelope proteins in hepatitis B virus assembly. Proc Natl Acad Sci U S A 1991;88(3):1059–63.

8. Tang R, Lei Z, Wang X, et al. Hepatitis B envelope antigen increases Tregs by converting CD4+CD25(-) T cells into CD4(+)CD25(+)Foxp3(+) Tregs. Exp Ther Med 2020;20(4):3679–86.

9. Shi B, Ren G, Hu Y, et al. HBsAg inhibits IFN-alpha production in plasmacytoid dendritic cells through TNF-alpha and IL-10 induction in monocytes. PLoS One 2012;7(9):e44900.

10. Wu J, Meng Z, Jiang M, et al. Hepatitis B virus suppresses toll-like receptor–mediated innate immune responses in murine parenchymal and nonparenchymal liver cells. Hepatology 2009;49(4):1132–40.

11. Loirat D, Mancini-Bourgine M, Abastado JP, et al. HBsAg/HLA-A2 transgenic mice: a model for T cell tolerance to hepatitis B surface antigen in chronic hepatitis B virus infection. Int Immunol 2003;15(10):1125–36.

12. Le Bert N, Gill US, Hong M, et al. Effects of hepatitis B surface antigen on virus-specific and global T cells in patients with chronic hepatitis B virus infection. Gastroenterology 2020;159(2):652–64.

13. Yuen MF, Chen DS, Dusheiko GM, et al. Hepatitis B virus infection. Nat Rev Dis Primers 2018;4:18035.

14. Svicher V, Salpini R, Piermatteo L, et al. Whole exome HBV DNA integration is independent of the intrahepatic HBV reservoir in HBeAg-negative chronic hepatitis B. Gut 2021;70(12):2337–48.

15. Riviere L, Quioc-Salomon B, Fallot G, et al. Hepatitis B virus replicating in hepatocellular carcinoma encodes HBx variants with preserved ability to antagonize restriction by Smc5/6. Antiviral Res 2019;172:104618.

16. Liu WC, Wu IC, Lee YC, et al. Hepatocellular carcinoma-associated single-nucleotide variants and deletions identified by the use of genome-wide high-throughput analysis of hepatitis B virus. J Pathol 2017;243(2):176–92.

17. Yuen MF, Wong DK, Fung J, et al. HBsAg Seroclearance in chronic hepatitis B in Asian patients: replicative level and risk of hepatocellular carcinoma. Gastroenterology 2008;135(4):1192–9.

18. Mak LY, Seto WK, Hui RW, et al. Fibrosis evolution in chronic hepatitis B e antigen-negative patients across a 10-year interval. J Viral Hepat 2019;26(7):818–27.

19. Anderson RT, Choi HSJ, Lenz O, et al. Association between seroclearance of hepatitis B surface antigen and long-term clinical outcomes of patients with chronic hepatitis B virus infection: systematic review and meta-analysis. Clin Gastroenterol Hepatol 2021;19(3):463–72.

20. Buti M, Gane E, Seto WK, et al. Tenofovir alafenamide versus tenofovir disoproxil fumarate for the treatment of patients with HBeAg-negative chronic hepatitis B virus infection: a randomised, double-blind, phase 3, non-inferiority trial. Lancet Gastroenterol Hepatol 2016;1(3):196–206.

21. Buti M, Tsai N, Petersen J, et al. Seven-year efficacy and safety of treatment with tenofovir disoproxil fumarate for chronic hepatitis B virus infection. Dig Dis Sci 2015;60(5):1457–64.

22. European Association For The Study Of The L. EASL clinical practice guidelines: management of chronic hepatitis B virus infection. J Hepatol 2012;57(1):167–85.

23. Hara T, Suzuki F, Kawamura Y, et al. Long-term entecavir therapy results in falls in serum hepatitis B surface antigen levels and seroclearance in nucleos(t)ide-naive chronic hepatitis B patients. J Viral Hepat 2014;21(11):802–8.

24. Ko KL, To WP, Mak LY, et al. A large real-world cohort study examining the effects of long-term entecavir on hepatocellular carcinoma and HBsAg seroclearance. J Viral Hepat 2020;27(4):397–406.

25. Lam YF, Seto WK, Wong D, et al. Seven-Year treatment outcome of entecavir in a real-world cohort: effects on clinical parameters, HBsAg and HBcrAg levels. Clin Transl Gastroenterol 2017;8(10):e125.

26. Wong VW, Wong GL, Yan KK, et al. Durability of peginterferon alfa-2b treatment at 5 years in patients with hepatitis B e antigen-positive chronic hepatitis B. Hepatology 2010;51(6):1945–53.

27. Cornberg M, Lok AS, Terrault NA, et al. Guidance for design and endpoints of clinical trials in chronic hepatitis B - Report from the 2019 EASL-AASLD HBV Treatment Endpoints Conference. Hepatology 2019. https://doi.org/10.1002/hep.31030.

28. Boulon R, Blanchet M, Lemasson M, et al. Characterization of the antiviral effects of REP 2139 on the HBV lifecycle in vitro. Antiviral Res 2020;183:104853.

29. Boulon R, Blanchet M, Vaillant A, Labonte P. The Hsp40 chaperone DnaJB12 is involved in the morphogenesis of HBV spherical subviral particles and is selectively targeted by nucleic acid polymers. presented at: The Liver Meeting 2020, The AASLD annual meeting; 13-16 November, 2020 2020; Digital Experience.

30. Al-Mahtab M, Bazinet M, Vaillant A. Safety and efficacy of nucleic acid polymers in monotherapy and combined with immunotherapy in treatment-naive Bangladeshi patients with HBeAg+ chronic hepatitis B infection. PLoS One 2016;11(6):e0156667.

31. Mata JE, Bishop MR, Tarantolo SR, et al. Evidence of enhanced iron excretion during systemic phosphorothioate oligodeoxynucleotide treatment. J Toxicol Clin Toxicol 2000;38(4):383–7.

32. Kao CC, Nie Y, Ren S, et al. Mechanism of action of hepatitis B virus S antigen transport-inhibiting oligonucleotide polymer, STOPS, molecules. Mol Ther Nucleic Acids 2022;27:335–48.

33. Gane E, Yuen MF, Jucov A, et al. Safety, Tolerability and Pharmacokinetics (PK) of Single and Multiple Doses of ALG-010133, an S-antigen Transport Inhibiting Oligonucleotide Polymer (STOPSTM), for the Treatment of Chronic Hepatitis B. presented at: The International Liver Congress; June 23–26, 2021 2021.

34. Bazinet M, Pantea V, Cebotarescu V, et al. Safety and efficacy of REP 2139 and pegylated interferon alfa-2a for treatment-naive patients with chronic hepatitis B virus and hepatitis D virus co-infection (REP 301 and REP 301-LTF): a non-randomised, open-label, phase 2 trial. Lancet Gastroenterol Hepatol 2017;2(12):877–89.

35. Bazinet M, Pantea V, Placinta G, et al. Safety and efficacy of 48 Weeks REP 2139 or REP 2165, tenofovir disoproxil, and pegylated interferon alfa-2a in patients with chronic HBV infection naive to nucleos(t)ide therapy. Gastroenterology 2020; 158(8):2180–94.

36. Durantel D, Asselah T. Nucleic acid polymers are effective in targeting hepatitis B surface antigen, but more trials are needed. Gastroenterology 2020;158(8): 2051–4.

37. Vaillant A, Stern C, de Freitas C, et al. Safety and efficacy of REP 2139-Mg in association with TDF in patients with chronic hepatitis delta and decompensated cirrhosis. presented at: The 32 annual meeting of APASL 2023; 15-19 February 2023, Taipei, Taiwan.

38. Zlotnick A, Venkatakrishnan B, Tan Z, et al. Core protein: a pleiotropic keystone in the HBV lifecycle. Antivir Res 2015;121:82–93.

39. Salfeld J, Pfaff E, Noah M, et al. Antigenic determinants and functional domains in core antigen and e antigen from hepatitis B virus. J Virol 1989;63(2):798–808.

40. Ceres P, Zlotnick A. Weak protein-protein interactions are sufficient to drive assembly of hepatitis B virus capsids. Biochemistry 2002;41(39):11525–31.

41. Zhao F, Xie X, Tan X, et al. The functions of hepatitis B virus encoding proteins: viral persistence and liver pathogenesis. Front Immunol 2021;12. https://doi.org/10.3389/fimmu.2021.691766.

42. Ryu DK, Ahn BY, Ryu WS. Proximity between the cap and 5' epsilon stem-loop structure is critical for the suppression of pgRNA translation by the hepatitis B viral polymerase. Virology 2010;406(1):56–64.

43. Kock J, Nassal M, Deres K, et al. Hepatitis B virus nucleocapsids formed by carboxy-terminally mutated core proteins contain spliced viral genomes but lack full-size DNA. J Virol 2004;78(24):13812–8.

44. Huovila AP, Eder AM, Fuller SD. Hepatitis B surface antigen assembles in a post-ER, pre-Golgi compartment. J Cell Biol 1992;118(6):1305–20.

45. Hui RW, Mak LY, Seto WK, et al. Role of core/capsid inhibitors in functional cure strategies for chronic hepatitis B. Curr Hepat Rep 2020;19(3):293–301.

46. Zlotnick A, Ceres P, Singh S, et al. A small molecule inhibits and misdirects assembly of hepatitis B virus capsids. J Virol 2002;76(10):4848–54.

47. Stray SJ, Bourne CR, Punna S, et al. A heteroaryldihydropyrimidine activates and can misdirect hepatitis B virus capsid assembly. Proc Natl Acad Sci U S A 2005; 102(23):8138–43.

48. Debing Y, Buh Kum D, Sanchez AA, et al. ALG-005398 is a potent non-HAP class I HBV capsid assembly modulator that strongly reduces HBsAg levels in vivo. Hepatology 2021;74:502A–3A.

49. Katen SP, Chirapu SR, Finn MG, et al. Trapping of hepatitis B virus capsid assembly intermediates by phenylpropenamide assembly accelerators. ACS Chem Biol 2010;5(12):1125–36.

50. Corcuera A, Stolle K, Hillmer S, et al. Novel non-heteroarylpyrimidine (HAP) capsid assembly modifiers have a different mode of action from HAPs in vitro. Antivir Res 2018;158:135–42.

51. Spunde K, Vigante B, Dubova UN, et al. Design and synthesis of hepatitis B virus (HBV) capsid assembly modulators and evaluation of their activity in mammalian cell model. Pharmaceuticals 2022;15(7). https://doi.org/10.3390/ph15070773.

52. Berke JM, Dehertogh P, Vergauwen K, et al. Capsid assembly modulators have a dual mechanism of action in primary human hepatocytes infected with hepatitis B virus. Antimicrob Agents Chemother 2017;61(8). https://doi.org/10.1128/aac.00560-17.

53. Guo F, Zhao Q, Sheraz M, et al. HBV core protein allosteric modulators differentially alter cccDNA biosynthesis from de novo infection and intracellular amplification pathways. PLoS Pathog 2017;13(9):e1006658.
54. Zhang H, Wang F, Zhu X, et al. Antiviral activity and pharmacokinetics of the hepatitis B virus (HBV) capsid assembly modulator GLS4 in patients with chronic HBV infection. Clin Infect Dis 2021;73(2):175–82.
55. Zhang M, Zhang J, Tan Y, et al. Efficacy and safety of GLS4/ritonavir combined with entecavir in HBeAg-positive patients with chronic hepatitis B: interim results from phase 2b, multi-center study. J Hepatol 2020;73:S878–80.
56. Yuen MF, Zhou X, Gane E, et al. Safety, pharmacokinetics, and antiviral activity of RO7049389, a core protein allosteric modulator, in patients with chronic hepatitis B virus infection: a multicentre, randomised, placebo-controlled, phase 1 trial. The lancet Gastroenterology & hepatology 2021;6(9):723–32.
57. Hou J, Gane EJ, Zhang W, et al. Hepatitis B virus antigen reduction effect of RO7049389 plus NUC with/without Peg-IFN in chronic hepatitis B patients. J Hepatol 2022;77:S299.
58. Yuen MF, Gane EJ, Kim DJ, et al. Antiviral activity, safety, and pharmacokinetics of capsid assembly modulator NVR 3-778 in patients with chronic HBV infection. Gastroenterology 2019;156(5):1392–403.e7.
59. Hui RW-H, Mak L-Y, Seto W-K, et al. RNA interference as a novel treatment strategy for chronic hepatitis B infection. Clin Mol Hepatol 2022;28(3):408–24.
60. Feld JJ, Lawitz E, Nguyen T, et al. EDP-514 in healthy subjects and nucleos(t)ide reverse transcriptase inhibitor-suppressed patients with chronic hepatitis B. Antivir Ther 2022;27(6). 13596535221127848.
61. Yuen MF, Chuang WL, Peng CY, et al. EDP-514, a Novel Pangenotypic Class II Hepatitis B Virus Core Inhibitor Demonstrates Significant HBV DNA and HBV RNA Reductions in a Phase 1b Study in Viremic, Chronic Hepatitis B Infected Patients presented at: Poster presentation at the AASLD The Liver Meeting; November 4-8 2022, 2022. Washington, DC, USA.
62. Sulkowski MS, Agarwal K, Ma X, et al. Safety and efficacy of vebicorvir administered with entecavir in treatment-naïve patients with chronic hepatitis B virus infection. J Hepatol 2022;77(5):1265–75.
63. Yuen MF, Agarwal K, Ma X, et al. Safety and efficacy of vebicorvir in virologically suppressed patients with chronic hepatitis B virus infection. J Hepatol 2022; 77(3):642–52.
64. Hui RW-H, Mak LY, Seto W-K, et al. Assessing the developing pharmacotherapeutic landscape in hepatitis B treatment: a spotlight on drugs in phase II clinical trials. Expet Opin Emerg Drugs 2022;27(2):127–40.
65. Yuen MF, Agarwal K, Ma X, et al. Antiviral activity and safety of the hepatitis B core inhibitor ABI-H0731 administered with a nucleos(t)ide reverse transcriptase inhibitor in patients with HBeAg-positive chronic hepatitis B infection in a long-term extension study. J Hepatol 2020;73:S140.
66. Mak LY, Cheung KS, Fung J, et al. New strategies for the treatment of chronic hepatitis B. Trends Mol Med 2022;28(9):742–57.
67. Janssen H, Hou J, Asselah T, et al. Efficacy and safety results of the phase 2 JNJ-56136379 JADE study in patients with chronic hepatitis B: interim week 24 data. J Hepatol 2020;73:S129–30.
68. Yuen MF, Agarwal K, Gane EJ, et al. Safety, pharmacokinetics, and antiviral activity of the class II capsid assembly modulator ALG-000184 in subjects with chronic hepatitis B. Poster Presentation (SAT835). J Hepatol 2022;77(S1): S835–6.

69. Yuen MF, Agarwal K, Gane EJ, et al. Safety, pharmacokinetics, and antiviral effects of ABI-H0731, a hepatitis B virus core inhibitor: a randomised, placebo-controlled phase 1 trial. The lancet Gastroenterology & hepatology 2020;5(2): 152–66.

70. Hou JL, Niu J, Ding Y, et al. Safety, pharmacokinetics (PK), and antiviral activity of the capsid assembly modulator (CAM) ALG-000184 in subjects with HBeAg positive chronic hepatitis B. presented at: Poster presentation at the AASLD The Liver Meeting, November 4-8 2022; 2022. Washington, DC, USA.

71. Amblard F, Boucle S, Bassit L, et al. Novel hepatitis B virus capsid assembly modulator induces potent antiviral responses in vitro and in humanized mice. Antimicrob Agents Chemother 2020;(2):64. https://doi.org/10.1128/aac.01701-19.

72. Unchwaniwala N, Pionek K, Loeb DD, et al. ABI-4334, a novel hepatitis B virus core inhibitor, accelerates capsid assembly and inhibits cccDNA formation via multiple pathways. Hepatology 2022;76(Suppl1):S248.

73. Agarwal K, Xu J, Gane EJ, et al. Safety, pharmacokinetics and antiviral activity of ABI-H2158, a hepatitis B virus core inhibitor: a randomized, placebo-controlled phase 1 study. J Viral Hepat 2022. https://doi.org/10.1111/jvh.13764.

74. Hui RW-H, Mak L-Y, Cheung K-S, et al. Novel combination strategies with investigational agents for functional cure of chronic hepatitis B infection. Curr Hepat Rep 2022;21(4):59–67.

75. Yuen MF, Locarnini S, Lim TH, et al. Combination treatments including the small-interfering RNA JNJ-3989 induce rapid and sometimes prolonged viral responses in patients with CHB. J Hepatol 2022;77(5):1287–98.

76. George J, Stefanova-Petrova D, Antonov K, et al. Evaluation of the vebicorvir, Nrtl and AB-729 combination in virologically suppressed patients with HBeAg negative chronic hepatitis B virus infection: Interim analysis from an open label Phase 2 study presented at: Presentation at the AASLD The Liver Meeting, November 4-8 2022; 2022.

Targeting Hepatitis B Virus DNA Using Designer Gene Editors

Henrik Zhang, BSc, Thomas Tu, PhD*

KEYWORDS

• Hepatitis B virus • ZFN • TALEN • CRISPR-Cas9 • cccDNA • Integrated DNA

KEY POINTS

• Gene editing technologies such as zinc finger nucleases (ZFNs), transcription activator-like effector nucleases (TALENS), and clustered regularly interspaced short palindromic repeats (CRISPR) have emerged as potential therapies for targeting HBV cccDNA and integrated DNA.
• These technologies have shown some efficacy in vitro and in vivo in inducing HBV DNA mutation and suppressing HBV antigen levels.
• Multilocus targeting also has potential to completely remove integrated HBV from host genome and excise select fragments from cccDNA.
• To ensure translation to the clinic, the field must reduce the risk of off-target effects and increase efficacy for different HBV genotypes and quasispecies.

INTRODUCTION

Chronic infection with hepatitis B virus (HBV) is a major cause of liver cirrhosis and cancer, accounting for approximately 650,000 deaths every year.[1] At present, there is no cure, and treatment consists of ongoing viral suppression via nucleos(t)ide analogue (NA) therapy.

Replication Strategy of Hepatitis B Virus

HBV initially attaches to the surface of hepatocytes via binding to heparan sulfate proteoglycans, followed by a stronger specific docking to hepatocyte specific sodium taurocholate cotransporting polypeptide (NTCP) via the HBV surface protein. Viral relaxed circular DNA (rcDNA) is delivered to the nucleus where host proteins convert it to covalently closed circular DNA (cccDNA), which is stable within the nucleus and produces all the downstream viral transcripts necessary for viral replication. These

Westmead Institute for Medical Research, University of Sydney School of Medicine and Health, 176 Hawkesbury Road, Westmead, NSW 2145, Australia
* Corresponding author.
E-mail address: t.tu@sydney.edu.au

Clin Liver Dis 27 (2023) 895–916
https://doi.org/10.1016/j.cld.2023.05.006
1089-3261/23/© 2023 Elsevier Inc. All rights reserved.

transcripts include pregenomic RNA, which is encapsidated by HBV core protein along with the viral polymerase. Reverse transcription of the pregenomic RNA occurs within the nucleocapsid, which is then enveloped by HBV surface antigen (HBsAg) and secreted from the cell as a virion. New virions generated by this process usually contain an rcDNA genome but in 5% to 10% of cases can result in virions with double-stranded linear DNA (dslDNA) genome. When HBV dslDNA is introduced to the nucleus, it can integrate into the host genome, forming a replication-incompetent form that can, nonetheless, express HBsAg.[2]

Both cccDNA and integrated DNA are important targets in the treatment of HBV infection. cccDNA drives chronicity through continual production of new virions. Integrated DNA can persist in cells, be conveyed to daughter cells, and contribute to the ongoing production of HBsAg (which drives immune evasion, likely by inducing B-cell tolerance).[3] Integrated HBV DNA is also strongly associated with cancer formation, possibly contributing through insertional mutagenesis and chromosomal instability.[4–6]

Current antiviral therapies

NAs such as lamivudine, entecavir, and tenofovir work via direct inhibition of HBV DNA polymerase reverse transcriptase activity. These drugs effectively suppress viral replication and thus decrease viral load. Interferon is also occasionally used in HBV treatment to induce or enhance antiviral immune responses, as well as inhibit viral replication.[7,8]

Although these treatments can suppress viral replication and reduce the risks of HBV-associated hepatic disease, cure of the infection is rare.[9] Direct targeting and destruction of HBV cccDNA is necessary for complete eradication of persistent infection, and gene editing technology is arising as a potential method of achieving this without destruction of the infected host cell.

MOLECULAR TOOLS FOR GENE EDITING

Custom-designed gene therapies have been gaining interest due to development of several technologies allowing for the specific modification of target DNA, including zinc finger nucleases (ZFNs), transcription activator-like effector nucleases (TALENs), and clustered regularly interspaced short palindromic repeats (CRISPRs). These technologies are essentially composed of 2 functional regions (**Fig. 1**): (1) a guide domain or motif (allowing for sequence-specific attachment to target DNA) and (2) an effector domain that edits the target DNA sequence in some manner (most commonly a nuclease, which will induce a double-stranded break [DSB]). Although broadly similar, each has its own idiosyncrasies, which affects its capabilities in HBV treatment (**Table 1**).

Zinc Finger Nucleases

ZFNs consist of an engineered zinc finger protein (ZFP) bound to the cleavage domain of the *FokI* restriction enzyme.

The ZFP region contains a tandem array of Cys2-His2 fingers, each of which can recognize and bind to a discrete DNA sequence 3 to 4 bp long. The number of fingers per ZFP determines its specificity; from 3 fingers for recognition of 9 bp per ZFP up to 6 fingers for an 18-bp recognition sequence. Designing these sequences, however, can be difficult and time consuming because of the variable specificity and binding affinity of each zinc finger, which depends on the neighboring units.[10]

Originally isolated from *Flavobacterium okeanokoites*, the *FokI* endonuclease catalytic domain requires dimerization for activity.[11] Thus, ZFNs work as a pair: 2 ZFNs

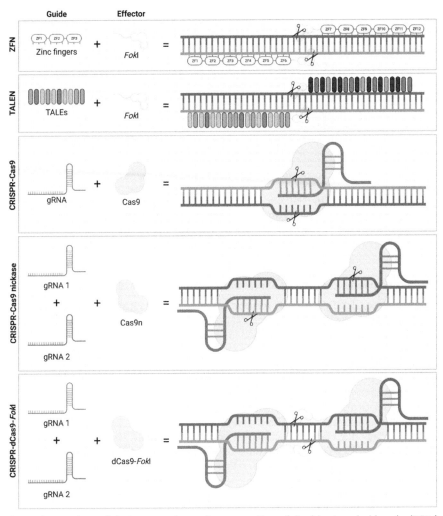

Fig. 1. Comparison of designer nucleases for generation of double-stranded breaks (DSBs). Designer nucleases consist of a guide and effector. The guide domain attaches specifically to the corresponding sequence in the genome, and the effector cleaves the DNA forming a DSB. *Fok*I and Cas9n only cleave a single strand each and must be paired to generate a DSB, whereas Cas9 does not, because it has 2 nuclease domains (RuvC and HNH). gRNA, guide RNA. (Created with BioRender.com.)

must be designed for each cleavage site, one each for the sense and antisense strands.[12]

Transcription Activator-Like Effector Nucleases

TALENs emerged as an alternative to ZFNs in genomic editing. Although they use the same *Fok*I nuclease domain as ZFNs, their DNA-binding domain is composed of repeated modules of transcription activator-like effectors (TALEs), derived from *Xanthomonas* spp bacteria originally for altering transcription in host plant cells.[13,14]

Table 1	
Limitations of gene editing technologies on targeting hepatitis B virus	
Tool	Restrictions on Targeting cccDNA/Integrated HBV DNA
ZFN	Difficult modular assembly of guide domain Cytotoxicity[69]
TALEN	Large size, more difficult to deliver and express protein
CRISPR-Cas9	Target site selection restricted to PAM sites
All	Small size of HBV genome limits target site selection Unintended cleavage of host DNA may result in host genome instability In vivo delivery is a challenge

Abbreviations: PAM, protospacer adjacent motif; ZFN, zinc finger nuclease.

These TALEs attach to DNA via an array of 33 to 35 amino acid tandem repeats, wherein each individual repeat binds to a single base pair of DNA, determined by 2 hypervariable residues at positions 12 and 13, called the repeat variable diresidues. Thus, functional TALEs are simpler to design and enable more flexibility compared with ZFPs.

Clustered Regularly Interspaced Short Palindromic Repeat-Cas9

The engineered CRISPR/CRISPR-associated protein 9 (Cas9) system consists of (1) a Cas9 nuclease; (2) a CRISPR RNA (crRNA), which provides sequence specificity via a 17- to 20-nucleotide spacer region; and (3) a transactivating CRISPR RNA (tracrRNA) that complexes and activates Cas9. The crRNA and tracrRNA can be combined into a single guide RNA (gRNA) without loss of activity. crRNA is complementary to the target region, upstream from the protospacer adjacent motif (PAM).[15] The PAM is a specific sequence typically 3 to 8 bp long and is used as a recognition signal by Cas9 to initially bind to target DNA. After recognition, the Cas9 protein cleaves target DNA strands with its 2 nucleolytic domains (RuvC and HNH) at a site 3 bp upstream of the PAM.

CRISPR/Cas9 has been proved to be a popular and widely used gene editing technology because of its simplicity and ease of use. Target site can be modified by generating an appropriate gRNA sequence, rather than having to design a completely new protein as with engineered ZFN and TALENs. The ability of Cas9 to cleave both strands of DNA means only a single construct for inducing double-stranded DNA breaks, further simplifying design and delivery. Additional orthologs and variants of the classic *Streptococcus pyogenes* Cas9 (SpCas9) have been developed, each with advantages and limitations (**Table 2**).

Cas9 Effector Domain Variants

Transcriptional regulators

By introducing 2 point mutations in the nucleolytic domains RuvC and HNH (D10A and H840A, respectively)[16] the nucleolytic activity of the Cas9 protein can be rendered inert, producing a dead Cas9 (dCas9) that can then be replaced by other functions.

Even without replacement of the effector domain, attachment of a catalytically inactive dCas9 can physically block transcription factors from attaching to the targeted DNA region resulting in gene suppression and is referred to as CRISPR interference.[16] Attachment of a transcriptional repressor domain such as Krüppel-associated box (KRAB) domain of Kox1 to the dCas9 can further improve transcriptional silencing through histone methylation.[17]

CRISPR activation uses an effector protein such as VP64 to upregulate transcription of target genes. This effector protein can be fused onto either the dCas9 protein or the

Table 2
Cas9 nuclease orthologs

Species	WT/ Variant	Size (Amino Acids)	PAM Recognition	Advantages	Limitations	Citations
Streptococcus pyogenes (SpCas9)	WT	1368	5'NGG	Most used Well studied	High off-target effects Large size	Cong et al,[54] 2013
	E voCas9 Cas9-HF1 eCas9			Higher specificity than WT	Lower targetable sites	Casini et al,[70] 2018 Zuo et al,[71] 2020 Slaymaker et al,[72] 2016
	xCas9 SpG SpRY		5'NG, 5'GAA, 5'GAT 5'NGN 5'NRN	Different PAM specificity	Lower activity than WT	Hu et al,[73] 2018 Vicencio et al,[74] 2022 Vicencio et al,[74] 2022
Staphylococcus aureus (SaCas9)	WT	1053	5'NNGRRT	High specificity Low size	Restrictive PAM	68,75–77
Streptococcus thermophilus (StCas9)	WT	1388	5'NNAGAAW, 5'NGGNG	High specificity	Large size Restrictive PAM	Kostyushev et al,[33] 2019 & Müller et al,[75] 2016
Neisseria meningitidis (NmCas9)	WT	1081	5'NNNNGATT	High specificity Low size Unique PAM-independent cleavage	Restrictive PAM	Lee et al,[76] 2016 & Zhang et al,[78] 2015
Francisella novicida (FnCas9)	WT	1629	5'NGG	RNA-targeting ability High specificity	Very large size	33,79,80

Abbreviation: WT, wild type.

gRNA[18,19]; this can be enhanced by recruitment of up to 24 copies of effector proteins to the target site, through a repeating peptide array called SunTag.[20]

Cas9 nickase

Mutant Cas9 with only one functional nuclease domain will induce a single-stranded DNA nick and is known as a Cas9 nickase (Cas9n). A Cas9 with only the D10A mutation will cleave only the target strand, whereas the H840A mutant will cleave only the nontarget strand. In mammalian cells, the HNH domain was found to have higher activity, and therefore D10A Cas9n is more efficient at cleavage.[21]

Cas9n can be paired to generate DSBs with higher specificity and lower off-target cleavage. Furthermore, by placing nicks at different sites, DNA overhangs can be generated, larger sections of the target site can be excised, and greater disruption to viral genome viability may be caused. The requirement for 2 nickases in DSB generation, however, reduces on-target efficiency compared with nucleases, demonstrated by the lowered HBV-inactivating capability of Cas9n.[22,23]

Nickases can also be engineered by fusing dCas9 with the *Fok*I nuclease (the same nuclease used in ZFNs and TALENs)[24] with increased specificity compared with baseline SpCas9 because the *Fok*I nuclease needs to dimerize to be activated. As such, the specificity of this hybrid enzyme is comparable to that of paired Cas9 nickases.[24]

Base editing and prime editing

Base editing refers to dCas9, which has been modified with attachment to either a cytidine or adenine base editor to allow for limited (C>T, G>A, A>G or T>C) point mutation in DNA without generation of DSBs.[25] Prime editing expands on this idea and allows for mutation of any base to any other base using a fusion of Cas9n and reverse transcriptase as well as a prime editing guide, which contains both the target site and desired edit sequence.[26] However, because these are recent technologies, there is much additional research to characterize safety, efficacy, and application.

RESULTS OF HEPATITIS B VIRUS DNA CLEAVAGE

Nuclease-mediated cleavage will result in a DSB at the target site, typically resulting in host machinery-induced repair via either error-prone nonhomologous end joining (NHEJ) or accurate but slower homology-directed repair (HDR) (**Fig. 2**). NHEJ is the primary pathway for DSB repair, in which the break ends are directly ligated without reference to a template, often resulting in an indel, frameshift mutation, and subsequent genomic loss of function.[27]

NHEJ-induced mutations in key open reading frames (ORFs) of cccDNA are associated with reduced levels in viral markers (**Box 1**). Multilocus targeting not only can induce these mutations multiple times at each target site but also can cause large deletions between target loci, and thus increase the chance of disruption.[23,28] These altered HBV episomes can be transcriptionally active, even with large deletions.[29,30]

Multi-gRNA strategies have also been shown to excise full-length integrated HBV from host genome with minimal reported off-target effects.[31] However, care must be taken when targeting host genome, considering that integration events may occur at or within fragile sites for tumor development and indel formation while excising may lead to genomic instability.[32]

Another pathway for HBV elimination is complete degradation of HBV DNA via host exonucleases. This pathway has been reported in multiple studies[27,28,33,34] because of rapid and numerous cleavage events overwhelming repair mechanisms, allowing for host exonuclease degradation; this is supported by studies showing CRISPR-

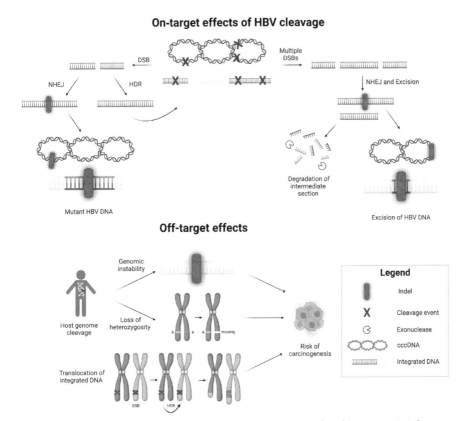

Fig. 2. Effects of nuclease-mediated cleavage on HBV-integrated and cccDNA. HBV cleavage by nucleases results in the formation of a DSB. This break can either be repaired by the faster error-prone NHEJ pathway or the error-free HDR pathway. NHEJ repair results in indel formation, resulting in mutant HBV, with potentially impaired transcriptional activity. Multiple DSBs may result in excision of the intermediate segment, which will be degraded by host exonucleases. Off-target effects for HBV cleavage include host genome cleavage, resulting in possible genomic instability and/or loss of heterozygosity. On-target cleavage of integrated DNA may also result in unintentional off-target translocation of other integrations as a function of HDR. These off-target effects result in increased risk of carcinogenesis. (Created with BioRender.com.)

Cas9 generation of DSBs in the presence of NHEJ pathway inhibition caused a reduction in cccDNA, rather than repair by slower HDR pathways.[35]

These approaches have been tested in various models of HBV (**Table 3**), and efficacy of these strategies has been quantified based on several parameters (see **Box 1**).

ANTIVIRAL EFFECT OF NUCLEASES AGAINST HEPATITIS B VIRUS

ZFNs, TALENs, and CRISPR-Cas9 systems have induced antiviral activity against HBV, with most studies showing a 1- to 2-log decrease in most viral measures (**Fig. 3**). In general, regardless of the underlying molecular tool, a greater effect is seen in reducing extracellular HBV DNA, and this may be due to its inherent sensitivity to changes in any of the viral proteins or the overlapping nature of the HBV genome causing compounding effects on viral reproduction (eg, targeting the S ORF may

---

Box 1
Measures of antiviral activity

HBeAg/HBsAg expression and secretion
  Measurement of downstream protein expression reflects inactivation of DNA transcripts by gene editing, whether that is inactivation or complete degradation. These are useful metrics, particularly if editors are designed to cleave at specific ORFs for targeted disruption of viral proteins (eg, cleaving at S ORF should not affect HBcAg).[62]

cccDNA copy number
  Because cccDNA is the transcriptional center of HBV, analyzing cccDNA for disruption is essential. Analysis of cccDNA levels after destructive gene editing indicates efficacy in either mutation of primer sites or complete degradation of cccDNA. Analysis of cccDNA levels may also be relevant as a measure of enhanced antiviral immunity, such as after activation of anti-HBV factors, resulting in clearance of HBV host cells. Indels and genomic excisions outside of primer sites, however, will result in detectable mutant cccDNA and therefore will not result in any change in copy number. Efficacy in these cases should be quantified through the other measures.

Target site editing
  Detection of target site editing remains crucial in gene editing for analysis of genomic sequences for potential sites of interest, to verify modification at target sites, and to check for off-target effects.
  These approaches are divided into biased and unbiased approaches. Biased methods depend on a priori knowledge of likely sites of editing and include direct PCR sequencing such as the T7 endonuclease 1 assay and deep sequencing. These approaches are simpler; however, they are likely to miss potential off-target effects that are not predicted. Whole genome sequencing (NGS)-based approaches are unbiased and are more sensitive, allowing for greater detection of affected sites, both on and off target.
  HBcAg, Hepatitis B virus core antigen; HBeAg, Hepatitis B virus e antigen; NGS, Next Generation Sequencing.

---

also affect reverse transcription through its simultaneous effect on the viral polymerase). The greatest reduction of extracellular HBV DNA (3-log decrease) was observed in the HepAD38 model,[36] which is an integrated HBV DNA model regulated by a Tet repressed promoter. CRISPR-Cas9 was delivered using a lentivirus vector, leading to high transduction efficiencies and likely a strong factor in the large effect.

In vivo, the 2 studies that reported the greatest reduction in secreted virus (2-log decrease) both used a hydrodynamic injection mouse model, wherein the gene editor and HBV plasmid were coinjected into the tail vein at high pressure to physically force the DNA into hepatocytes.[37,38] These studies do not replicate treatment after a chronic infection has already been established. Also, the HBV DNA templates in these models do not represent true cccDNA and are more akin to a transfection model.

Overall, transfection models (in which a plasmid construct is introduced into the cells to represent infection) are most sensitive to these gene editing tools, followed by integration models (in which a stable cell line containing an integrated HBV DNA genome is cleaved). Infection models (in which true cccDNA is formed) are the least sensitive to designer nucleases. This difference in sensitivity could be due accessibility to the HBV genome—HBV plasmids and integrations are in a relatively open conformation and can be edited by nucleases without issue, whereas cccDNA may be tightly bound to histones preventing access and cleavage.[39]

The highest in vitro reduction in cccDNA, at a 2-log change, was observed in a HepG2-hNTCP-C4-iCas9 model, which is an infection model with a stable inducible cas9 expression,[35] which meant that all cells were expressing high levels of Cas9,

Table 3
Hepatitis B virus models

	Definition	Advantages	Disadvantages
In Vitro			
Integrated HBV	Hepatoma cell lines with stable integration of HBV DNA into host genome	Ease of use High viral replication High viral markers	No modeling of viral entry cccDNA likely in a different confirmation and activity is not likely comparable
Transfection	HBV plasmid transfection into hepatoma cell lines	High viral markers. eg, HBsAg, HBeAg	Not true infection model High viral copy number not true to natural infection
Infection: hepatoma	Cultured cell lines infected with HBV inoculum	True infection model	Low infectivity Cannot analyze carcinogenic off-target effects of gene editing
Infection: primary	Primary human hepatocytes infected with HBV inoculum	True infection model Closest in vitro model to natural infection	Cannot be subcultured Expensive
In vivo			
HDI	Rapid injection of HBV plasmid in solution into mouse tail vein	Simple Effective Cheap Immune competent	High viral copy number not true to natural infection
AAV	Engineered virus to deliver HBV plasmid to target cells	Low toxicity Ease of use Immune competent	Viral vehicle Potential transient antigenemia
Transgenic HBV integration	Genetically modified mouse model with HBV genome integration	High viral markers	Not true infection model
Humanized chimeric mouse	Mouse model with transplanted human hepatocytes	True infection model	Requires source of human hepatocytes Immunodeficient
Nonhuman primates	Chimpanzees, recombinant macaques	Closest model to human infection	Restriction on use Expensive

Abbreviations: AAV, adeno-associated virus; HBeAg, Hepatitis B Virus e antigen; HDI, hydrodynamic injection.

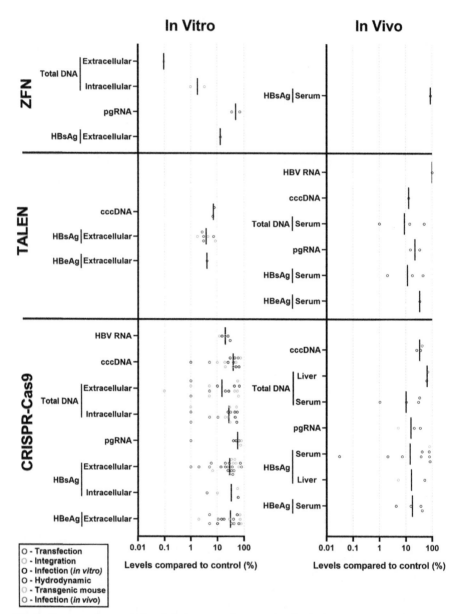

Fig. 3. Comparative analysis of designer nuclease technologies in anti-HBV activity. Data from 33 studies were consolidated on effect of nucleases on HBV antigen levels in vitro (*A*) and in vivo (*B*) and graphed with geometric mean indicated by the vertical line. Included studies are detailed in **Table 4**. Each point represents a study and is colored by the underlying model: HBV transfection model, red; integrated HBV model, green; HBV infection model, blue; HBV hydrodynamic injection model, purple; transgenic HBV mouse model, gold; HBV infection of humanized mouse model, orange.

Table 4
Comparative analysis of designer nuclease technologies in anti-HBV activity

Model	Editing Strategy	Study	Cell/Mouse Line	HBeAg Intracellular (% of Control)	HBeAg Extracellular (% of Control)	HBsAg Intracellular (% of Control)	HBsAg Extracellular (Serum In Vivo) (% of Control)	pgRNA (% of Control)	cccDNA (% of Control)	Total Intracellular DNA (% of Control)	Total Extracellular DNA (Serum In Vivo) (% of Control)	HBV RNA (% of Control)
In vitro — Transfection cell line HBV plasmid	TALEN	Bloom et al, [62] 2013	Huh7				20		69			
		Chen[81] Mol Ther 2014	Huh7		30		65	55	60			
		Dreyer et al, [44] 2016	Huh7				20		60			
		Smith et al, [38] 2021	Huh7				17	71				
	ZFN	Cradick[82], Mol Ther 2010	Huh7/pTHBV2 HBV									
	CRISPR/Cas9	Lin[86], Mol Ther Nucleic Acids 2014	Huh7			4	36					
		Dong et al, [34] 2015	Huh7		41.6		41.6		60			
		Liu et al, [51] 2015	HepG2							1	1	
		Ramanan et al, [27] 2015	HepG2				34	1	5	5	5	
		Wang[89], World J Gastroenterol 2015	HuH-7		5		1					
		Zhu[94], Virus Res 2016	Huh7 + HepG2		40		37.5					
		Liu et al, [52] 2018	Huh7 and HepG2.2.15		5		2	65	40			
		Yan[92], Frontiers Microbiol 2021	Huh7		34		25			1	1	
		Scott[87], Sci Rep 2017	Huh7				5					
	CRISPR/Cas9 nickase	Jiang[83], Cell Res 2017	HepAD38				80					
		Sakuma et al, [23] 2016	HepG2		10.52		5.8			31.25	62.5	
		Kurihara[85], Sci Rep 2017	Huh7				34			10.41		
Cell lines harboring the integrated HBV genome	TALEN	Bloom et al, [62] 2013	HepG2.2.15									
		Dreyer et al, [44] 2016	HepG2.2.15				10					

(continued on next page)

Table 4
(continued)

Model	Editing Strategy	Study	Cell/Mouse Line	HBeAg Intracellular (% of Control)	HBeAg Extracellular (% of Control)	HBsAg Intracellular (% of Control)	HBsAg Extracellular (Serum In Vivo) (% of Control)	pgRNA (% of Control)	cccDNA (% of Control)	Total Intracellular DNA (% of Control)	Total Extracellular DNA (Serum In Vivo) (% of Control)	HBV RNA (% of Control)
	ZFN	Smith et al,[38] 2021; Weber[90], Plos One 2014	HepG2.2.15 AD38				81.8			3.400000000000001	0.0999999999999943	
	CRISPR/Cas9	Dong et al,[34] 2015; Wang[89], World J Gastroenterol 2015	HepG2.2.15 AD38		70	57.1	50		50		58	
		Zhen[93], Gene Ther 2015	HepG2.2.15				39		20			
		Liu et al,[52] 2018	AD38		2			80				
			HepG2.2.15		76.9			75				
		Li et al,[37] 2016	HepG2.A64						75	52.6	45	
		Ramanan et al,[27] 2015	HepG2.2.15		28.5		34				5	12
		Kennedy et al,[36] 2015	AD38		71.4		29.6		10	1	0.0999999999999943	
		Kayesh[84], Virus Res 2020	HepG2.2.15				64.3		39.4	29	56.8	
		Scott[87], Sci Rep 2017	HepG2.2.15			10						20
		Kayesh[84], Virus Res 2020	HepG2.2.15							30	1	
	CRISPR/Cas9 nickase	Karimova et al,[50] 2015	HepG2.2.15 and HepG2-H1.3				6.5999999999999					
		Kurihara[85], Sci Rep 2017	HepG2.2.15.7							25.8		
		Schiwon et al,[28] 2018	HepG2.2.15				45		19.2	20	5	
HBV infection system	CRISPR/Cas9	Ramanan et al,[27] 2015	Hep-NTCP						45	45		15
		Seeger[88], Mol Ther Nucleic Acids 2014	NTCP/cas9									
		Kennedy et al,[36] 2015	HepaRG		17.6		27.7		30	53.5	26.6	
		Murai et al,[35] 2022	HepG2-hNTCP-C4-iCas9		14.2		13.5	40	1		20	
		Scott[87], Sci Rep 2017	hNTCP-HepG2			60			25		10	
			HepG2-hNTCP-30						65	55.5	43.3	

Category	Method	Reference	Model						
		Kayesh[84], Virus Res 2020							
		Murai et al,[35] 2022	PHH	63.6	72.7	50	50	67	30
		Schiwon et al,[28] 2018	HepG2-NTCP	55		25	25		25
		Martinez et al,[30] 2022	HepG2-NTCP	10	20	20		1	25
	CRISPR/Cas9 nickase	Karimova et al,[50] 2015	HepG2hNTCP		20				
		Kurihara[85], Sci Rep 2017	HepG2-hNTCP-C4				46.5		100
In vivo mouse	HDI with HBV-expressing plasmid or pre-ccDNA — TALEN	Bloom et al,[62] 2013	NMRI		17.8	13		14.2	
		Chen[81], Mol Ther 2014	C3H/HeN	34	45	34		50	
		Smith et al,[38] 2021	NMRI		2	15		1	
	ZFN	Xirong[91], Biochemistry 2014	M-TgHBV		88				
	CRISPR/Cas9	Lin[86], Mol Ther Nucleic Acids 2014	C57BL/6		73.9				
		Dong et al,[34] 2015	BALB/c	14.8	79.5				
		Liu et al,[51] 2015	BALB/c	4.0999999999999	2	35		10	
		Ramanan et al,[27] 2015	NRG		75.7			29.2	
		Zhen[93], Gene Ther 2015	BALB/c		7	25			
		Li et al,[37] 2016	C57BL/6	50	0.030000000000011				
		Jiang[83], Cell Res 2017	C57BL/6	40	40	20	60	1	
		Yan[92], Frontiers Microbiol 2021	C57BL/6	35.71	36.37	34		32.1	
HBV transgenic mice	CRISPR/Cas9	Zhen[93], Gene Ther 2015	HBV-Tg BALB/c	5					
		Zhu[94], Virus Res 2016	M-TgHBV C57BL/6J		77.7				
HBV infection system	CRISPR/Cas9	Stone[95], Mol Ther Methods Clin Dev. 2021	Liver-humanized chimeric FRG mice			40	66		

Abbreviations: HBeAg, Hepatitis B virus e antigen; HDI, hydrodynamic injection.

likely a limiting factor for cleavage. Supporting this, in the same study, transduction of the same CRISPR-Cas9 system in a PHH model resulted in only a 50% reduction in cccDNA levels, more in line with other studies.[35]

Together, the overall picture around designer nucleases against HBV suggests that both the expression level of effectors and the target being assessed have a large contribution to the reported efficacy. To treat people with chronic HBV infections, the field will need to develop appropriate mechanisms to overcome low expression and delivery, as well as enhance their targeting to cccDNA in particular.

ALTERNATE APPROACHES TO TARGET HEPATITIS B VIRUS DNA
Transcriptional Silencing

Transcriptional silencing of the HBV genome has been investigated as a method to alter expression without the removal of viral DNA and may be safer for inactivation of integrated DNA considering generation of DSBs in host genome may result in genomic instability and lesions.

ZFP and TALEs fused with KRAB have been used to silence HBV DNA, causing short-term viral silencing.[40,41] Base editing CRISPRs have been studied for permanent alteration of HBV genome by introducing nonsense mutations and thus pre-emptive termination of downstream protein synthesis. Base editing has been used for inactivation of HBsAg, resulting in reduction of up to 95%,[42] as well as decreased expression of Pol, in both cccDNA and integrated DNA.[43]

HDR has been exploited to introduce anti-HBV primary microRNAs into viral target DNA, via TALENs. Using this combined approach, there was increased inhibition of HBsAg secretion compared with using TALENs alone in HepG2.2.15 cells, and with hepatitis B core antigen (HBcAg)-targeting TALEN in a Huh7 transfection model but not with HBsAg-targeting TALEN.[44]

TARGETING CELLULAR GENES

Instead of directly editing the viral genome, some groups have targeted cellular genes as an antiviral approach. Mutant NTCP (NTCP-S267F) does not support HBV entry. Although mutant is reported to be nonfunctional with respect to its physiologic role of bile acid transport,[45] individuals with this mutation are not known to have altered phenotype possibly indicating compensatory mechanisms. CRISPR-Cas9 base editing has been used to induce formation of this mutation and was effective in preventing viral entry in cells with homozygous, but not heterozygous, mutations.[46]

BARRIERS AND SOLUTIONS TO USING NUCLEASES FOR THERAPY
Efficacy

Mutational evasion
High rates of viral replication combined with the inability to proofread reverse transcription results in high potential for HBV to mutate and develop quasispecies.[47] Although Cas9 is able to tolerate mismatching to an extent, this ability may vary based on proximity of these deviations to target sequence from the PAM region, with more mismatches being tolerated the more distal they are.[48]

Moreover, some Cas9 orthologs such as NmCas9 have higher specificity and thus are less tolerant of mismatches. StCas9 can tolerate single nucleotide mismatches; however, 2 and 3 mismatches cause significant impairment of HBV antiviral potency (see **Table 2**).[33]

Genotypic differences—targeting more or conserved targets

The high heterogeneity of HBV genomes presents a technical challenge in designing nucleases for effective targeting of several or all HBV genotypes. Targeting highly conserved areas of the HBV genome is necessary for broad coverage, as well as multiplexing treatment to target multiple sites.

These design limitations are compounded if these nucleases are to be used in vivo, because a balance is required between minimizing off-target effects and targeting the range of viral quasispecies. Moreover, because most studies on designer nuclease-based treatment of HBV only use a single HBV clone for analyzing treatment efficacy, the results need to be validated in multiple genotypes for translation into a clinical setting. This fine line between specificity and mutant recognition is difficult to overcome, especially when considering finding specific sites in the small (3.2-kb) HBV genome.[33]

A solution to targeting varied genomic sequences within a common genome is to focus on highly conserved target sites, which are not or are seldom altered for CRISPR-Cas9 treatment.[27,31,49,50] Several have been identified between HBV genotypes, in spCas9, saCas9, and stCas9.[33,51,52] Efficacy can also be enhanced by targeting multiple sites, for example, by multiplexing gRNAs.[16,51–54] Using these strategies together, antiviral activity can be maximized.

Safety

Off-target activity

Off-target activity is defined as nonspecific cleavage at DNA sites outside of the target sequences. This cleavage results in unintended mutations in the host genome, which are difficult to repair, increasing the risk of cellular dysregulation and carcinogenesis.[55] Off-target activity is of particular concern in species with large genomes such as humans, which may contain thousands of potential sites for off-target activity, rendering target site selection a challenge.

Nonspecific *Fok*I activity is a major contributor to off-target activity in ZFN, TALEN, and *Fok*I-dCas9 systems. Designed as left and right monomers for canonical heterodimeric cleavage, functional left/left and right/right homodimers may also be assembled, resulting in cleavage at unintended sites. To solve this, obligate heterodimerizing *Fok*I mutants have been developed, preventing homodimer cleavage.[56,57] Reducing the levels of nuclease can reduce off-target effects because canonical binding sequences will be prioritized over nonspecific binding. *Fok*I mutants with enhanced cleavage activity can allow for lower concentrations of nuclease with the same efficacy and with improved specificity[58]; however, this has been reported to decrease effective HBV silencing.[38]

SpCas9 is known to have the largest potential for off-target activity compared with other Cas9 orthologs. Thus, orthologs with improved specificities (such as StCas9) have been recommended for progression into clinical trials considering safety concerns.[33] SpCas9, however, remains the most used and studied Cas9, and other methods of mitigating off-target activity have been developed. As discussed previously, nickases and *Fok*I-dCas9 chimeric fusions require paired activity to induce DSBs, improving precision and specificity. Several engineered SpCas9 variants have been developed with the primary goal of destabilizing the CRISPR-Cas9 complex leading to reduced efficiency during off-target binding, including evoCas9, Cas9-HF1, and eCas9 (see **Table 2**).[59]

In general, the longer a nuclease is present in a cell, the greater the potential to develop off-target effects.[60] Transient delivery of Cas9 protein through vehicles such as ribonucleoprotein complexes (**Box 2**) limits Cas9 activity time, reducing

---

Box 2
Delivery

Lipid nanoparticle
A benefit of delivery of RNA is low off-target effect and improved safety due to transient expression of Cas9 protein; however, these compounds are susceptible to degradation by RNase activity, necessitating protective delivery methods, such as with ZALs codelivery.[63] Direct delivery of CRISPR/Cas9 system as a packaged RNP complex has the benefits of being faster due to not requiring translation into protein, and with minimal off-target activity or immunogenicity; however, delivery of these compounds remains a challenge.

Lentiviral
The main advantages of lentiviral-based transduction are a high rate of transfection when compared with nonviral methods, as well as their ability to modify both dividing and nondividing cells.[64] Integrating lentiviruses can cause insertional mutagenesis, as well as concerns for sustained Cas9 expression, and thus are not appropriate for therapeutic function. Integrase-deficient lentiviral vectors are a promising vehicle for delivery in vivo because they lack this disadvantage and retain activity in quiescent and other nondividing cells.

Adenovirus-associated vectors
rAAV have a low level of immunogenicity, are not pathogenic, and have the ability transduce both dividing and nondividing cells. However, a limitation in using them as a vehicle for CRISPR/Cas9 components is the tight packaging limits, at approximately 4.4 kb, which can barely fit spCas9 (4.14 kb) and its gRNA. Although it is technically feasible, this does limit the length of other elements such as expression vectors, and gene knockins, and cannot deliver larger transgenes such as base editors or prime editors. The most common method of solving this is to split the package into 2 AAV packages.[65–67] Smaller Cas9 sequence, such as saCas9, may also used if a single package is desired.[68]
rAAV, recombinant adenovirus-associated vector; RNP, ribonucleoprotein; ZALs, zwitterionic amino lipids.

---

potential capability for off-target effects. However, this may directly affect the efficacy of the nuclease treatment: as mentioned earlier, sufficient expression levels of the effectors are likely to have a large impact on antiviral activity.

Detection of these off-target effects is critical in ensuring the safety of gene editors. Detection can be done in tandem with verifying on-target cleavage through the use of genomic tools (see **Box 1** — target site editing).

Risk of increasing mutation or cancer
Owing to integration of linearized HBV DNA into host genome, concerns have been raised on cleavage of these HBV fragments causing chromosomal rearrangement of the host genome, which can subsequently lead to altered expression of local oncogenes.[32] Expression of Cas9 per se has also been associated with disruption of DSB repair pathways,[61] which may contribute to genomic instability, especially under constitutive expression. Within the context of nuclease-mediated DSB formation, NHEJ will remove the recognition site, whereas HDR will restore it, potentially resulting in continual cleavage. Considering the presence of integrated HBV within the host genome, this may cause chromosomal translocation of integrated HBV, increasing genomic instability.

What is safe enough?
Chronic HBV, despite causing long-term deleterious health outcomes in the form of cirrhosis and liver cancer, can be asymptomatic for many decades. As such, the risk calculation of any treatment is different to that of other diseases that have been

successfully treated with gene editing, many if not all of which have much more imme-diate deleterious consequences. As such for any therapy using gene therapy, it is crit-ical for mass adoption for their safety to be paramount and any potential negative risks to be smaller than the positive outcomes. This calculation may alter on a case-by-case basis, with the main consideration being risk of HCC development.

SUMMARY

Development of gene editing technologies has advanced at breakneck speed in the last decade, opening the door to novel treatments of diseases that were previously untreatable. In this age of more personalized medicine, bespoke design of gene edi-tors tailored to a patient's individual circumstances seems just around the corner. With these new technologies, however, does come new challenges, and care must be taken to prevent unforeseen consequences of gene editing and to make sure that the cure is not worse than the disease.

CLINICS CARE POINTS

- The persistence of covalently closed circular DNA and integrated HBV DNA maintains chronic Hepatitis B virus infections, necessitating ongoing suppressive antiviral therapies.
- Gene editing technologies provide hope for curative treatments by excising or inactivating these persistent forms of the virus, freeing patients from ongoing antiviral therapy.
- However, due to limited effect size and technological limitations, these approaches remain in pre-clinical phases, but may eventually lead to clinical trials if these barriers can be overcome.

DISCLOSURE

The authors have no commercial or financial conflicts of interest to declare.

FUNDING

Work on this manuscript was in part supported by Ideas grants 2002565 and 2021586 from the National Health and Medical Research Council (NHMRC) of Australia, The University of Sydney, and by the Robert W Storr bequest to the Sydney Medical Foun-dation, University of Sydney. Thomas Tu is supported by the Paul and Valeria Ains-worth Fellowship.

REFERENCES

1. Lozano R, Naghavi M, Foreman K, et al. Global and regional mortality from 235 causes of death for 20 age groups in 1990 and 2010: a systematic analysis for the Global Burden of Disease Study 2010. Lancet 2012;380(9859):2095–128.
2. Tu T, Zhang H, Urban S. Hepatitis B virus DNA integration: in vitro models for investigating viral Pathogenesis and persistence. Viruses 2021;13(2):180.
3. Huang L-R, Wu H-L, Chen P-J, et al. An immunocompetent mouse model for the tolerance of human chronic hepatitis B virus infection. Proc Natl Acad Sci USA 2006;103(47):17862–7.
4. Tu T, Budzinska MA, Shackel NA, et al. Conceptual models for the initiation of hepatitis B virus-associated hepatocellular carcinoma. Liver Int 2015;35(7): 1786–800.

5. Tu T, Budzinska MA, Shackel NA, et al. HBV DNA integration: molecular mechanisms and clinical implications. Viruses 2017;9(4).
6. Tu T, Bühler S, Bartenschlager R. Chronic viral hepatitis and its association with liver cancer. Biol Chem 2017;398(8):817–37.
7. van Zonneveld M, Flink HJ, Verhey E, et al. The safety of pegylated interferon alpha-2b in the treatment of chronic hepatitis B: predictive factors for dose reduction and treatment discontinuation. Aliment Pharmacol Ther 2005;21(9):1163–71.
8. Perrillo R. Benefits and risks of interferon therapy for hepatitis B. Hepatology 2009;49(5 Suppl):S103–11.
9. EASL 2017 Clinical Practice Guidelines on the management of hepatitis B virus infection. J Hepatol 2017;67(2):370–98.
10. Ramirez CL, Foley JE, Wright DA, et al. Unexpected failure rates for modular assembly of engineered zinc fingers. Nat Methods 2008;5(5):374–5.
11. Bitinaite J, Wah DA, Aggarwal AK, et al. FokI dimerization is required for DNA cleavage. Proc Natl Acad Sci U S A 1998;95(18):10570–5.
12. Urnov FD, Rebar EJ, Holmes MC, et al. Genome editing with engineered zinc finger nucleases. Nat Rev Genet 2010;11:636+.
13. Mussolino C, Morbitzer R, Lütge F, et al. A novel TALE nuclease scaffold enables high genome editing activity in combination with low toxicity. Nucleic Acids Res 2011;39(21):9283–93.
14. Joung JK, Sander JD. TALENs: a widely applicable technology for targeted genome editing. Nat Rev Mol Cell Biol 2013;14(1):49–55.
15. Pickar-Oliver A, Gersbach CA. The next generation of CRISPR–Cas technologies and applications. Nat Rev Mol Cell Biol 2019;20(8):490–507.
16. Qi LS, Larson MH, Gilbert LA, et al. Repurposing CRISPR as an RNA-guided platform for sequence-specific control of gene expression. Cell 2013;152(5):1173–83.
17. Thakore PI, D'Ippolito AM, Song L, et al. Highly specific epigenome editing by CRISPR-Cas9 repressors for silencing of distal regulatory elements. Nat Methods 2015;12(12):1143–9.
18. Perez-Pinera P, Kocak DD, Vockley CM, et al. RNA-guided gene activation by CRISPR-Cas9-based transcription factors. Nat Methods 2013;10(10):973–6.
19. Zalatan Jesse G, Lee ME, Almeida R, et al. Engineering complex synthetic transcriptional Programs with CRISPR RNA scaffolds. Cell 2015;160(1):339–50.
20. Tanenbaum ME, Gilbert LA, Qi LS, et al. A protein-tagging system for signal amplification in gene expression and fluorescence imaging. Cell 2014;159(3):635–46.
21. Gopalappa R, Suresh B, Ramakrishna S, et al. Paired D10A Cas9 nickases are sometimes more efficient than individual nucleases for gene disruption. Nucleic Acids Res 2018;46(12):e71.
22. Mali P, Aach J, Stranges PB, et al. CAS9 transcriptional activators for target specificity screening and paired nickases for cooperative genome engineering. Nat Biotechnol 2013;31(9):833–8.
23. Sakuma T, Masaki K, Abe-Chayama H, et al. Highly multiplexed CRISPR-Cas9-nuclease and Cas9-nickase vectors for inactivation of hepatitis B virus. Gene Cell 2016;21(11):1253–62.
24. Guilinger JP, Thompson DB, Liu DR. Fusion of catalytically inactive Cas9 to FokI nuclease improves the specificity of genome modification. Nat Biotechnol 2014;32(6):577–82.

25. Komor AC, Kim YB, Packer MS, et al. Programmable editing of a target base in genomic DNA without double-stranded DNA cleavage. Nature 2016;533(7603):420–4.
26. Anzalone AV, Randolph PB, Davis JR, et al. Search-and-replace genome editing without double-strand breaks or donor DNA. Nature 2019;576(7785):149–57.
27. Ramanan V, Shlomai A, Cox DBT, et al. CRISPR/Cas9 cleavage of viral DNA efficiently suppresses hepatitis B virus. Sci Rep 2015;5(1):10833.
28. Schiwon M, Ehrke-Schulz E, Oswald A, et al. One-vector system for multiplexed CRISPR/Cas9 against hepatitis B virus cccDNA utilizing high-capacity adenoviral vectors. Mol Ther Nucleic Acids 2018;12:242–53.
29. Kostyushev D, Kostyusheva A, Brezgin S, et al. Suppressing the NHEJ pathway by DNA-PKcs inhibitor NU7026 prevents degradation of HBV cccDNA cleaved by CRISPR/Cas9. Sci Rep 2019;9(1):1847.
30. Martinez MG, Combe E, Inchauspe A, et al. CRISPR-Cas9 targeting of hepatitis B virus covalently closed circular DNA generates transcriptionally active episomal variants. mBio 2022;13(2):e0288821.
31. Li H, Sheng C, Wang S, et al. Removal of integrated hepatitis B virus DNA using CRISPR-cas9. Front Cell Infect Microbiol 2017;7:91.
32. Feitelson MA, Lee J. Hepatitis B virus integration, fragile sites, and hepatocarcinogenesis. Cancer Lett 2007;252(2):157–70.
33. Kostyushev D, Brezgin S, Kostyusheva A, et al. Orthologous CRISPR/Cas9 systems for specific and efficient degradation of covalently closed circular DNA of hepatitis B virus. Cell Mol Life Sci 2019;76(9):1779–94.
34. Dong C, Qu L, Wang H, et al. Targeting hepatitis B virus cccDNA by CRISPR/Cas9 nuclease efficiently inhibits viral replication. Antiviral Res 2015;118:110–7.
35. Murai K, Kodama T, Hikita H, et al. Inhibition of nonhomologous end joining-mediated DNA repair enhances anti-HBV CRISPR therapy. Hepatol Commun 2022;6(9):2474–87.
36. Kennedy EM, Bassit LC, Mueller H, et al. Suppression of hepatitis B virus DNA accumulation in chronically infected cells using a bacterial CRISPR/Cas RNA-guided DNA endonuclease. Virology 2015;476:196–205.
37. Li H, Sheng C, Liu H, et al. An effective molecular target site in hepatitis B virus S gene for Cas9 cleavage and mutational inactivation. Int J Biol Sci 2016;12(9):1104–13.
38. Smith T, Singh P, Chmielewski KO, et al. Improved specificity and safety of anti-hepatitis B virus TALENs using obligate heterodimeric FokI nuclease domains. Viruses 2021;13(7):1344.
39. Bock CT, Schwinn S, Locarnini S, et al. Structural organization of the hepatitis B virus minichromosome. J Mol Biol 2001;307(1):183–96.
40. Zhao X, Zhao Z, Guo J, et al. Creation of a six-fingered artificial transcription factor that represses the hepatitis B virus HBx gene integrated into a human hepatocellular carcinoma cell line. J Biomol Screen 2012;18(4):378–87.
41. Bloom K, Kaldine H, Cathomen T, et al. Inhibition of replication of hepatitis B virus using transcriptional repressors that target the viral DNA. BMC Infect Dis 2019;19(1):802.
42. Zhou H, Wang X, Steer CJ, et al. Efficient silencing of hepatitis B virus S gene through CRISPR-mediated base editing. Hepatology Communications 2022;6(7):1652–63.
43. Yang YC, Chen YH, Kao JH, et al. Permanent inactivation of HBV genomes by CRISPR/Cas9-Mediated non-cleavage base editing. Mol Ther Nucleic Acids 2020;20:480–90.

44. Dreyer T, Nicholson S, Ely A, et al. Improved antiviral efficacy using TALEN-mediated homology directed recombination to introduce artificial primary miR-NAs into DNA of hepatitis B virus. Biochem Biophys Res Commun 2016;478(4):1563–8.

45. Hu H-H, Liu J, Lin Y-L, et al. The rs2296651 (S267F) variant on NTCP (SLC10A1) is inversely associated with chronic hepatitis B and progression to cirrhosis and hepatocellular carcinoma in patients with chronic hepatitis B. Gut 2016;65(9):1514–21.

46. Uchida T, Park SB, Inuzuka T, et al. Genetically edited hepatic cells expressing the NTCP-S267F variant are resistant to hepatitis B virus infection. Molecular Therapy - Methods & Clinical Development 2021;23:597–605.

47. Revill PA, Tu T, Netter HJ, et al. The evolution and clinical impact of hepatitis B virus genome diversity. Nat Rev Gastroenterol Hepatol 2020;17(10):618–34.

48. Hsu PD, Scott DA, Weinstein JA, et al. DNA targeting specificity of RNA-guided Cas9 nucleases. Nat Biotechnol 2013;31(9):827–32.

49. Seeger C, Sohn JA. Complete spectrum of CRISPR/Cas9-induced mutations on HBV cccDNA. Mol Ther 2016;24(7):1258–66.

50. Karimova M, Beschorner N, Dammermann W, et al. CRISPR/Cas9 nickase-mediated disruption of hepatitis B virus open reading frame S and X. Sci Rep 2015;5(1):13734.

51. Liu X, Hao R, Chen S, et al. Inhibition of hepatitis B virus by the CRISPR/Cas9 system via targeting the conserved regions of the viral genome. J Gen Virol 2015;96(8):2252–61.

52. Liu Y, Zhao M, Gong M, et al. Inhibition of hepatitis B virus replication via HBV DNA cleavage by Cas9 from Staphylococcus aureus. Antivir Res 2018;152:58–67.

53. Wang H, Yang H, Shivalila CS, et al. One-step generation of mice carrying mutations in multiple genes by CRISPR/Cas-Mediated genome engineering. Cell 2013;153(4):910–8.

54. Cong L, Ran FA, Cox D, et al. Multiplex genome engineering using CRISPR/cas systems. Science 2013;339(6121):819–23.

55. Rasul MF, Hussen BM, Salihi A, et al. Strategies to overcome the main challenges of the use of CRISPR/Cas9 as a replacement for cancer therapy. Mol Cancer 2022;21(1):64.

56. Doyon Y, Vo TD, Mendel MC, et al. Enhancing zinc-finger-nuclease activity with improved obligate heterodimeric architectures. Nat Methods 2011;8(1):74–9.

57. Ramalingam S, Kandavelou K, Rajenderan R, et al. Creating designed zinc-finger nucleases with minimal cytotoxicity. J Mol Biol 2011;405(3):630–41.

58. Guo J, Gaj T, Barbas CF. Directed evolution of an enhanced and highly efficient FokI cleavage domain for zinc finger nucleases. J Mol Biol 2010;400(1):96–107.

59. Bak SY, Jung Y, Park J, et al. Quantitative assessment of engineered Cas9 variants for target specificity enhancement by single-molecule reaction pathway analysis. Nucleic Acids Res 2021;49(19):11312–22.

60. Liang X, Potter J, Kumar S, et al. Rapid and highly efficient mammalian cell engineering via Cas9 protein transfection. J Biotechnol 2015;208:44–53.

61. Xu S, Kim J, Tang Q, et al. CAS9 is a genome mutator by directly disrupting DNA-PK dependent DNA repair pathway. Protein Cell 2020;11(5):352–65.

62. Bloom K, Ely A, Mussolino C, et al. Inactivation of hepatitis B virus replication in cultured cells and in vivo with engineered transcription activator-like effector nucleases. Mol Ther 2013;21(10):1889–97.

63. Miller JB, Zhang S, Kos P, et al. Non-viral CRISPR/cas gene editing in vitro and in vivo enabled by synthetic nanoparticle Co-delivery of Cas9 mRNA and sgRNA. Angew Chem Int Ed Engl 2017;56(4):1059–63.

64. Segal DJ, Gonçalves J, Eberhardy S, et al. Attenuation of HIV-1 replication in primary human cells with a designed zinc finger transcription factor. J Biol Chem 2004;279(15):14509–19.

65. Yang Y, Wang L, Bell P, et al. A dual AAV system enables the Cas9-mediated correction of a metabolic liver disease in newborn mice. Nat Biotechnol 2016;34(3):334–8.

66. Chew WL, Tabebordbar M, Cheng JK, et al. A multifunctional AAV-CRISPR-Cas9 and its host response. Nat Methods 2016;13(10):868–74.

67. Swiech L, Heidenreich M, Banerjee A, et al. In vivo interrogation of gene function in the mammalian brain using CRISPR-Cas9. Nat Biotechnol 2015;33(1):102–6.

68. Ran FA, Cong L, Yan WX, et al. In vivo genome editing using Staphylococcus aureus Cas9. Nature 2015;520(7546):186–91.

69. Cornu TI, Cathomen T. Quantification of zinc finger nuclease-associated toxicity. Methods Mol Biol 2010;649:237–45.

70. Casini A, Olivieri M, Petris G, et al. A highly specific SpCas9 variant is identified by in vivo screening in yeast. Nat Biotechnol 2018;36(3):265–71.

71. Zuo W, Depotter JR, Doehlemann G. Cas9HF1 enhanced specificity in Ustilago maydis. Fungal Biol 2020;124(3–4):228–34.

72. Slaymaker IM, Gao L, Zetsche B, et al. Rationally engineered Cas9 nucleases with improved specificity. Science 2016;351(6268):84–8.

73. Hu JH, Miller SM, Geurts MH, et al. Evolved Cas9 variants with broad PAM compatibility and high DNA specificity. Nature 2018;556(7699):57–63.

74. Vicencio J, Sánchez-Bolaños C, Moreno-Sánchez I, et al. Genome editing in animals with minimal PAM CRISPR-Cas9 enzymes. Nat Commun 2022;13(1):2601.

75. Müller M, Lee CM, Gasiunas G, et al. Streptococcus thermophilus CRISPR-cas9 systems enable specific editing of the human genome. Mol Ther 2016;24(3):636–44.

76. Lee CM, Cradick TJ, Bao G. The Neisseria meningitidis CRISPR-cas9 system enables specific genome editing in mammalian cells. Mol Ther 2016;24(3):645–54.

77. Friedland AE, Baral R, Singhal P, et al. Characterization of Staphylococcus aureus Cas9: a smaller Cas9 for all-in-one adeno-associated virus delivery and paired nickase applications. Genome Biol 2015;16(1):257.

78. Zhang Y, Rajan R, Seifert HS, et al. DNase H activity of Neisseria meningitidis Cas9. Mol Cell 2015;60(2):242–55.

79. Price AA, Sampson TR, Ratner HK, et al. Cas9-mediated targeting of viral RNA in eukaryotic cells. Proc Natl Acad Sci USA 2015;112(19):6164–9.

80. Acharya S, Mishra A, Paul D, et al. Francisella novicida Cas9 interrogates genomic DNA with very high specificity and can be used for mammalian genome editing. Proc Natl Acad Sci USA 2019;116(42):20959–68.

81. Chen J, Zhang W, Lin J, et al. An efficient antiviral strategy for targeting hepatitis B virus genome using transcription activator-like effector nucleases. Mol Ther 2014;22(2):303–11. https://doi.org/10.1038/mt.2013.212.

82. Cradick TJ, Keck K, Bradshaw S, et al. Zinc-finger nucleases as a novel therapeutic strategy for targeting hepatitis B virus DNAs. Mol Ther 2010;18(5):947–54. https://doi.org/10.1038/mt.2010.20.

83. Jiang C, Mei M, Li B, et al. A non-viral CRISPR/Cas9 delivery system for therapeutically targeting HBV DNA and pcsk9 in vivo. Cell Res 2017;27(3):440–3. https://doi.org/10.1038/cr.2017.16.

84. Kayesh MEH, Amako Y, Hashem MA, et al. Development of an in vivo delivery system for CRISPR/Cas9-mediated targeting of hepatitis B virus cccDNA. Virus Res 2020;290:198191. https://doi.org/10.1016/j.virusres.2020.198191.

85. Kurihara T, Fukuhara T, Ono C, et al. Suppression of HBV replication by the expression of nickase- and nuclease dead-Cas9. Sci Rep 2017;7(1):6122. https://doi.org/10.1038/s41598-017-05905-w.

86. Lin SR, Yang HC, Kuo YT, et al. The CRISPR/Cas9 system facilitates clearance of the intrahepatic HBV templates in vivo. Mol Ther Nucleic Acids 2014;3(8):e186. https://doi.org/10.1038/mtna.2014.38.

87. Scott T, Moyo B, Nicholson S, et al. ssAAVs containing cassettes encoding Sa-Cas9 and guides targeting hepatitis B virus inactivate replication of the virus in cultured cells. Sci Rep 2017;7(1):7401. https://doi.org/10.1038/s41598-017-07642-6.

88. Seeger C, Sohn JA. Targeting hepatitis B virus with CRISPR/Cas9. Mol Ther Nucleic Acids 2014;3:e216. https://doi.org/10.1038/mtna.2014.68.

89. Wang J, Xu ZW, Liu S, et al. Dual gRNAs guided CRISPR/Cas9 system inhibits hepatitis B virus replication. World J Gastroenterol 2015;21(32):9554–65. https://doi.org/10.3748/wjg.v21.i32.9554.

90. Weber ND, Stone D, Sedlak RH, et al. AAV-mediated delivery of zinc finger nucleases targeting hepatitis B virus inhibits active replication. PLoS One 2014;9(5): e97579. https://doi.org/10.1371/journal.pone.0097579.

91. Xirong L, Rui L, Xiaoli Y, et al. Hepatitis B virus can be inhibited by DNA methyltransferase 3a via specific zinc-finger-induced methylation of the X promoter. Biochemistry (Mosc) 2014;79(2):111–23. https://doi.org/10.1134/s0006297914020047.

92. Yan K, Feng J, Liu X, et al. Inhibition of hepatitis B virus by AAV8-derived CRISPR/SaCas9 expressed from liver-specific promoters. Original research. Front Microbiol 2021;12. https://doi.org/10.3389/fmicb.2021.665184.

93. Zhen S, Hua L, Liu YH, et al. Harnessing the clustered regularly interspaced short palindromic repeat (CRISPR)/CRISPR-associated Cas9 system to disrupt the hepatitis B virus. Gene Ther 2015;22(5):404–12. https://doi.org/10.1038/gt.2015.2.

94. Zhu W, Xie K, Xu Y, et al. CRISPR/Cas9 produces anti-hepatitis B virus effect in hepatoma cells and transgenic mouse. Virus Res 2016;217:125–32. https://doi.org/10.1016/j.virusres.2016.04.003.

95. Stone D, Long KR, Loprieno MA, et al. CRISPR-Cas9 gene editing of hepatitis B virus in chronically infected humanized mice. Molecular Therapy Methods Clinical Development 2021;20:258–75. https://doi.org/10.1016/j.omtm.2020.11.014.

Delta Hepatitis

Maternal-to-Child Transmission of Hepatitis B Virus and Hepatitis Delta Virus

Lital Aliasi-Sinai, BSc[a], Theresa Worthington, BSBA[b],
Marcia Lange, BSc[c], Tatyana Kushner, MD, MSCE[b],*

KEYWORDS

- Pregnancy • Hepatitis D virus • Hepatitis B virus • Mother-to-child transmission
- Vertical transmission

KEY POINTS

- The overall rates of chronic hepatitis B in women of childbearing age within the United States has declined, with some increases seen in Appalachian states possibly related to injection drug use. Meanwhile the prevalence of hepatitis delta virus (HDV) in the pregnant population in the United States is largely unknown as HDV testing is underused, including during pregnancy care.
- There are important considerations when caring for pregnant individuals with hepatitis B virus (HBV) which includes the risk of HBV flare, HBV-associated adverse pregnancy outcomes, concern for vertical transmission, and interventions needed to optimize pregnancy outcomes.
- Individuals with hepatitis B and high HBV viral loads are at high risk of maternal-to-child transmission of HBV, but effective interventions exist to decrease risk. Maternal-to-child transmission of hepatitis D is exceptionally rare.

INTRODUCTION

Hepatitis B is a major public health threat, responsible for approximately 820,000 deaths in 2019 alone.[1] It is estimated that approximately 262 million people are living with hepatitis B virus (HBV) infection globally,[2] which includes an estimated 65 million women of childbearing age,[3] with highest prevalence in the Western Pacific Region and African region.[4] In addition, among the reproductive-aged population in certain parts of the United States, there has been an increase in incidence of HBV since

[a] Sackler School of Medicine, Tel Aviv University, Tel Aviv, Israel; [b] Division of Liver Diseases, Icahn School of Medicine at Mount Sinai, New York, USA; [c] Icahn School of Medicine at Mount Sinai, New York, USA
* Corresponding author.
E-mail address: tatyana.kushner@mssm.edu

Clin Liver Dis 27 (2023) 917–935
https://doi.org/10.1016/j.cld.2023.05.007
1089-3261/23/© 2023 Elsevier Inc. All rights reserved.

2009 possibly related to emergent risk factors among young individuals, such as injection drug use (IDU).[5,6]

Hepatitis delta virus (HDV) infection causes the most severe viral hepatitis and rapid progression to cirrhosis and hepatocellular carcinoma (HCC).[7–9] Data on the prevalence of HDV are variable, because HDV screening is largely underused and not widely available in developing regions across the globe,[10] and as a result, there is very scarce data on HDV specifically in women of childbearing age or in the pregnancy setting.

Most cases of chronic hepatitis B (CHB) are contracted under the age of 5 years old, with the majority of cases spread perinatally in endemic regions.[11] In fact, maternal-to-child transmission (MTCT) is responsible for almost half of the chronic HBV infections globally.[12] In the absence of prophylactic treatment, approximately 90% of infants exposed to HBV during delivery develop CHB.[13] Therefore, the World Health Organization (WHO) has placed significant emphasis on the reduction of MTCT to meet their goal of eliminating viral hepatitis as a major public health threat by 2030.[13] Although maternal-to-child co-transmission of HDV is rare, some cases have been reported.[14] Given the severity of the sequela of both HBV and HDV (eg, HCC and cirrhosis), perinatal transmission of HBV and co-transmission of HBV/HDV must be avoided to reduce the global burden of disease of HBV and HDV.

It is important to be aware of HBV and HDV in pregnant patients to effectively reduce the MTCT of these infections. Pregnancy is a critical time to diagnose HBV and HDV and counsel patients on the associated risks. This review evaluates the epidemiology and implications of HBV and HDV in pregnancy, MTCT of HBV and HDV, and the management of HBV and HDV in pregnancy.

EPIDEMIOLOGY OF HEPATITIS B VIRUS AND HEPATITIS DELTA VIRUS IN WOMEN OF CHILDBEARING AGE AND IN PREGNANCY
Hepatitis B Virus

MTCT accounts for approximately half of the CHB cases globally.[12] In 2015, an estimated 65 million women of childbearing age worldwide were chronically infected with HBV.[3] Globally, there are an estimated 4.5 million women with chronic HBV who give birth annually, mostly in African regions and Western Pacific Regions.[15]

Within the United States, there are approximately 1000 cases of MTCT of HBV in the United States each year.[16] The hepatitis B surface antigen (HBsAg) prevalence in pregnant people within the United States between 1990 and 1993 varied from 0.2% to 6%. The highest rates of HBV were found in Asian American (6%) and Black (1%) women while lowest in White (0.6%) and Hispanic (0.14%) women.[17] In a more recent retrospective analysis of HBV in women of childbearing age (15–44 years old) using the national Quest laboratory database from 2011 to 2017, the prevalence of new, chronic HBV (CHB) diagnosis was 0.19% in 2017, which declined significantly from 0.83% in 2011. However, there was an increase in CHB cases in Mississippi, Kentucky, and West Virginia. Rates of acute HBV were stable over time in the country as whole, though Kentucky, Alabama, and Indiana had significant increases (P < 0.03).[6] The increase in HBV cases in these particular states is thought to be possibly related to IDU, which also led to previously established increases in HCV rates.

Hepatitis D Virus

Globally, hepatitis D virus affects almost 5% of people with chronic HBV infection.[18] It is estimated that about 12 million people have serological evidence of HDV infection, with the highest concentration in Mongolia, Pakistan, upper Amazonia and Orinoco

River valley, Republic of Moldova, and countries in Western and Middle Africa.[18,19] The true prevalence of HDV in the obstetric population is not entirely clear, as HDV testing is not widely available in resource-limited areas and is not routinely checked in the pregnancy context in developed countries.

However, few studies have shed light on the prevalence of HDV coinfection in pregnant people with HBV in countries in Africa and South Asia (**Table 1**). Within Africa, the prevalence of HDV-antibodies (HDV-Abs) in pregnant women with HBsAg in the public health care setting in Nouakchott, Mauritania, from 2008 to 2009 was found to be 14.7%,[20] whereas another study conducted in five major cities in Gabon (Libreville, Port Gentil, Lambaréné, Oyem, and Franceville) found that HDV-Ab prevalence in HBsAg-positive pregnant women was 15.6%.[21] In another study conducted in Central Africa Republic, 18.8% of HBsAg-positive pregnant women from six different public health maternity wards in Bangui were found to have HDV-Abs.[22] In South Asia, HDV-Abs were found in 20.3% of HBsAg-positive pregnant women in public sector hospitals in Lahore, Pakistan, between 2016 and 2017.[23]

The prevalence of HDV infection in pregnant persons within the United States is unknown, as HDV testing is not routinely conducted in patients with HBV. In a US Midwestern population of 1007 HBsAg-positive nonpregnant people, it was found that only 121 were actually tested for HDV-Abs.[10] In the general US population, there are mixed findings for the prevalence of HDV-Abs among HBV-infected individuals.[24] According to one study conducted with NHANES data from 2011 to 2016, 42% of adult HBsAg carriers had HDV-Abs.[25] Meanwhile, in a retrospective chart review done in Northern California, 8% of patients with CHB were found to have HDV infection.[26] A large study looking at United States and Puerto Rican American Red Cross Blood services in 1985 found that 3.8% of HBsAg-positive individuals were positive for HDV infection, with significantly higher rates in San Jose and California (12.1%) and significantly lower rates in Alabama, Kentucky, Mississippi, and Tennessee.[27] In a nationwide retrospective study of all veterans who were HBsAg-positive from October 1999 to December 2013, 3.4% had HDV-Abs present.[28] High-quality studies need to be conducted to estimate the true prevalence of HDV in the United States and within the obstetric population in the country. Given that routine HBV screening is recommended in pregnancy, this may be an opportune time to delineate prevalence of HDV among those who screen positive for HBV during pregnancy.

Risk Factors for Transmission of Hepatitis B and D Viruses

Both HBV and HDV are transmitted through exchange of bodily fluids (eg, blood, semen) via percutaneous and mucosal routes.[29] The major risk factors for HBV include perinatal transmission, sexual activity, intravenous (IV) drug use, and occupational exposure. Notable risk factors in endemic regions include household contacts, hemodialysis, transmission from a surgeon,[30] and receipt of organs or blood products.[31]

To become infected with HDV, there must be a preexisting HBV infection. Major risk factors for HDV include IV drug use, history of human immunodeficiency virus (HIV) or hepatitis C virus infection, exposure to infected blood or bodily fluids, and intrafamilial and iatrogenic transmission in more highly endemic areas.[32–37] Although sexual transmission and MTCT are major risk factors for HBV, it is relatively rare to transmit HDV sexually and/or perinatally.[38]

HEPATITIS B VIRUS IN PREGNANCY

There are important factors to consider when taking care of pregnant people with HBV, as summarized in **Box 1**. These include the impact of pregnancy on the course

Table 1
Studies evaluating prevalence of hepatitis delta virus-antibodies in pregnant population

Author and Year	Country	Number of HBsAg-Positive Pregnant Individuals Identified	Prevalence Estimate of HDV-Ab in HBsAg-Positive Pregnant Individuals	Notes
Mansour et al,[20] 2012	Mauritania	109	14.7%	• Prospective study on 1966 subjects and 1020 pregnant people ages 14–47 in Sabkha public health care setting in Nouakchott • HDV-Ab positivity was significantly correlated with age ≥44 y
Makuwa et al,[21] 2008	Gabon	109	15.6%	• Cross-sectional study on 1186 pregnant people ages 14–40 in five main cities of Gabon • HDV-Ab percentage was found to be the lowest in women ages 14–20
Komas et al,[22] 2018	Central Africa Republic	69	18.8%	• Cross-sectional study with historical comparison of 2172 subjects and 874 pregnant people in six public health structures with maternity wards in Bangui • Age, transfusion, tendency to tattoo, and absence of condom use were found to be significant risk factors for HDV infection
Aftab et al,[23] 2019	Pakistan	63	20.3%	• Cross-sectional study of 1394 pregnant people ages 20–40 y old in public sector hospitals in Lahore district • Prevalence of HDV-Ab highest in pregnant women ages 26–30

Abbreviations: HBsAg, hepatitis B surface antigen; HDV-Ab, hepatitis D virus-antibodies.

Box 1
Counseling considerations in hepatitis B virus in pregnancy
Risk of HBV flare
Association of HBV with pregnancy outcomes
Concern for vertical transmission
Interventions needed to optimize pregnancy outcomes

of HBV as well as the impact of HBV on the pregnancy course. There is evidence that changes to the immune system that occur during pregnancy may cause hepatitis flares both during pregnancy and in the postpartum period. Rates of hepatitis flares, loosely defined as an elevation in liver aminotransferase levels above the upper limit of normal, have been reported to range from 6% to 14% during pregnancy and 4% to 50% after delivery.[39–44] In the absence of HDV coinfection or advanced fibrosis, these HBV flares are generally asymptomatic and self-limiting, with very few progressing to jaundice or hepatic decompensation.[39] There is conflicting evidence of risk factors for HBV flares, whereas some studies identified the presence of hepatitis B evelope antigen (HBeAg), younger maternal age,[39,45] and decreased parity[42] as risk factors for HBV flares, others did not.[40] Postpartum HBV flares have also been documented after the discontinuation of antiviral treatment.[46]

There are mixed findings in literature regarding the impact of HBV on the pregnancy course. CHB may increase risk for adverse pregnancy outcomes such as gestational diabetes,[47] antepartum hemorrhage, postpartum hemorrhage, placental abruption,[48] threatened preterm labor,[49,50] intrahepatic cholestasis of pregnancy,[51,52] and miscarriage.[53] In contrast, some studies failed to find correlations between CHB and placenta previa, placental abruption,[54] preterm labor,[47,55] or gestational diabetes.[56] The literature on the effect of HBV infection on infertility is also mixed, with some studies suggesting HBV infection negatively impacts cumulative live birth rates and implantation rates during in vitro fertilization (IVF),[57] whereas others did not find an association between HBV infection and fertility treatment outcomes.[58–60] Interestingly, a few studies found a negative correlation between HBV infection in pregnancy and preeclampsia, suggesting a possible protective effect of pregnancy on preeclampsia.[47,61]

MATERNAL-TO-CHILD TRANSMISSION OF HEPATITIS B VIRUS

MTCT is a leading cause of CHB in endemic areas of the world and thus is of critical focus in the strategy to eliminate hepatitis B, a goal the WHO has set to reach by 2030.[62] Vertical transmission can occur at any stage of pregnancy, though most of the cases occur during the peripartum period due to exposure to infected maternal blood and secretions during delivery.[63]

Rates of HBV vertical transmission vary. Without intervention, rates of MTCT vary from 70% to 90% in HBeAg-positive mothers and from 10% to 40% in HBeAg-positive mothers.[63] When implemented correctly, preventive interventions have proven to be effective in drastically reducing MTCT rates. With interventions—such as prenatal screening, antiviral therapy, and vaccination of newborns—transmission can be reduced from 90% to 21% in HBeAg + women and from 30% to 2.6% in HBeAg− women.[63]

Risk Factors for Transmission

There are a few important risk factors to consider for HBV vertical transmission (summarized in **Table 2**). A high HBV viral load, indicated by the presence of HBeAg in

Table 2 Risk factors for maternal-to-child transmission of hepatitis B	
Potential Risk Factors for MTCT	**Increases Transmission**
Biological	
High viral load (HBeAg+)	Yes
Mode of delivery	Inconclusive
Breastfeeding	No
Invasive fetal testing	Potentially for patients with high viral load
PROM	No (with proper prophylaxis)
Social/environmental	
Lack of maternal knowledge	Yes
Lack of formal hospital policies	Yes
High cost/other barriers to access	Yes
Perceived stigma (particularly in developing countries)	Yes

serum, high HBV DNA level, and high quantitative HBsAg levels, increases the risk of vertical transmission.[62,64] Despite studies demonstrating the presence of HBeAg and HBV DNA in a high percentage of HBV-infected mothers' breast milk, breastfeeding does not seem to be a risk factor for transmission. The mechanism remains unclear; however, lactoferrin in breast milk may serve a protective role by inhibiting the amplification of HBV DNA.[65]

There have also been a number of studies conducted evaluating whether mode of pregnancy delivery affects transmission. Given that the risk of MTCT is largely due to infant exposure to vaginal blood and secretions at the time of delivery, cesarean sections should theoretically reduce risk of vertical transmission. A systematic review from 2008 showed that elective cesarean delivery (ECD) could prevent MTCT, with no instances of postpartum morbidity as a result of the ECD, though the review noted bias and lack of quality in all the included studies.[66] However, other studies showed that cesarean delivery did not affect the risk of transmission or that the reduction was not significant.[67] Given the paucity of research pertaining to this issue, the conflicting results of the studies that have been conducted, and the fact that cesarean delivery comes with its own risks, the Society for Maternal-Fetal Medicine does not advise clinicians to recommend cesarean delivery for the sole purpose of reducing the risk of vertical HBV transmission.[68]

Similarly, researchers have speculated whether premature rupture of membranes (PROM) in delivery increases the risk of HBV vertical transmission. Studies have found no increased risk of transmission when prophylaxis strategies are implemented.[69]

Another potential risk factor to consider is invasive fetal testing, such as amniocentesis or chorionic villus sampling. Although many earlier studies showed no increase in risk, newer studies demonstrate risk for infected mothers with viral load greater than 7 log 10 copies/mL.[70]

From a socioeconomic and environmental perspective, the lack of maternal knowledge regarding HBV infection, management, and transmission poses a significant risk for MTCT, particularly in endemic countries. For example, in Nigeria, 76% of mothers had suboptimal HBV knowledge. In North America, higher percentages of mothers asserted knowledge, though knowledge gaps do exist.[71] Similar challenges have been reported in Uganda—only 8.3% of women were screened for HBV in their current pregnancy and only 15.6% were aware of HBV screenings; age of respondents, partners' education, perceived risk, and access to screening services were positively associated with HBV screening.[72] A study conducted in Ghana also showed that social stigma impedes testing.[73] A lack of formal hospital policies regarding HBV prophylaxis represents another risk factor. A 2006 survey across 242 delivery hospitals in the United States found significant gaps in hospital policies and practices regarding HBV vaccination and hepatitis B immunoglobulin (HBIG). Among infants who were born to HBsAg-positive women, only 62.1% received hepatitis B vaccine and HBIG within 12 hours.[74] Cost and access are other barriers to effective implementation of interventions—providing pregnant individuals with free HBsAg screening, HBV vaccination if nonimmune, and administration of HBIG for newborns is important.

EFFECTS ON INFECTED INFANTS

The implications of transmission of hepatitis B to infants are profound—according to the Center for Disease Control and Prevention, infants infected with HBV have a 90% chance of progressing to chronic infection, and when left untreated, 25% will die of liver-related complications.[75] Increasing the rates of infection in infants contributes to greater risk of horizontal transmission among children as well.

Reducing MTCT is a major priority in eliminating hepatitis B worldwide by 2030 and thereby reducing the burden of chronic liver disease and HCC. Although comprehensive guidelines to minimize MTCT have been developed, access to care and effective implementation remain a challenge worldwide.

HEPATITIS DELTA VIRUS IN PREGNANCY

Data regarding maternal hepatitis D infection in pregnancy are scarce. Similar to HBV infection, hepatitis D infection in pregnancy is generally well tolerated. However, hepatitis D virus is associated with more severe liver disease, including higher chance of progression to cirrhosis within 5 years and HCC within 10 years. Cirrhosis is known to lead to adverse pregnancy outcomes such as increased risk for preterm delivery and low birth weight.[76] Thus, while not included as part of current recommendations for the management of HBV or HBV/HDV infections during pregnancy, prenatal screening for HDV in HBsAg-positive mothers is crucial.[77]

Vertical transmission of HDV is rare. A study from 1988 showed that with prophylaxis, 0 of 16 infants exhibited serological evidence of HBV and HDV infection at 7 months.[78] A more recent study from 2004 to 2015 revealed similar results.[38] This rarity could be due in part to the fact that HBV load levels have been found to be lower in HBV/HDV coinfected patients. In addition, a cross-sectional study showed that both viruses were only active in about 40% of coinfected patients, and HDV alone was only active in about 30%.[79] **Box 1 Table 3**, for overview of these studies.

The same strategies used to prevent MTCT of HBV are effective in preventing transmission of HDV as well.

Table 3 Studies investigating efficacy of maternal-to-child transmission of hepatitis D		
Study	Results	Takeaway
Ramia et al,[78] 1988	No infants exhibited serological evidence of HBV and HDV infection at 7 months follow-up	HDV MTCT is exceptional
Sellier et al,[38] 2017	HDV Ab was negative in 36 children	HDV MTCT is exceptional

MANAGEMENT OF HEPATITIS B VIRUS AND HEPATITIS DELTA VIRUS IN PREGNANCY

HBV infection during pregnancy presents with special considerations and management issues for both the mother and the fetus. The prevention of MTCT is at the forefront, especially as vertical transmission is responsible for approximately half of chronic HBV infections worldwide.[12] Screening prenatally, early linkage to care with a hepatologist, monitoring for hepatitis flares, antiviral treatment for mothers with high HBV DNA levels, and administering passive–active immunization to newborns are all important components of effective disease management in pregnancy. Clinic care points can be found in **Table 4.**

Table 4
Recommendations for management of hepatitis B and hepatitis D viruses in pregnancy

	Overview of Recommendations
Screening	• All pregnant patients should be screened at initial prenatal visit for HBsAg • In high-risk populations[a], additionally screen for anti-HBs and anti-HBc to determine immune status
Vaccination	All nonimmune pregnant patients should be vaccinated against HBV
Initial testing	In newly HBsAg-positive pregnant patients, obtain and test for: • HBV DNA • Anti-HBs • Anti-HBc • Anti-HBe • Liver panel (ALT, AST, total bilirubin) • HCV • HIV • HDV antibody
Referral to hepatology	Refer pregnant patient to hepatologist if HBV DNA >200 000 IU/L, liver tests are elevated, HBeAg is positive, or coinfected with HCV or HDV
Monitoring	• Obtain a liver panel every 3 months during pregnancy and up to 6 months postpartum ○ If elevated, follow-up with HBV DNA levels • At 26 to 28 wk gestation, measure HBV DNA levels to determine whether to initiate peripartum antiviral therapy
Initiation of antiviral therapy	Initiate antiviral therapy with TDF if HBV DNA > 200 000 IU/mL or HBeAg-positive
Discontinuation of antiviral therapy	Discontinue antiviral therapy at the time of delivery or within 4 wk postpartum
Newborn immunoprophylaxis	Within 12 hours of birth: • Active immunization with birth dose of HBV vaccine • Passive immunization with 100 IU HBIG Following birth: • Completion of HBV vaccine series
Lactation	If a newborn has received immunoprophylaxis, breastfeeding is safe

Abbreviations: anti-HBc, hepatitis B core antibody; anti-HBs, hepatitis B surface antibody; anti-HBe, hepatitis B evelope antibody; HBIG, hepatitis B immunoglobulin; HBsAg, hepatitis B surface antigen; HBeAg, hepatitis B envelope antigen; HBV, hepatitis B virus; ALT, alanine aminotransferase; AST, aspartate aminotransferase; TDF, tenofovir disoproxil fumarate.
[a] High-risk populations include IV drug users, pregnant individuals with sexual partners, or household contacts with hepatitis B infection, those with multiple sexual partners in the last 6 months, or those recently evaluated for or treated for a sexually transmitted infection.

Screening and Surveillance

All pregnant women presenting for their first prenatal visit should be tested for HBsAg. The presence of HBsAg establishes the diagnosis of HBV infection. Although universal neonatal HBV vaccination has been implemented in many countries including the United States, universal screening for HBV during pregnancy allows for additional preventative measures. Any patient not tested prenatally should be tested at the time of hospital admission for delivery.[80] In addition to screening for HBsAg, in high-risk populations (eg, IV drug users, sexual partners, or household contacts with CHB, multiple sexual partners in the past 6 months, or recently evaluated or treated for a sexually transmitted infection), testing for hepatitis B surface antibody (anti-HBs) and hepatitis B core antibody (anti-HBc) is recommended as it helps determine immune status. HBV vaccination should be offered during pregnancy for those not immune.

If a pregnant individual is found to be positive for HBsAg, additional testing should be conducted, including HBV DNA, anti-HBs, anti-HBc, HBeAg, anti-HBe, and baseline liver panel. Patients should be referred to a hepatologist to determine the need for early initiation of antiviral therapy if HBV DNA greater than 200 000 IU/L, liver tests are elevated, or HBeAg is positive. Furthermore, screening for HDV, hepatitis C virus, and HIV infections should also be conducted as coinfection can significantly worsen outcomes.[24] HDV testing should start with screening for anti-HDV-Abs in serum; if positive, verify for active disease with HDV RNA (qualitative or quantitative).[24] Sexual partners of HBsAg-positive patients should also be assessed for HBV infection or immunity and receive the HBV vaccine if appropriate.

If HBsAg-negative without evidence of prior HBV infection (negative for anti-HBs or anti-HBc) or HBsAg-negative but only anti-HBc-positive, the patient should be vaccinated.[77] For those with the evidence of prior HBV infection, HBsAg screening should be repeated again at 26 to 28 weeks gestation. If at that time HBV DNA $\geq$ 200 000 IU/mL, prompt antiviral treatment should be initiated.[77]

Monitoring Hepatitis B Virus Infection During Pregnancy

Although acute HBV infection during pregnancy is generally mild and not associated with an increased risk of mortality or teratogenicity,[81,82] there is still a risk of MTCT, particularly if the infection is acquired later in pregnancy.[83] In those with CHB, pregnancy can precipitate hepatitis flares, particularly in pregnant individuals without indication for antiviral therapy. For both acute and chronically HBV-infected patients, serial monitoring should be performed throughout pregnancy. Liver biochemical tests should be obtained every 3 months during pregnancy and up to 6 months postpartum. HBV DNA should be measured whenever there is an elevation in alanine aminotransferase (ALT). At the end of the second trimester (26–28 weeks), DNA and aminotransferase levels should be tested to determine the need for initiation of antiviral therapy before delivery.

Recommendations for Initiation and Choice of Antiviral Therapy

In addition to passive–active immunization of newborns, antiviral therapy during pregnancy further reduces the risk of perinatal transmission of HBV.[84–87] The duration of therapy and choice of antiviral medication are important considerations when deciding to initiate antiviral therapy.

Pregnant patients who meet standard indications for HBV therapy should be treated (eg, ALT > 2 times the upper limit of normal, HBV DNA > 20000 IU/mL if HBeAg-positive, HBV DNA > 200000 IU/mL if HBeAg-negative, acute liver failure, or cirrhosis).[77] For those without active or advanced CHB and who do not meet indications, the decision to initiate antiviral therapy should be deferred until the end of the second trimester when HBV DNA is retested.[84] If HBV DNA greater than 200000 IU/mL on retesting at 26 to 28 weeks gestation, antiviral therapy should be offered.[88] This HBV DNA level threshold is based on an increased risk of transmission at these high viral loads, despite passive–active immunization in infants.[89,90] In areas where HBV DNA may not be available, screening for HBeAg is a suitable alternative to assess eligibility for antiviral prophylaxis.[15,91] Other considerations for starting antiviral therapy before delivery include threatened preterm labor, prolonged uterine contractions, and a child who failed immunoprophylaxis previously.[92]

The choice of antiviral therapy should weigh risk of teratogenicity, adverse effects, and safety profile as well as risk of resistance. Lamivudine, telbivudine, and tenofovir disoproxil fumarate (TDF) have all been shown to effectively reduce the MTCT of HBV.[88,93] A major concern for lamivudine is however its lower barrier of resistance.[94] Although human studies support its safety in pregnancy, adverse events have been observed in some animal studies. There is no evidence of teratogenicity for TDF or telbivudine. Renal and bone toxicity are among the concerns for TDF use. Although a study of HIV-infected pregnant mothers given TDF antiviral prophylaxis saw 12% lower whole body bone mineral content in exposed infants as compared with unexposed infants,[95] a subsequent study with 2 year follow-up showed no significant differences in bone growth.[96] This suggests that any impact on bone toxicity may be transient. Two randomized controlled trials of MTCT with TDF prophylaxis demonstrated no significant differences in the rates of prematurity, congenital malformations, or Apgar scores between exposed and unexposed infants.[85,97] A network meta-analysis also showed that tenofovir is more effective than lamivudine and telbivudine in preventing MTCT.[98] Overall, due its efficacy, safety profile, and lower risk of resistance, TDF is the preferred agent for antiviral therapy during pregnancy.[85,88,97,99] Lamivudine may be a good option in special circumstances, such as if cost is a barrier or if treatment will definitely last less than 3 months.

Tenofovir alafenamide fumarate (TAF) is a new, more stable formulation of TDF that delivers active metabolite more efficiently to hepatocytes. This allows for similar antiviral activity at a lower dose, meaning less systemic exposure and thus decreased renal and bone toxicity.[77] Emerging literature on the use of TAF during pregnancy is promising; TAF is equally as effective as TDF in blocking MTCT of HBV while also being superior with regard to renal safety and breastfeeding.[100–104] **Table 5** provides a summary of studies of TAF use during pregnancy in HBV-infected mothers. More safety data for pregnancy are needed, and HBsAg-positive patients on TAF should switch to TDF when they become pregnant.[94]

If not already on TDF during pregnancy, TDF antiviral prophylaxis should begin at 28 to 30 weeks gestation to allow sufficient time for viral load to decline to less than 200 000 IU/mL.[94] If antiviral therapy is initiated during third trimester to decrease the risk of MTCT, The American Association for the Study of Liver Diseases recommends cessation of antiviral therapy occurs at the time of delivery or within 4 weeks, given that studies have not shown a reduction in the frequency of hepatitis flares with longer duration regimens.[44,77] If cessation of therapy occurs, there should be close monitoring for HBV flares thereafter.

For patients who become pregnant while already receiving antiviral therapy, the risks and benefits of continuing treatment need to be weighed. Patients who need to continue treatment during pregnancy and are on another antiviral medication should be switched to TDF and monitored closely during the transition period to ensure viral suppression.

Table 5
Summary of studies evaluating the safety of tenofovir alafenamide fumarate during pregnancy in hepatitis B surface antigen-positive mothers

Study	Design	Summary of Findings
Han et al,[102] 2022	Initiation of TAF at 24–28 wk gestation (n = 89)	• TAF therapy prevented MTCT with no safety concerns for mothers and infants
Chen et al,[103] 2021	Group 1 (n = 31): TAF initiated during early pregnancy Group 2 (n = 57): TAF initiated during middle pregnancy	• Initiation of pregnancy in early and middle pregnancy seems to be safe for both mothers and infants • TAF blocks MTCT of HBV and controls maternal infection
Li et al,[100] 2021	Initiation of TAF or TDF at 24–25 wk gestation Group 1 (n = 36): TDF Group 2 (n = 36): TAF	• TAF was superior to TDF with regard to renal safety and breastfeeding • Both TAF and TDF block MTCT of HBV • No significant differences in ALT, total bilirubin, serum creatinine, or BUN levels
Zeng et al,[104] 2021	Initiation of TDF or TAF at 24–35 wk gestation Group 1 (n = 115): TAF Group 2 (n = 116): TDF	• Use of TAF during pregnancy reduced MTCT of HBV and is safe for both mothers and infants • TDF group had safety profiles comparable to TAF group
Ding et al,[101] 2020	Initiation of TAF at 24–30 wk gestation (n = 71)	• TAF for highly viremic mothers prevents MTCT of HBV • No safety concerns for either mothers or infants at 24–28 wk follow-up

Abbreviations: BUN, blood urea nitrogen; HBsAg, hepatitis B surface antigen; HBV, hepatitis B virus; MTCT, maternal-to-child transmission; TAF, tenofovir alafenamide fumarate; TDF, tenofovir disoproxil fumarate.

There are currently no HDV-specific guidelines or treatment options for pregnant patients coinfected with HBV/HDV. The recent approval of bulevirtide for treatment of HDV infection in Europe and ongoing trials on its safety and efficacy in adults gives hope for possible future HDV-specific interventions in pregnancy. Given that vertical transmission of HDV is rare and more likely to occur if HBV levels are high,[105] antiviral therapy for HBV, as well as infant immunoprophylaxis, should minimize the risk of MTCT of HDV.

Recommendations for Interventions in Infants to Prevent Maternal-to-Child Transmission

All infants of HBsAg-positive mothers should receive both active and passive immunization at two different sites within the first 12 hours of life.[106,107] Current recommendations include 100 IU of HBIG and a birth dose of HBV vaccine (administered regardless of infant birth weight). This combination effectively reduces the rate of vertical transmission from 90% to 10% in infants whose mothers HBV DNA levels less than 200 000 IU/mL. However, there are emerging data that suggest that HBIG may not be necessary for prevention of MTCT if tenofovir antiviral therapy is initiated at least 4 weeks before birth.[108] Conversely, there is contrasting evidence demonstrating that if active and passive immunization are provided within less than 2 hours of life (rather than 12 hours), antiviral therapy may not be necessary.[109] Regardless, in conjunction with interventions at birth, close follow-up with a pediatrician and completion of the HBV vaccine series are vital. In the United States, all HBsAg-positive pregnant individuals should be referred to their jurisdiction's perinatal hepatitis B prevention program for case management to ensure that their infants receive timely prophylaxis and follow-up.[77] Given the rarity of vertical transmission of HDV and that routine immunization for HBV also protects against HDV, there are no special considerations for infants of HBsAg-positive mothers coinfected with HDV.

Infants who receive active and passive immunization at birth can be breastfed.[87,110,111] Breastfeeding does not seem to increase the risk of HBV transmission.[87] For patients on antiviral therapy while breastfeeding, studies support the safety of breastfeeding. For instance, only levels of TDF have been detected in the breast milk of women receiving TDF, and given the low levels, it is unlikely that there is any biological effect on the infant.[112–115] Even in HBV/HDV coinfected mothers,[116] decision to breastfeed should ultimately be based on the patient preference and discussion of benefits of breastfeeding, availability of alternatives, and need to continue antiviral treatment after delivery.[116] Mothers should prevent bleeding from cracked nipples and should not participate in donating breast milk.

SUMMARY

Despite significant public health efforts to combat HBV, it remains an important contributor to the global burden of disease and has required special attention to certain subpopulations, such as women of childbearing age. Pregnant individuals living with CHB are at increased risk for hepatitis flares and adverse pregnancy outcomes. Reducing maternal-to-child transmission of HBV is also a major priority, particularly given that almost half the cases of CHB worldwide occur due to perinatal transmission. Management of hepatitis B infection in pregnancy is complex, requiring clinicians to balance the well-being of both the mother and the infant. However, with a careful individualized treatment plan that considers the use of antiviral therapy perinatally and ensures passive–active immunization, successful pregnancy with healthy offspring can be achieved. In contrast to the robust data on the prevalence of HBV, its impact on pregnancy outcomes, and guidelines for its management during pregnancy, there remains a paucity of literature on HDV in pregnancy. To better inform guidelines, future studies should investigate pregnancy course in those infected with HDV, its possible association with adverse pregnancy outcomes in comparison to HBV, and safety of HDV-specific antiviral treatment during pregnancy.

DISCLOSURE

Tatyana Kushner—advisory for Gilead, Abbvie, Advisory for Eiger and Bausch; research support from Gilead. Theresa Worthington, Marcia Lange, Lital Aliasi-Sinai—do not have any disclosures to report.

CLINICS CARE POINTS

- All pregnant patients should be screened at initial prenatal visit for HBsAg.
- All non-immune pregnant patients should be vaccinated against HBV.

- In pregnant patients that are newly HBsAg positive, obtain and test for: HBV DNA, anti-HBs, anti-HBc, anti-HBe, HCV, HIV and HDV antibody, and a liver panel.
- Pregnant patients with HBV DNA > 200,000 IU/L, elevated liver tests, positive HBeAg or co-infection with HCV or HDV should be referred to a hepatologist.
- Liver function should be monitored every 3 months during pregnancy and up to 6 months post partum; elevations should prompt follow up with HBV DNA levels.
- Pregnant patients with HBV DNA > 200,000 IU/ml or positive HBeAg should be started on antiviral therapy with TDF, which should be discontinued at time of delivery or within 4 weeks postpartum.
- Within 12 hours of birth, active immunization (HBV vaccine) and passive immunization (HBIG) should be initiated.
- Newborns who received immunoprophylaxis are safe to breastfeed.

REFERENCES

1. Global progress report on HIV, viral hepatitis and sexually transmitted infections, 2021. Accountability for the global health sector strategies 2016–2021: actions for impact, 2021, Geneva: World Health Organization.
2. Polaris Observatory Member Access. Available at: https://cdafound.org/premium-dashboard/. Accessed April 10, 2023.
3. Global Hepatitis Report 2017. Geneva: World Health Organization; 2017. Licence: CC BY-NC-SA 3.0 IGO
4. Nelson NP, Easterbrook PJ, McMahon BJ. Epidemiology of hepatitis B virus infection and impact of vaccination on disease. Clin Liver Dis 2016;20(4): 607–28.
5. Harris AM, Iqbal K, Schillie S, et al. Increases in acute hepatitis B virus infections — Kentucky, Tennessee, and West Virginia, 2006–2013. MMWR Morbidity and Mortality Weekly Report 2016;65(3):47–50.
6. Kushner T, Chen Z, Tressler S, et al. Trends in Hepatitis B infection and immunity among women of childbearing age in the United States. Clin Infect Dis 2020; 71(3):586–92.
7. Fattovich G, Giustina G, Christensen E, et al. Influence of hepatitis delta virus infection on morbidity and mortality in compensated cirrhosis type B. The European Concerted Action on Viral Hepatitis (Eurohep). Gut 2000;46(3):420–6.
8. Saracco G, Rosina F, Brunetto MR, et al. Rapidly progressive HBsAg-positive hepatitis in Italy. The role of hepatitis delta virus infection. J Hepatol 1987; 5(3):274–81.
9. Fattovich G, Boscaro S, Noventa F, et al. Influence of hepatitis delta virus infection on progression to cirrhosis in chronic hepatitis type B. JID (J Infect Dis) 1987;155(5):931–5.
10. Hepatitis D diagnostics:Utilization and testing in the United States. Virus Res 2018;250:114–7.
11. Beasley RP, Trepo C, Stevens CE, et al. The e antigen and vertical transmission of hepatitis B surface antigen. Am J Epidemiol 1977;105(2):94–8.
12. WHO., World Health Organization. Guidelines for the Prevention Care and Treatment of Persons with Chronic Hepatitis B Virus Infection: Mar-15.; 2015.
13. Organization WH, *others. Global health sector Strategy on viral hepatitis 2016-2021. Towards ending viral hepatitis*, 2016, Geneva, World Health Organization,

Available at: https://apps.who.int/iris/bitstream/handle/10665/246177/who?sequence=1. Accessed February 1, 2023.

14. Zanetti AR, Ferroni P, Magliano EM, et al. Perinatal transmission of the hepatitis B virus and of the HBV-associated delta agent from mothers to offspring in northern Italy. J Med Virol 1982;9(2):139–48.

15. Prevention of mother-to-child transmission of hepatitis B Virus (HBV): guidelines on antiviral prophylaxis in pregnancy, Geneva: World Health Organization, 2020.

16. Office of Infectious Disease, HIV/AIDS Policy (OIDP). Hepatitis B Basic Information. HHS.gov. Published April 20, 2016. Available at: https://www.hhs.gov/hepatitis/learn-about-viral-hepatitis/hepatitis-b-basics/index.html. Accessed April 3, 2023.

17. Gambarin-Gelwan M. Hepatitis B in pregnancy. Clin Liver Dis 2007;11(4):945–63.

18. Stockdale AJ, Kreuels B, Henrion MYR, et al. The global prevalence of hepatitis D virus infection: systematic review and meta-analysis. J Hepatol 2020;73(3):523–32.

19. Gish R. Delta virus infection: epidemiology and initiatives to intercept it. Gastroenterol Hepatol 2013;9(9):589.

20. Mansour W, Malick FZF, Sidiya A, et al. Prevalence, risk factors, and molecular epidemiology of hepatitis B and hepatitis delta virus in pregnant women and in patients in Mauritania. J Med Virol 2012;84(8):1186–98.

21. Makuwa M, Caron M, Souquière S, et al. Prevalence and genetic diversity of hepatitis B and delta viruses in pregnant women in Gabon: molecular evidence that hepatitis delta virus clade 8 originates from and is endemic in central Africa. J Clin Microbiol 2008;46(2):754–6.

22. Komas NP, Ghosh S, Abdou-Chekaraou M, et al. Hepatitis B and hepatitis D virus infections in the Central African Republic, twenty-five years after a fulminant hepatitis outbreak, indicate continuing spread in asymptomatic young adults. PLoS Neglected Trop Dis 2018;12(4):e0006377.

23. Aftab M, Naz S, Aftab B, et al. Characterization of hepatitis delta virus among pregnant women of Pakistan. Viral Immunol 2019;32(8):335–40.

24. Lange M, Zaret D, Kushner T. Hepatitis delta: current knowledge and future directions. Gastroenterol Hepatol 2022;18(9):508–20.

25. Patel EU, Thio CL, Boon D, et al. Prevalence of hepatitis B and hepatitis D virus infections in the United States, 2011-2016. Clin Infect Dis 2019;69(4):709–12.

26. Gish RG, Yi DH, Kane S, et al. Coinfection with hepatitis B and D : epidemiology, prevalence and disease in patients in Northern California. J Gastroenterol Hepatol 2013;28(9):1521–5.

27. Nath N, Mushahwar IK, Fang CT, et al. Antibodies to delta antigen in asymptomatic hepatitis B surface antigen-reactive blood donors in the United States and their association with other markers of hepatitis B virus. Am J Epidemiol 1985;122(2):218–25.

28. Kushner T, Serper M, Kaplan DE. Delta hepatitis within the veterans affairs medical system in the United States: prevalence, risk factors, and outcomes. J Hepatol 2015;63(3):586–92.

29. Alter MJ. Epidemiology and prevention of hepatitis B. Semin Liver Dis 2003;23(1):039–46.

30. Harpaz R, Von Seidlein L, Averhoff FM, et al. Transmission of hepatitis B virus to multiple patients from a surgeon without evidence of inadequate infection control. N Engl J Med 1996;334(9):549–54.

31. Lee WM. Hepatitis B virus infection. N Engl J Med 1997;337(24):1733–45.

32. Miao Z, Zhang S, Ou X, et al. Estimating the global prevalence, disease progression, and clinical outcome of hepatitis delta virus infection. J Infect Dis 2020;221(10):1677–87.

33. Chen HY, Shen DT, Ji DZ, et al. Prevalence and burden of hepatitis D virus infection in the global population: a systematic review and meta-analysis. Gut 2019; 68(3):512–21.

34. Pascarella S, Negro F. Hepatitis D virus: an update. Liver Int 2011;31(1):7–21.

35. Wasuwanich P, Striley CW, Kamili S, et al. Hepatitis D-associated hospitalizations in the United States: 2010–2018. J Viral Hepat 2022;29(3):218–26.

36. Cross TJS, Rizzi P, Horner M, et al. The increasing prevalence of hepatitis delta virus (HDV) infection in South London. J Med Virol 2008;80(2):277–82.

37. Niro GA, Casey JL, Gravinese E, et al. Intrafamilial transmission of hepatitis delta virus: molecular evidence. J Hepatol 1999;30(4):564–9.

38. Sellier PO, Maylin S, Brichler S, et al. Hepatitis B virus-hepatitis D virus mother-to-child co-transmission: a retrospective study in a developed country. Liver Int 2018;38(4):611–8.

39. Kushner T, Shaw PA, Kalra A, et al. Incidence, determinants and outcomes of pregnancy-associated hepatitis B flares: a regional hospital-based cohort study. Liver Int 2018;38(5):813–20.

40. Chang CY, Aziz N, Poongkunran M, et al. Serum alanine aminotransferase and hepatitis B DNA flares in pregnant and postpartum women with chronic hepatitis B. Am J Gastroenterol 2016;111(10):1410–5.

41. ter Borg MJ, Leemans WF, de Man RA, et al. Exacerbation of chronic hepatitis B infection after delivery. J Viral Hepat 2008;15(1):37–41.

42. Giles M, Visvanathan K, Lewin S, et al. Clinical and virological predictors of hepatic flares in pregnant women with chronic hepatitis B. Gut 2015;64(11): 1810–5.

43. Liu J, Wang J, Qi C, et al. Baseline hepatitis B virus titer predicts initial postpartum hepatic flare. J Clin Gastroenterol 2018;52(10):902–7.

44. Nguyen V, Tan PK, Greenup AJ, et al. Anti-viral therapy for prevention of perinatal HBV transmission: extending therapy beyond birth does not protect against post-partum flare. Aliment Pharmacol Ther 2014;39(10):1225–34.

45. Lu J, Wang X, Zhu Y, et al. Clinical and immunological factors associated with postpartum hepatic flares in immune-tolerant pregnant women with hepatitis B virus infection treated with telbivudine. Gut Liver 2021;15(6):887–94.

46. Bzowej NH, Tran TT, Li R, et al. Total alanine aminotransferase (ALT) flares in pregnant north american women with chronic hepatitis B infection: results from a prospective observational study. Am J Gastroenterol 2019;114(8): 1283–91.

47. Chen B, Wang Y, Lange M, et al. Hepatitis C is associated with more adverse pregnancy outcomes than hepatitis B: a 7-year national inpatient sample study. Hepatol Commun 2022;6(9):2465–73.

48. Zhang Y, Chen J, Liao T, et al. Correction to: maternal HBsAg carriers and pregnancy outcomes: a retrospective cohort analysis of 85,190 pregnancies. BMC Pregnancy Childbirth 2021;21(1):131.

49. Tse KY, Ho LF, Lao T. The impact of maternal HBsAg carrier status on pregnancy outcomes: a case-control study. J Hepatol 2005;43(5):771–5.

50. Sirilert S, Traisrisilp K, Sirivatanapa P, et al. Pregnancy outcomes among chronic carriers of hepatitis B virus. Int J Gynecol Obstet 2014;126(2):106–10.

51. Zhang Y, Chen J, Liao T, et al. Maternal HBsAg carriers and pregnancy outcomes: a retrospective cohort analysis of 85,190 pregnancies. BMC Pregnancy Childbirth 2020;20(1). https://doi.org/10.1186/s12884-020-03257-4.
52. Jiang R, Wang T, Yao Y, et al. Hepatitis B infection and intrahepatic cholestasis of pregnancy: a systematic review and meta-analysis. Medicine 2020;99(31): e21416.
53. Cui AM, Cheng XY, Shao JG, et al. Maternal hepatitis B virus carrier status and pregnancy outcomes: a prospective cohort study. BMC Pregnancy Childbirth 2016;16(1). https://doi.org/10.1186/s12884-016-0884-1.
54. Huang QT, Chen JH, Zhong M, et al. The risk of placental abruption and placenta previa in pregnant women with chronic hepatitis B viral infection: a systematic review and meta-analysis. Placenta 2014;35(8):539–45.
55. Huang QT, Wei SS, Zhong M, et al. Chronic hepatitis B infection and risk of preterm labor: a meta-analysis of observational studies. J Clin Virol 2014;61(1):3–8.
56. Kong D, Liu H, Wei S, et al. A meta-analysis of the association between gestational diabetes mellitus and chronic hepatitis B infection during pregnancy. BMC Res Notes 2014;7(1). https://doi.org/10.1186/1756-0500-7-139.
57. Cantalloube A, Ferraretto X, Lepage J, et al. [Outcomes of cumulative transfers of fresh and frozen embryos in in vitro fertilization in women infected by hepatitis B virus]. Gynecol Obstet Fertil Senol 2021;49(6):529–37.
58. Mak JSM, Lao TT. Assisted reproduction in hepatitis carrier couples. Best Pract Res Clin Obstet Gynaecol 2020;68:103–8.
59. Farsimadan M, Riahi SM, Muhammad HM, et al. The effects of hepatitis B virus infection on natural and IVF pregnancy: a meta-analysis study. J Viral Hepat 2021;28(9):1234–45.
60. Mak JSM, Leung MBW, Chung CHS, et al. Presence of Hepatitis B virus DNA in follicular fluid in female Hepatitis B carriers and outcome of IVF/ICSI treatment: a prospective observational study. Eur J Obstet Gynecol Reprod Biol 2019; 239:11–5.
61. Huang QT, Chen JH, Zhong M, et al. Chronic hepatitis B infection is associated with decreased risk of preeclampsia: a meta-analysis of observational studies. Cell Physiol Biochem 2016;38(5):1860–8.
62. Liu JF, Chen TY, Zhao YR. Vertical transmission of hepatitis B virus: propositions and future directions. Chin Med J 2021;134(23):2825–31.
63. Veronese P, Dodi I, Esposito S, et al. Prevention of vertical transmission of hepatitis B virus infection. World J Gastroenterol 2021;27(26):4182–93.
64. Liaw YF. Clinical utility of hepatitis B surface antigen quantitation in patients with chronic hepatitis B: a review. Hepatology 2011;54(2):E1–9.
65. Petrova M, Kamburov V. Breastfeeding and chronic HBV infection: clinical and social implications. World J Gastroenterol 2010;16(40):5042–6.
66. Yang J, Zeng XM, Men YL, et al. Elective caesarean section versus vaginal delivery for preventing mother to child transmission of hepatitis B virus–a systematic review. Virol J 2008;5:100.
67. Levy MT, Terrault NA. Caesarean section or non-breastfeeding for prevention of MTCT-beware of sending the wrong message. J Viral Hepat 2021;28(3):575–6.
68. Society for Maternal-Fetal Medicine (SMFM), Dionne-Odom J, Tita ATN, et al. #38: hepatitis B in pregnancy screening, treatment, and prevention of vertical transmission. Am J Obstet Gynecol 2016;214(1):6–14.
69. Cheung KW, Seto MTY, So PL, et al. The effect of rupture of membranes and labour on the risk of hepatitis B vertical transmission: prospective multicentre observational study. Eur J Obstet Gynecol Reprod Biol 2019;232:97–100.

70. Guo Z, Shi XH, Feng YL, et al. Risk factors of HBV intrauterine transmission among HBsAg-positive pregnant women. J Viral Hepat 2013;20(5):317–21.

71. Lisker-Melman M, Khalili M, Belle SH, et al. Maternal knowledge of the risk of vertical transmission and offspring acquisition of hepatitis B. Ann Hepatol 2020;19(4):388–95.

72. Katamba PS, Mukunya D, Kwesiga D, et al. Prenatal hepatitis B screening and associated factors in a high prevalence district of Lira, northern Uganda: a community based cross sectional study. BMC Public Health 2019;19(1):1004.

73. Adjei CA, Stutterheim SE, Bram F, et al. Correlates of hepatitis B testing in Ghana: the role of knowledge, stigma endorsement and knowing someone with hepatitis B. Health Soc Care Community 2022;30(6):e4564–73.

74. Willis BC, Wortley P, Wang SA, et al. Gaps in hospital policies and practices to prevent perinatal transmission of hepatitis B virus. Pediatrics 2010;125(4):704–11.

75. HBV. Published September 6, 2022. Available at: https://www.cdc.gov/nchhstp/pregnancy/effects/hbv.html. Accessed February 6, 2023.

76. Terrault NA, Levy MT, Cheung KW, et al. Viral hepatitis and pregnancy. Nat Rev Gastroenterol Hepatol 2021;18(2):117–30.

77. Terrault NA, Lok ASF, McMahon BJ, et al. Update on prevention, diagnosis, and treatment of chronic hepatitis B: AASLD 2018 hepatitis B guidance. Hepatology 2018;67(4):1560–99.

78. Ramia S, Bahakim H. Perinatal transmission of hepatitis B virus-associated hepatitis D virus. Ann Inst Pasteur Virol 1988;139(3):285–90.

79. Negro F. Hepatitis D virus coinfection and superinfection. Cold Spring Harb Perspect Med 2014;4(11):a021550.

80. Schillie S, Vellozzi C, Reingold A, et al. Prevention of Hepatitis B Virus Infection in the United States: recommendations of the advisory committee on immunization practices. MMWR Recomm Rep (Morb Mortal Wkly Rep) 2018;67(1):1–31.

81. Sookoian S. Liver disease during pregnancy: acute viral hepatitis. Ann Hepatol 2006;5(3):231–6.

82. Hieber JP, Dalton D, Shorey J, et al. Hepatitis and pregnancy. J Pediatr 1977;91(4):545–9.

83. Jonas MM. Hepatitis B and pregnancy: an underestimated issue. Liver Int 2009;29(Suppl 1):133–9.

84. Terrault NA, Bzowej NH, Chang KM, et al. AASLD guidelines for treatment of chronic hepatitis B. Hepatology 2016;63(1):261–83.

85. Pan CQ, Duan Z, Dai E, et al. Tenofovir to prevent hepatitis B transmission in mothers with high viral load. N Engl J Med 2016;374(24):2324–34.

86. Pan CQ, Han GR, Jiang HX, et al. Telbivudine prevents vertical transmission from HBeAg-positive women with chronic hepatitis B. Clin Gastroenterol Hepatol 2012;10(5):520–6.

87. Dionne-Odom J, Tita AT, Silverman NS. Hepatitis B in pregnancy screening, treatment, and prevention of vertical transmission. Obstet Anesth Digest 2016;36(4):184.

88. Brown RS Jr, McMahon BJ, Lok ASF, et al. Antiviral therapy in chronic hepatitis B viral infection during pregnancy: a systematic review and meta-analysis. Hepatology 2016;63(1):319–33.

89. Zou H, Chen Y, Duan Z, et al. Virologic factors associated with failure to passive-active immunoprophylaxis in infants born to HBsAg-positive mothers. J Viral Hepat 2012;19(2):e18–25.

90. Liu Y, Wang M, Yao S, et al. Efficacy and safety of telbivudine in different trimesters of pregnancy with high viremia for interrupting perinatal transmission of hepatitis B virus. Hepatol Res 2016;46(3):E181–8.

91. Boucheron P, Lu Y, Yoshida K, et al. Accuracy of HBeAg to identify pregnant women at risk of transmitting hepatitis B virus to their neonates: a systematic review and meta-analysis. Lancet Infect Dis 2021;21(1):85–96.

92. Pan CQ, Duan ZP, Bhamidimarri KR, et al. An algorithm for risk assessment and intervention of mother to child transmission of hepatitis B virus. Clin Gastroenterol Hepatol 2012;10(5):452–9.

93. Funk AL, Lu Y, Yoshida K, et al. Efficacy and safety of antiviral prophylaxis during pregnancy to prevent mother-to-child transmission of hepatitis B virus: a systematic review and meta-analysis. Lancet Infect Dis 2021;21(1):70–84.

94. Kushner T, Sarkar M. Chronic hepatitis B in pregnancy. Clin Liver Dis 2018; 12(1):24–8.

95. Siberry GK, Jacobson DL, Kalkwarf HJ, et al. Lower newborn bone mineral content associated with maternal use of tenofovir disoproxil fumarate during pregnancy. Clin Infect Dis 2015;61(6):996–1003.

96. Jacobson DL, Patel K, Williams PL, et al. Growth at 2 years of age in HIV-exposed uninfected children in the United States by trimester of maternal antiretroviral initiation. Pediatr Infect Dis J 2017;36(2):189–97.

97. Chen HL, Lee CN, Chang CH, et al. Efficacy of maternal tenofovir disoproxil fumarate in interrupting mother-to-infant transmission of hepatitis B virus. Hepatology 2015;62(2):375–86.

98. Jia F, Deng F, Tong S, et al. Efficacy of oral antiviral drugs to prevent mother-to-child transmission of hepatitis B virus: a network meta-analysis. Hepatol Int 2020;14(3):338–46.

99. Lee YS, Lee HS, Kim JH, et al. Role of tenofovir disoproxil fumarate in prevention of perinatal transmission of hepatitis B virus from mother to child: a systematic review and meta-analysis. Korean J Intern Med 2021;36(1):76–85.

100. Li B, Liu Z, Liu X, et al. Efficacy and safety of tenofovir disoproxil fumarate and tenofovir alafenamide fumarate in preventing HBV vertical transmission of high maternal viral load. Hepatol Int 2021;15(5):1103–8.

101. Ding Y, Cao L, Zhu L, et al. Efficacy and safety of tenofovir alafenamide fumarate for preventing mother-to-child transmission of hepatitis B virus: a national cohort study. Aliment Pharmacol Ther 2020;52(8):1377–86.

102. Han G, Zhou G, Sun T, et al. Tenofovir alafenamide in blocking mother-to-child transmission of hepatitis B virus: a multi-center, prospective study. J Matern Fetal Neonatal Med 2022;35(26):10551–8.

103. Chen R, Zou J, Long L, et al. Safety and efficacy of tenofovir alafenamide fumarate in early-middle pregnancy for mothers with chronic hepatitis B. Front Med 2021;8:796901.

104. Zeng QL, Yu ZJ, Ji F, et al. Tenofovir alafenamide to prevent perinatal hepatitis B transmission: a multicenter, prospective, observational study. Clin Infect Dis 2021;73(9):e3324–32.

105. Seto MTY, Cheung KW, Hung IFN. Management of viral hepatitis A, C, D and E in pregnancy. Best Pract Res Clin Obstet Gynaecol 2020;68:44–53.

106. Weinbaum CM, Williams I, Mast EE, et al. Recommendations for identification and public health management of persons with chronic hepatitis B virus infection. MMWR Recomm Rep (Morb Mortal Wkly Rep) 2008;57(RR-8):1–20.

107. Mast EE, Weinbaum CM, Fiore AE, et al. A comprehensive immunization strategy to eliminate transmission of hepatitis B virus infection in the United States:

recommendations of the Advisory Committee on Immunization Practices (ACIP) Part II: immunization of adults. MMWR Recomm Rep (Morb Mortal Wkly Rep) 2006;55(RR-16):1–33 [quiz CE1-CE4].

108. Segeral O, Dim B, Durier C, et al. Immunoglobulin-free strategy to prevent HBV mother-to-child transmission in Cambodia (TA-PROHM): a single-arm, multi-centre, phase 4 trial. Lancet Infect Dis 2022;22(8):1181–90.

109. Jourdain G, Ngo-Giang-Huong N, Harrison L, et al. Tenofovir versus placebo to prevent perinatal transmission of hepatitis B. N Engl J Med 2018;378(10):911–23.

110. Kimberlin D, Faap MAJ, Jackson MA, American Academy of Pediatrics Committee, American Academy of Pediatrics Committee on Infectious Diseases. Red book 2015: 2015 report of the committee on infectious diseases. Elk Grove Village, IL, American Academy of Pediatrics; 2015.

111. Benaboud S, Pruvost A, Coffie PA, et al. Concentrations of tenofovir and emtricitabine in breast milk of HIV-1-infected women in Abidjan, Cote d'Ivoire, in the ANRS 12109 TEmAA Study, Step 2. Antimicrobial Agents Chemother 2011; 55(3):1315–7.

112. Cundy KC, Sueoka C, Lynch GR, et al. Pharmacokinetics and bioavailability of the anti-human immunodeficiency virus nucleotide analog 9-[(R)-2-(phosphono-methoxy)propyl]adenine (PMPA) in dogs. Antimicrobial Agents Chemother 1998;42(3):687–90.

113. Waitt C, Olagunju A, Nakalema S, et al. Plasma and breast milk pharmacokinetics of emtricitabine, tenofovir and lamivudine using dried blood and breast milk spots in nursing African mother-infant pairs. J Antimicrob Chemother 2018;73(4):1013–9.

114. Van Rompay KKA, Hamilton M, Kearney B, et al. Pharmacokinetics of tenofovir in breast milk of lactating rhesus macaques. Antimicrobial Agents Chemother 2005;49(5):2093–4.

115. Ehrhardt S, Xie C, Guo N, et al. Breastfeeding while taking lamivudine or tenofovir disoproxil fumarate: a review of the evidence. Clin Infect Dis 2015;60(2):275–8.

116. Sanghi V, Lindenmeyer CC. Viral hepatitis in pregnancy: an update on screening, diagnosis, and management. Clin Liver Dis 2021;18(1):7–13.

State of the Art
Test all for Anti-Hepatitis D Virus and Reflex to Hepatitis D Virus RNA Polymerase Chain Reaction Quantification

Emuejevuoke Umukoro, DO[a], Joseph J. Alukal, MD[b],
Kevin Pak, MD[c], Julio Gutierrez, MD[d],*

KEYWORDS

- Hepatitis D virus • Acute and chronic HDV infection • RT-qPCR • HDV genotype
- Pegylated interferon-alfa • Droplet digital PCR

KEY POINTS

- HDV is diagnosed by clinical assays for Hepatitis D antigen, anti-hepatitis D antibody, and hepatitis D RNA.
- RT-PCR is the gold standard of diagnosis for assessing HDV RNA but is limited by the genetic variability of the virus.
- Pegylated interferon alfa-2 is the main medication used for HDV treatment and the endpoint is a decrease in HDV RNA levels in the United States.
- In the future, droplet digital PCR (ddPCR) could provide more accurate quantification of HDV viral load and rapid test for HDV detection could improve HDV testing in resource-limited areas.

INTRODUCTION/HISTORY/DEFINITION/BACKGROUND
General Background of Hepatitis D Virus

The most severe form of viral hepatitis is caused by hepatitis D virus (HDV), with an estimated 12 million people infected globally.[1] HDV infection is endemic among those with hepatitis B and is transmitted predominantly via parenteral exposure.[2] HDV is one of the smallest viruses that can cause human disease. It is an RNA virus dependent on HBV for transmission, using HBsAg as a viral envelope and sharing the same

Funding: None.
[a] Scripps Mercy Hospital, 435 H Street, Chula Vista, CA 91910, USA; [b] University of California, School of Medicine, 3390 University Avenue, Riverside, CA 92501, USA; [c] Naval Medical Center, 34800 Bob Wilson Drive, San Diego, CA 92134, USA; [d] Center for Organ Transplant, Scripps Clinic, Scripps MD Anderson Center, Scripps Green Hospital, 10666 N. Torrey Pines Road (N-200), La Jolla, CA 92037, USA
* Corresponding author.
E-mail address: gutierrez.julio@scrippshealth.org

Clin Liver Dis 27 (2023) 937–954
https://doi.org/10.1016/j.cld.2023.05.008
1089-3261/23/© 2023 Elsevier Inc. All rights reserved.

hepatocyte cell entry receptor – sodium taurocholate cotransporter polypeptide (NTCP) receptor.[3,4] HDV is about 35 to 36 nm in diameter and is made up of the RNA genome, Hepatitis D antigen (HDAg) and the lipoprotein envelope.[5] The genome is a circular single-stranded RNA of 1.7kilobases and the HDAg is expressed in large and small forms. The genome and antigen together make up the ribonucleoprotein (RNP), which is packaged in the viral envelope of HBV.[5]

Transmission of HDV occurs in 2 patterns - coinfection with HBV or superinfection in chronic HBV. Concurrent infection with HBV, which can progress to fulminant hepatitis. However, in most individuals, both viruses are cleared spontaneously. Conversely, acute HDV superinfection in patients with chronic HBV infection leads to chronic HBV/HDV infection, which accelerates liver cirrhosis and increases the risk of HCC compared to chronic HBV infection alone.[3,4]

DISEASE STATES OF HEPATITIS D VIRUS
Diagnosis of Hepatitis D Virus Infection

The current diagnostic strategies for HDV infection consist of hepatitis B and D serology, biomarkers, and assessment of liver fibrosis and cirrhosis. The serum serologies and biomarkers include HBV/HDV antigens and antibodies (IgM and total antibody that include IgM and IgG), as well as HBV DNA quantification and HDV RNA quantificaiton.[4] The serum levels of these markers vary based on whether the infection is acute or chronic. There are new biomarkers and noninvasive tests, which have been integrated into the diagnostic algorithm and management of viral liver disease and have transformed the landscape of viral hepatitis.[1] These will be discussed in detail later in the article.

Individuals with hepatitis D infection can manifest as acutely or chronically infected. Acute HDV infection has been described in two major patterns – coinfection and superinfection, while chronic infection usually develops after an acute superinfection in a patient with chronic HBV. A third minor pattern or helper independent HDV infection has been reported in the setting of liver transplants, but its existence is still being questioned.[6] Acute HDV occurs after an incubation time of 1-2 months, and is marked by nonspecific symptoms such as fatigue, lethargy, anorexia, and nausea, as well as elevated biochemical markers (ALT, AST, and bilirubin).[6]

ACUTE HEPATITIS D VIRUS: COINFECTION PATTERN

Concurrent infection of a susceptible patient with both HBV and HDV causes acute HBV and HDV, which is clinically indistinguishable from an acute HBV mono-infection.[6] The clinical expression of HBV/HDV can vary from mild to severe or even fulminant hepatitis.[7] This variability in expression is due to complex interplay between both viruses. HDV infection is reliant and limited by the virulence of the simultaneous HBV infection. A limited expression of HbsAg may result in unsuccessful HDV infection, whereas a florid expression allows for the full expression of HDV's pathogenicity.[7] Usually, HBV/HDV coinfection is transient and self-limited, with less than 5% progression to chronicity.[6] In the early phase of infection, a transient increase in serum HbsAg and HDAg is expected. There are also elevated levels of HBV DNA and HDV RNA indicating active disease. As antibodies develop to the antigens, increased levels of anti-HDV and anti-HBV IgM will be noted initially, with subsequent increases in anti-HDV and anti-HBc IgG later (**Fig. 1**).

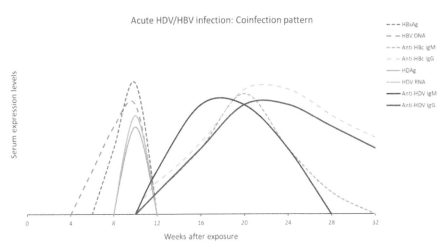

Fig. 1. Serum markers in Acute HDV/HBV coinfection over the duration of infection.

ACUTE HEPATITIS D VIRUS: SUPERINFECTION PATTERN

Superinfection occurs when an individual chronically infected with HBV develops a new infection with HDV. The preexisting HBV infection provides the perfect conditions for HDV, which uses the preexisting HBsAg to cause immediate infection.[7] Clinically, it may manifest as an exacerbation of the chronic HBV infection, causing liver decompensation, or as a new hepatitis in an asymptomatic HBsAg carrier.[7] Serologic studies will likely show elevated levels of HDAg (in the early phase of infection), HDV RNA and anti-HDV IgM (initially). Anti-HDV IgG levels will increase in the later phase of infection (see **Fig. 1**). As for hepatitis B, anti-HBV IgG will likely be the only elevated serum markers because the hepatitis B infection is chronic (**Fig. 2**). HDV superinfection progresses to chronic hepatitis D in greater than 90% of cases. However, a minority of superinfected carriers has a self-limited hepatitis and clear the HBV infection.[8]

CHRONIC HEPATITIS D INFECTION

Chronic hepatitis D infection is a frequent sequela of the superinfection pattern of acute HDV infection.[7] Dual infection induces a severe and rapidly progressive form

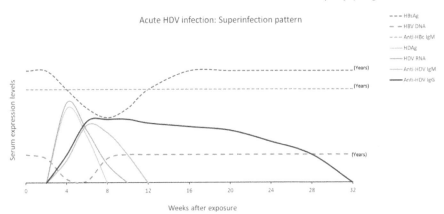

Fig. 2. Serum markers in acute HDV superinfection over the duration of infection.

of chronic viral hepatitis, which results in cirrhosis in more than 50% of cases. Usually, it exacerbates the preexisting liver disease associated with HBV infection.[6,7] Serology will likely show anti-HDV IgM and total (including IgM and IgG) antibodies. Since there is no active infection, anti-HBV IgM will likely be low or undetected. In most patients infected with chronic hepatitis D, ALT and AST levels are usually elevated. Splenomegaly is also common amongst those with chronic infection, a notable clinical feature of the disease.[7] **Table 1** shows the serologic markers in acute and chronic HDV infection.

FEATURES OF HEPATITIS D ANTIGEN

The HDV virion consists of a ribonucleoprotein (RNP) complex inside and a coat protein (envelope) derived from pre-S and S antigens of the hepatitis B virus (HBV) on the outside.[4,9] The RNP complex in turn is made up of the of HDV genome (1672–1697 nucleotides) and the delta antigen (HDAg) which exists in two isoforms: the small delta antigen (S-HDAg, 195 amino acids, 24 kDa) and the large delta antigen (L-HDAg, 214 amino acids, 27 kDa). HDAg is the only protein that is encoded by the HDV genome. The N-terminal sequence of the two isoforms are the same and they differ by only 19 amino acids at the C-terminus of the L-HDAg. While S-HDAg plays a key role in initiating and maintaining viral replication, L-HDAg is a negative regulator of viral replication and is involved in virion morphogenesis by triggering the envelopment of the virus into the HBV surface proteins.[4,9,10] The envelope contains three HBV coat proteins: small-HBsAg (S-HBsAg), medium-HBsAg (M-HBsAg) and large-HBsAg (L-HBsAg) that is necessary for completing the viral life cycle and producing infectious HDV virions. Although M-HBsAg and L-HBsAg have a similar sequence to that of S-HBsAg, they contain additional N-terminal extensions: preS2 for M-HBsAg and preS1 plus preS2 for L-HBsAg. While S-HBsAg proteins are required for HDV assembly and release of HDV particles, the preS1 domain of L-HBsAg is critical for binding to the hepatocyte receptor-sodium taurocholate co-transporting polypeptide (NTCP) and in the absence of HBsAg-L preS1 domain, HDV remain non-infectious.[11,12]

The HDV genome is a single-stranded (ss) negative-sense circular RNA that contains about 200 molecules of HDAg per genome and has a peculiar structure similar to a DNA double helix, whereby the genome owing to a high degree of self-complementarity (74% intramolecular base-pairing) can fold into an unbranched,

Table 1
Serologic patterns in HDV infection

	Acute HDV/HBV Infection	Acute HDV Superinfection in Chronic HBV	Chronic HDV/ HBV Infection	Resolved HDV/HBV Infection
HDV Ag	+ (transient)	+ (transient)	−/+	-
Anti-HDV IgM	+	+	+	-
HDV RNA	+	+	+	-
Anti-HDV Total	+ (- in early phase)	+	+	+
HBsAg	+	+	+	-
Anti-HBc IgM	+	-	-	-
HBV DNA	+	+	+	-
Anti-HBc Total	+ (- in early phase)	+	+	+

rod-like structure.[9-13] Although the genome has many open reading frames (ORF), only one ORF located between position 962 and 1606 on the anti-genomic strand encodes for HDAg.[14] Owing to its defective nature, HDV lacks the protein-coding capacity and therefore hijacks the host DNA-dependent RNA polymerases (DdRp) to facilitate RNA-directed RNA synthesis.[4,9,15] HDV enters the hepatocyte by interaction between L-HBsAg and the NTCP receptor and loses the envelope protein. The RNP complex is then mediated toward the nucleus of the infected hepatocyte by HDAg through a nuclear localization signal, after which replication is initiated by a double rolling circle mechanism using DdRp (RNA polymerases I and II).[16] During this process, the negative sense genomic RNA is used to generate its complement, the positive sense anti-genomic RNA which subsequently serves as a replication intermediate for the synthesis of de novo genomic RNA. These newly synthesized molecules undergo self-cleaving by intrinsic ribozymes into monomers which are then ligated to form circular RNA.[16,17] The open reading frame of the anti-genomic strand undergoes transcription into mRNA and translates to produce S-HDAg followed by post-transcriptional modification by adenosine deaminase-1, whereby the stop codon UAG at position 196 of the mRNA is replaced by tryptophan codon UGG leading to the encoding of L-HDAg.[4,9,10] Finally, L-HDAg undergoes post-translational prenylation of the cysteine residue at the C-terminus by cellular enzyme farnesyltransferase which helps mediate direct binding between L-HDAg and HBV envelope protein thereby facilitating HDV virion assembly.[18,19]

HEPATITIS D VIRUS TESTING AND DIAGNOSIS

There are two serum tests that are currently being used to screen for delta virus in those who test positive for HBsAg. They include anti-HDV total antibody and HDV RNA. However, a positive total anti-HDV antibody test is unable to distinguish between previous, chronic, and active infections, and therefore the quantitative detection of HDV RNA by reverse transcription polymerase chain reaction (RT-PCR) is used as the gold standard for diagnosis of current infection. Quantifying HDV RNA levels are important not only to measure therapeutic responses, but HDV viremia has been associated with increased risk of complications such as hepatic decompensation, hepatocellular carcinoma (HCC), and liver-related death.[20] Over the past 2 decades numerous commercial and in-house assays have been developed to detect HDV RNA via real-time RT-PCR, but currently there is no standardized HDV-RNA quantification assay. Moreover, due to the high genetic variability of HDV (8 genotypes and numerous sub-genotypes) some assays may underestimate HDV viral load and in some cases even fail to detect RNA despite high viremia (**Fig. 3**).[21]

REVERSE TRANSCRIPTION-POLYMERASE CHAIN REACTION ASSAYS

Real-time (RT) PCR utilizes primers and probes to either target the sequences coding for the conserved regions of the ribozyme domain or the HDAg. One of the first PCR assays to quantify HDV RNA was developed in Japan and this technique targeted a highly conserved sequence within the HDAg-coding region using primer 1164 (5′-CCGGCTACTCTTCTTTCCCTTCTCTCGTC-3′; positions 1164–1192) and primer 1297 (5′-CACCGAAGAAGGAAGGCCCTGGAGAACAA-3′; positions 1297–1268). This assay had a linearity of 1 to 106 copies of RNA/μL and could detect genotypes 1, 2a and 2b.[23] In 2005, another real-time RT-PCR based on TaqMan technology (Applied Biosystems, Courtaboef, France) was developed which was capable of detecting genotypes 1 to 7 with a sensitivity of 100 copies/ml of serum.[23] The assay used a forward primer (Delta -F, 5′-GCATGGTCCCAGCCTCC-3′) to target the

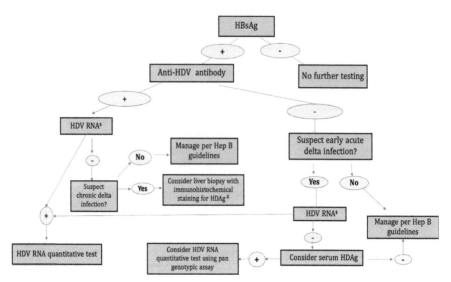

Fig. 3. Testing algorithm for hepatitis D virus. [a] HDV RNA may be false negative if the assay is unable to detect certain genotypes accurately. [$] Chronic delta infection should be suspected if ALT is persistently high, and HBV DNA is low/undetectable in those who test positive for HDV Ab.[22].

ribozyme region of the genome, a reverse primer (Delta-R, 5′-TCTTCGGGT CGGCATGG-3′) to target region I of the antigenome ribozyme, and a probe (Delta-P, 5′-FAM-ATGCCCAGGTCGGAC-MGB-3′) that was designed to anneal to the antigenomic sequence to avoid base pairing with the reverse primer, and this technology was found to be 100% specific.[24]

Mederacke and colleagues developed an assay using the Cobas TaqMan apparatus (Roche Diagnostics, Germany), a PCR platform that has been widely used to detect hepatitis C virus (HCV) RNA and hepatitis B virus (HBV) DNA.[25] This assay used primers to target a conserved region of the genome that encodes for HDAg and had an automated extraction system which not only reduced the risk of contamination, but also had a high degree of reproducibility. The primers and probes were as follows; forward primer 1.

(5′ TGGACGTkCGTCCTCCT-3′, positions 837–853), forward primer 2 (5′-TGGACG TCTGTCCTCCTT-3′, positions 837–854), reverse primer (5′-TCTTCGG GTCGGCATGG (positions 891–907) and the probe at positions 858 to 872. Moreover, the authors found that this test was 100% specific with a wide range of linearity from 3×10^2 to 10^7 copies/ml. In 2010, a novel real-time RT-PCR quantification assay was developed in Spain that combined amplification with fluorescence monitoring that had a specificity of 95% and a linear range from 10^3 to 10^7 HDV-RNA equivalent/ml.[26] The assay used primers DP1 5′ -TGGCTCTCCCTTAGCCATCCGA-3′ (position 887), DP2 5′-TCCTTCTTTCCTCTTCGGGT-3′ (position 993), fluorescent probe, HDV-FL 5′-TCCTCCTTCGGATGCCCAGGTCG-3′ (position 921), and HDV-LC 5′ -LC640-CCGCGAGGAGGTGGAGATGCCATp-3′ (position 947) to target a 107-bp fragment that was located in a highly conserved region of HDV-RNA between the autocatalytic cleavage sites. One of the limitations of this assay was that it was studied only in those with genotype 1. Most laboratories currently utilize the TaqMan probes in their real-time RT-PCR techniques. In 2017, investigators from France developed a pangenotypic commercial assay (Eurobioplex HDV kit) that was tested on 611 clinical samples and was found to have excellent sensitivity, specificity, and reproducibility.[27] While there are no consensus from professional societies (AASLD, EASL) on which assay is best suited for HDV RNA detection, based on its performance metrics, the authors suggest that the Eurobioplex kit should be used for RNA testing. **Table 2** shows a list of available assays for HDV RNA quantification.

RELIABILITY OF REVERSE TRANSCRIPTION-POLYMERASE CHAIN REACTION AND ISSUES WITH GENETIC HETEROGENEITY

HDV exists in 8 distinct genotypes that have a very specific geographic distribution. Genotype 1 has a worldwide distribution and is the predominant strain in North America, whereas genotypes 2 and 4 are found in Asia (Japan, Taiwan), genotype 3 in South America (Amazon Basin), and genotypes 5 to 8 are mainly restricted to west and central Africa. Genotype 1 is further divided into 4 sub-genotypes. Of these, sub-genotypes 1a and 1b are prevalent in sub-Saharan Africa, while sub-genotype 1d has been identified both in Europe and Asia. However, due to migration and immigration, it is possible that many of these strains now have a more global distribution.

The ideal assay should be 100% sensitive, reproducible, and capable of detecting all 8 genotypes. The currently available assays have excellent specificity anywhere between ~ 95 to 100%; however, issues with sensitivity still exist. Unfortunately, due to the due the high level of genetic heterogeneity and mutations, the HDV genome may diverge as much as 37% at the nucleotide sequence level, and such variability makes the development of a universallysensitive assay technically quite challenging.[11] A recent study in France demonstrated that some of the commercially available RT-PCR assays are unable to detect certain genotypes.[21] In that study, the in-house assay, TaqMan RT-PCR that is sensitive against all 8 genotypes was compared with 3 commercial assays: the Lightmix HDV kit (Roche, France) designed to quantify genotype 1, the RoboGene (Aj-Roboscreen, Germany) and the DiaPro HDV RNA assays (DiaPro, Italy) that are theoretically designed to quantify all genotypes. The study analyzed 128 HDV samples consisting of all 8 genotypes, majority of which belonged to genotype1 (33 samples from European or Asian patients and 33 samples from African patients). The authors found that compared to the in-house RT-PCR, many samples were under the limit of quantification (LOQ) for the commercial assays:11.7% for Lightmix Roche, 18.8% for Aj-Roboscreen, and 47.7% for DiaPro. All 3 commercial assays had excellent concordance for genotype 1 from European or Asian patients and the viral load (VL) value differences were 0.3 log10 copies/mL. However, for genotype 1 from Africa, the Roche assay underestimated VL values by 0.5 to 1 log10 copies/mL and failed to detect 1 sample, while DiaPro failed to amplify 4 samples with VLs ranging from 2 to 8 log10 copies/mL and underestimated 4 others by more than 2 log10. Also, the commercial kits greatly underestimated VLs in almost all non-genotype-1 strains by about 2 to 3 log10 and was unable to detect genotypes 7 and 8 in certain samples despite having a high viral concentration.

In 2013, the world health organization (WHO) developed an international standard (IS) for HDV RNA quantification that standardized results into IU/ml which made it possible to compare results and performance metrics of various assays that are currently available.[31] Investigators from France conducted a comprehensive international quality-control study that consisted of 28 laboratories from 17 different countries to analyze nearly all available commercial and in-house assays and found significant discrepancies.[32] Two panels of samples were sent to the various laboratories, where Panel A was made up of 20 clinical samples of different genotypes (1, 2, and 5–8)

Table 2
Currently available RT-PCR assays for HDV RNA quantification

RT-PCR Technique	Country and year	Target Site for Primers and Probes	HDV Genotypes Detected	Linearity	Comments
Light Cycler DNA Master SYBR Green I[22]	Japan, 2004	Target- HDAg coding region Primer:1164 (nt positions 1164–1192) Primer:1297 (nt positions 1297–1268)	1, 2a and 2b	1–10^6 copies of RNA/μL	• Unable to detect genotypes 3–8
TaqMan Universal PCR master mix[23]	France, 2005	Target: Ribozyme region of genome Forward primer: Delta-F Reverse primer: Delta-R Probe: Delta-P	1–7	10^3 to 10^9 copies/ml	• Sensitive to detect 100 HDV RNA copies/ml. • 100% specific
Cobas TaqMan[24]	Germany, 2010	Target: HDAg coding region Forward primer 1 (nt positions 837–853) Forward primer 2 (nt positions 837–854) Reverse primer (nt positions 891–907) Probe (nt positions 858–872)	Does not mention	3×10^2 to 10^7 copies/ml.	• Automated extraction system reduces the risk of contamination. • 100% specific
Light Cycler system[25]	Spain, 2010	Target: HDAg coding region Primer: DP1 at position 887 Primer: DP2 position 993 Probe: HDV-FL at position 921 Probe: HDV-LC at position 947	1	10^3 to 10^7 HDV-RNA equivalent/ml	• 95% specificity

Assay	Country	Details	Genotypes	Linear range	Notes
Robo Gene HDV RNA quantification kit[28] (commercial)	Germany	Target: HDAg coding region	1–8	10–108 copies/reaction	• Used to establish WHO HDV RNA standard. • 100% specificity
Droplet digital PCR[29] (commercial)	USA	Target: Ribozyme region of genome Forward Primer: HDVA1 (nt positions 818–837) Reverse Primer: HDVA2 (nt positions 902–920) Probe: (nt positions 876–894)	1–8	$10–1 \times 10^6$ IU/mL	• Allows absolute quantification of RNA • 100% specific • Linear range slightly lower than traditional RT-PCR.
Cobas 6800[30] (commercial)	Germany	Target: HDAg coding region	1 1–8	10^1 to 10^8 IU/mL	• Highly automated technique that allows the dynamic scaling of test capacity.
Eurobioplex HDV kit[27] (commercial)	France	Target: HDAg coding region	1–8	2.75–8.5 log IU/ml	• Demonstrated excellent specificity (100%), sensitivity (98.5%), and reproducibility

including two negative controls, while Panel B was composed of dilutions of the WHO-HDV-IS that permitted conversion of results from copies/mL into IU/mL for HDVL standardization. The authors found that less than half the laboratories (46%) properly quantified all 18 positive samples, while 57% failed to detect one to up to 10 samples. Several laboratories either failed to detect or dramatically underestimated African genotypes (strain 1 and strains 5–8) as well as the Asian genotype (strain 2). The study concluded that the significant discrepancies were likely due to the high level of genetic variability of the HDV genome that resulted in mismatches between the forward primers/probes and their potential target (ribozyme), as well as due to the complicated secondary structure of the HDV RNA.

GENOTYPING ASSAYS

Identifying the strain of HDV by genotyping assays is important, as it has implications for the prognosis of liver disease. However, these specialized assays are often available only at research laboratories and require direct sequencing and extensive phylogenetic analysis of the HDAg R0 region of the genome.[33] Therefore, routine testing for genotypes in clinical practice is currently not recommended. Nonetheless, it is worth noting that certain genotypes may impact the natural history of the disease more than others. For instance, a study in Taiwan found that patients infected with HDV genotype-1 were at increased risk of developing cirrhosis, HCC, or mortality compared to those with HDV genotype-2, whereas a more recent study showed that African patients with HDV genotype 5 had a higher risk of cirrhosis compared to other genotypes.[33,34] The 10-year cumulative risk of cirrhosis in African patients infected with HDV-5 was 40%, while it was only 26% in other Africans infected with genotypes 1, 6, 7, and 8. It has also been shown that Europeans with HDV-1 are more susceptible to cirrhosis than African patients with HDV-5, and some reports have linked genotype-3 with outbreaks of fulminant hepatitis in South America.[35,36] In another prospective study that looked at therapeutic outcomes, 24 patients with HDV (10 with HDV-1 and 15 with HDV-5) were treated with pegylated interferon-alfa (peg-IFN), and those with HDV-5 demonstrated a significantly higher treatment response compared to HDV-1 (64% vs 10%, $P = .013$).[37] There are no commercial assays for HDV genotyping and this remains a research laboratory based test.

BARRIERS TO TESTING

There is a significant gap in screening individuals who are positive for HBsAg. Reasons for the underutilization of HDV testing are multifactorial and may be from limited access to testing, cost factors, and poor knowledge regarding screening indications in patients with positive HBsAg. Of note, universal screening for HDV in HBsAg individuals is recommended according to the European (EASL) and Asia Pacific (APASL) guidelines.[22,38,39] However, in the US (AASLD), testing for HDV is only recommended in patients with positive HBsAg at risk for HDV.[40] These include persons born in regions with high HDV endemicity, persons who ever injected drugs, men who have sex with men, individuals infected with HCV or HIV, persons with multiple sexual partners or any history of sexually transmitted disease, and individuals with elevated ALT or AST with low or undetectable HBV DNA.[40] It is unclear to what degree the lack of a universal testing recommendation for HBsAg positive individuals in the US has had on overall testing rates. However, in Europe, even with a universal screening strategy, there seems to be a large gap in screening.

In a study carried out in Barcelona, Palom, and colleagues set out to assess and quantify adherence to the EASL screening guidance for HDV.[41] In the retrospective portion, of the study, the authors found that 1492 HBsAg-positive samples had been ordered between January 2018 and December 2020.[41] HDV testing was performed in 114 of the cases (7.6%). 11 of the 114 cases were found to have positive anti-HDV.[41] Breakdown of the orders revealed that 23% of 390 samples from academic hospitals had requested anti-HDV testing, whereas only 2% of 1102 samples from primary care centers had requested anti-HDV testing.41 In the prospective portion of the study, reflex anti-HDV testing was established (January 2021).41Data was collected from January 2021 to December 2021. 93% of HBsAg positive samples were tested for anti-HDV.[41] 100% of the primary care samples requested anti-HDV and 91% of the academic hospital samples had requested anti-HDV.[41] Additionally, the authors reported that the HDV testing rate had a slight increase after the new EASL guidelines had emerged which had recommended screening for HDV in all HBsAg positive individuals.[41]

Thus, a barrier to HDV testing is perhaps a knowledge gap among clinicians, particularly those practicing in the primary care setting. Some strategies that can be considered to overcome this gap include clinician education, encouraging and supporting a universal screening recommendation for all patients with HBsAg, and implementation of anti-HDV reflex testing in patients who test positive for HBsAg(**Table 3**). One study showed that in the Midwestern US, HDV testing was performed mainly by gastroenterology or hepatology providers.[42] Access to see subspecialty providers, particularly in resource-limited settings may also hinder appropriate screening.

Although the current guidelines recommend HDV testing in only high-risk individuals, the authors recommend reflex delta test using HDV antibody should be considered in all individuals who are positive for HBsAg (**Box 1**). Similarly, the current guidelines for initiating treatment for HBV are stringent and cumbersome and according to a recent WHO report only 16.7% of individuals with chronic hepatitis B (CHB) were on treatment with nucleoside/nucleotide (NA) analogue agents.[43] It has been shown that patients with CHB with persistent viremia and normal ALT levels are at increased risk of liver fibrosis.[44] Similarly, a more recent study from South America demonstrated that even low levels of HBV DNA burden were associated with chronic hepatocyte injury resulting in HCC.[45] Therefore, some experts recommend that HBV treatment guidelines should be expanded to include all patients who are positive for HBV DNA or those who persistently test positive for HBsAg $\geq$ 6 months.[46–48]

Table 3
Barriers to testing

Barriers to Testing	Potential Solutions
Differing screening recommendations across multiple societies	Adoption of a universal screening recommendation Implementation of HDV reflex testing
Knowledge gap among physicians	Provider education – with a focus on the primary care providers – regarding HDV and indications for testing
Patient knowledge of HDV	Provide educational resources to patients regarding HDV
Access to HDV testing	Improve general access to care among high-risk patients

---

Box 1
Five simplified guidelines for HBV screening and management

1. Test all adults for HBV using the triple panel test: HBsAg, Anti-HBs, and total antibody to hepatitis B core antigen (total anti-HBc).

2. Adults who are triple panel negative should be vaccinated against HBV.

3. Those who test positive for HBsAg should have a reflex link to both HBV quantitative DNA and anti-HDV antibody.

4. HBV treatment is recommended for all adults with positive HBV DNA irrespective of ALT levels and HBeAg status.

5. HBsAg individuals with cirrhosis should be screened for HCC using ultrasound ± AFP every 6 months. Surveillance against other chronic liver diseases such as NAFLD and alcohol-related liver disease is also recommended.

ENDPOINTS IN CLINICAL TRIALS AND DISEASE MONITORING

The HIDIT-1 study (2011) was a landmark trial in HDV therapy and compared treatment efficacy among peginterferon alfa-2a plus adefovir, peginterferon alone, and adefovir alone. The primary endpoints utilized in this study were achievement of undetectable levels of HDV RNA and normal levels of alanine aminotransferase (ALT) at week 48.[49] At week 48, 23% of the 31 individuals treated with peginterferon alf-2a plus adefovir and 24% of the 29 individuals treated with peginterferon alfa-2a alone had undetectable HDV RNA levels.[49] None of the patients who were treated with adefovir alone met this endpoint.[49] Among all patients who received peginterferon alfa-2a, a total of 23% of 60 patients had undetectable HDV-RNA levels at week 48.[49] 28% of 60 patients who received peginterferon alfa-2a had undetectable HDV-RNA levels at week 72.[49] However, in a long-term follow-up (median time of 4.5 years), 56% of the patients who had tested negative for HDV-RNA at 6 months had detectable HDV-RNA levels at least once during the follow-up period.[50,51]

In the HIDIT-1 study, ALT was also utilized as an endpoint. The median ALT among the three treatment groups in this study ranged from 88 to 111 IU/L.[49] In the peginterferon alfa-2a plus adefovir group, ALT normalized in 32% of 31 patients at week 48.[49] In the peginterferon alfa-2a alone group, 28% of 29 patients achieved the normalization of ALT at week 48.[49] Two patients of 30 (7%) receiving adefovir alone had normalization of ALT.[49] During long-term follow-up, (Heidrich and colleagues, 2014), the patients who received peginterferon alfa-2a had significantly lower median ALT levels than patients who received adefovir alone.[50] The median ALT in the peginterferon alfa-2a groups was 47.0 ± 35.9, whereas the median ALT was 99.5 ± 50.3 in the adefovir alone group.[50] At long-term follow-up, patients with long-term virological response had no ALT elevations.[50] However, there were a few patients who had ALT elevations at long-term follow-up despite having negative HDV-RNA.[50] The HIDIT-1 study also examined HBsAg as an endpoint. A decline of more than 1 $\log_{10}$ IU/mL in HBsAg levels at week 48 was observed in 10 patients receiving combination therapy and in 2 patients receiving only peginterferon alfa-2a.[49] Interestingly, the authors reported no association between a decline in HBsAg and ALT or HDV-RNA.[49]

The HIDIT-2 study was conducted to see if a longer duration of treatment would yield greater success. The HIDIT-2 study (2019) was a multicenter, randomized controlled trial assessing the efficacy of prolonged therapy with peginterferon alfa-2a plus tenofovir (TDF) or placebo for 96 weeks. The primary endpoint in the HIDIT-

2 study was the percentage of patients with undetectable HDV-RNA.[52] Secondary outcomes in HIDIT-2 were HBsAg loss, HBsAg decline (of more than 0.5 $\log_{10}$), and ALT normalization.[52] At week 96, a negative HDV-RNA was achieved in 48% of patients in the combination therapy arm as opposed to 33% in the placebo arm.[52] At week 96, HBsAg decline of at least 0.5 $\log_{10}$ was achieved in 28.8% of patients in the combination arm versus 19.7%.[52] Lastly, at week 96, normalization of ALT was achieved in 44% of patients in the combination arm versus 38%.[52]

Thus, a well-established treatment endpoint for HDV has been HDV RNA levels.[53] This is important because a decline in HDV RNA levels with peginterferon alfa-2a is associated with improved survival in patients with chronic HDV.[51] However, the measurement of HDV RNA levels has its limitations. This is due to the varying sensitivities of the current assays being used and the threshold level of HDV RNA is undefined.[53,54] Of note, a panel of experts had recommended using a decline of $\geq$ 2log in HDV RNA levels as a surrogate marker for treatment efficacy.[51] Sustained virologic response (SVR) for chronic hepatitis D (CHD) has previously been defined as undetectable HDV RNA 6 months after therapy.[53] SVR rates for CHD is estimated to be 25% which is considered low.[53,55] Given the low rates of reported SVR and high rates of HDV relapse in these individuals meeting treatment endpoints,[53] it is also important to consider alternative endpoints which have, as aforementioned, been utilized in clinical trials. These endpoints include HBsAg clearance and HBsAg decline.[54] Other potential endpoints that can also be implemented in clinical trials are biochemical response (normalization of ALT), histologic response, liver stiffness, and non-invasive serum fibrosis biomarkers.[54]

Similarly to chronic hepatitis B (CHB), the aspirational endpoint for hepatitis D treatment is HBsAg clearance.[53,54] Studies have shown that HBsAg clearance is associated with improved survival in patients treated with interferon therapy.[54] Overall, however, achieving HBsAg is rare and difficult – as can be appreciated from the interferon studies, the bulevirtide clinical trials, and the lonafarnib clinical trials.[53,54] The only class of medications that have had some success with achieving HBsAg clearance is REP 2139, the HBsAg secretion inhibitor. In a clinical trial assessing the safety and efficacy of REP 2139 and pegylated interferon alfa-2a in the treatment of patients with HBV/HDV coinfection, 6 of 12 patients had HBsAg clearance.[56] Four of the 12 patients had persistent clearance at 3.5 years.[57] Thus, HBsAg clearance can be a reasonable aspirational endpoint in individuals receiving a REP 2139 based treatment regimen.

Another endpoint in therapy is HBsAg decline. This seems to be a reasonable endpoint since complete clearance of HBsAg is difficult to achieve. In a post hoc analysis, a decline in quantitative HBsAg was used as one of the endpoints in the HIDIT-II study.[58] They used HBsAg less than 100 IU/mL at 24 weeks after the end of treatment.[58] In the HIDIT-II study, 14 of 120 individuals (12%) met this endpoint.[58] It is a reachable goal. By extension, it also parallels the CHB paradigm of predicting HBsAg clearance.[54] Regarding HBeAg seroconversion, Heidrich and colleagues carried out a study to investigate the role of HBeAg in patients with HDV coinfection using a cohort of 534 patients with positive anti-HDV. Between the patients with positive HBeAg and those who lost HBeAg, there was no difference in HBsAg, HBV DNA, and HDV RNA levels.[59] Additionally, patients with positive HBeAg did not have a worse long-term outcome than patients with HBeAg negative.[59] As such, based on this data, using HBeAg seroconversion as a potential endpoint may not be helpful.

Overall, ideal primary endpoints in clinical trials include undetectable HDV RNA, a decrease in HDV RNA by $\geq$ 2log, clearance of HBsAg, and a decrease in HBsAg levels to less than 100 IU/mL. Other endpoints include the normalization of liver enzymes (ALT), no worsening of fibrosis, improvement in histology, and liver stiffness measurements.[51,54]

ASSAYS PREDICTING THERAPEUTIC RESPONSE

Hepatitis B core-related antigen (HBcrAg) is a biomarker for intrahepatic covalently closed circular DNA (cccDNA) and is a surrogate marker of active HDV infection.[1] Sandmann and colleagues showed that HBcrAg could be used as a predictive marker for patients undergoing treatment with peg-IFNα-based therapies. The authors found that 30% of patients with a baseline HBcrAg level greater than 4.5 log U/mL were HDV RNA negative at 96 weeks after therapy.[58] 49% of patients with a baseline HBcrAg level between 3.0 and 4.5 log U/mL were HDV RNA negative.[58] And 59% of patients with HBcrAg levels ≤ 3.0 log U/mL were HDV RNA negative at 96 weeks.58 The authors assessed the predictive relationship using on-treatment HBcrAg values as well at week 48. 53% of patients with HBcrAg levels ≤ 3.0 log U/mL at 48 weeks had an undetectable HDV RNA at 96 weeks, 51% of patients with HBcrAg levels between 3.0 and 4.5 log U/mL had an undetectable HDV RNA at 96 weeks, and 20% of patients with HBcrAg levels greater than 4.5 log U/mL at 48 weeks had an undetectable HDV RNA at 96 weeks.[58] Furthermore, HBcrAg levels also had predictive quality for HBsAg decline: a HBcrAg level greater than 3.0 U/mL had an NPV of 91.7% for getting HBsAg less than 100 IU/mL at 24 weeks.[58]

Another predictor of virological response is the HBsAg. Niro and colleagues (2016) conducted a study to assess the role of HBsAg in the clearance of HDV RNA in patients treated with interferon therapy. The authors of the study found that a HBsAg level less than 1000 IU/mL after 6 months of interferon therapy was able to discriminate responders and partial responders from non-responders ($P < .001$).[55] They concluded that a reduction of serum HBsAg was necessary for a sustained HDV response and that a low titer of HBsAg at baseline predicted favorable response.[55]

FUTURE DIAGNOSTIC TESTS FOR HEPATITIS D VIRUS

A precise and accurate HDV RNA measurement is an elusive goal for HDV RNA testing. A couple of novel technologies are being developed to better quantify RNA. Currently, RT-qPCR is the most common method to evaluate HDV RNA viral load.[29] Unfortunately, as discussed previously, this method has shown high variability due to a multitude of factors.29 Droplet digital PCR (ddPCR) is a third-generation PCR technology that promises absolute quantification.[29] Olivero and colleagues developed a ddPCR assay for HDV-RNA viral load quantification. DdPCR had a conversion factor of 0.97 and a lower limit of detection (LOD) of 9.2 IU/mL.[29] Pfluger and colleagues developed a new quantitative HDV PCR assay on a fully automated platform called cobas6800.[30] RT-PCR is flawed by having considerable "run-to-run" and "inter-laboratory" variability.[30] The cobas6800 platform attempts to bypass these excesses and obtain a stream-lined result that is reliable.30 The cobas6800 had a lower LOD of 3.86 IU/mL.[30]

An accurate and expedient diagnosis of HDV coinfection is highly important. As aforementioned, there is a pervasive gap in HDV testing. A rapid HDV test for the detection of anti-HDV was developed by Lempp and colleagues in 2021. This rapid HDV test allows for the detection of anti-HDV within 20 minutes.[60] This test is based on a pan-genotypic, large HDV antigen (L-HDAg) and can detect anti-HDV of all genotypes (except type 4).[60] Lempp and colleagues tested its performance on a cohort of 474 patient samples. The sensitivity of this rapid test was determined to be 94.6% and its specificity was 100% when compared to ELISA.[60] This test can be useful in resource-limited settings where access to HDV testing is a challenge.

SUMMARY AND CONCLUSION

HDV is the most severe form of viral hepatitis and affects only those with hepatitis B infection. Identification of infected individuals by clinical suspicion alone is inadequate; instead, it is recommended that all individuals with acute or chronic hepatitis B be assessed for HDV. The best approach and the current standard of care is total anti-HDV that include IgG/IgM with reflex to HDV RNA RT-PCR quantitative in those with positive HDV serologies. Owing to the genetic heterogeneity of HDV, not all assays will efficiently measure or detect HDV RNA. Therefore, primers with pan-genotypic primers should be utilized when possible. When there is a high suspicion of HDV infection but negative HDV RNA, assessing liver tissue with staining for HDAg or serum HDAg testing can be employed. Currently, barriers to the identification of those with hepatitis delta involve the education of providers and access to already available testing. Emerging treatments have the potential to profoundly affect the natural history of HDV infection. HBV vaccination will be another path to ultimately control HDV (and HBV) infection.

CLINICS CARE POINTS

- Assess all individuals with acute or chronic HBV for concomitant HDV infection.
- The current standard of care is anti-HDV total (includes IgM/IgG) with reflex to HDV RNA RT-PCR quantitative, utilizing pan-genotypic primers when possible.
- Identifying HDV-infected individuals is limited by provider education and access to available testing.
- The main treatment for chronic HDV infection is pegylated interferon alfa-2a or telbivudine.
- Virologic response to treatment can be assessed using RT-PCR.
- The best way to ultimately control HDV (and HBV) infection is via HBV vaccination.

DISCLOSURE

The authors have no commercial or financial conflicts of interest or funding sources to disclose.

REFERENCES

1. Koffas A, Mak LY, Kennedy PTF. Hepatitis delta virus: disease assessment and stratification. J Viral Hepat 2023. https://doi.org/10.1111/jvh.13777.
2. Jameson J, Fauci AS, Kasper DL, et al. 20th edition. Harrison's principles of internal medicine, vol. 2. New York, USA: McGraw Hill; 2018.
3. Stockdale AJ, Kreuels B, Henrion MYR, et al. The global prevalence of hepatitis D virus infection: systematic review and meta-analysis. J Hepatol 2020;73(3):523.
4. Urban S, Neumann-Haefelin C, Lampertico P. Hepatitis D virus in 2021: virology, immunology and new treatment approaches for a difficult-to-treat disease. Gut 2021;70(9):1782–94.
5. Vogt A, Wohlfart S, Urban S, et al. Medical advances in hepatitis D therapy: molecular targets. Int J Mol Sci 2022;23(18).
6. Negro F. Hepatitis D virus coinfection and superinfection. Cold Spring Harb Perspect Med 2014;4(11):a021550.
7. Farci P, Niro G. Clinical features of hepatitis D. Semin Liver Dis 2012;32(3): 228–36.

8. Niro GA, Gravinese E, Martini E, et al. Clearance of hepatitis B surface antigen in chronic carriers of hepatitis delta antibodies. Liver 2001;21(4):254–9.
9. Hughes SA, Wedemeyer H, Harrison PM. Hepatitis delta virus. Lancet 2011; 378(9785):73–85.
10. Gilman C, Heller T, Koh C. Chronic hepatitis delta: a state-of-the-art review and new therapies. World J Gastroenterol 2019;25(32):4580–97.
11. Netter HJ, Barrios MH, Littlejohn M, et al. Hepatitis delta virus (HDV) and delta-like agents: insights into their origin. Front Microbiol 2021;12:652962.
12. Sureau C, Guerra B, Lanford RE. Role of the large hepatitis B virus envelope protein in infectivity of the hepatitis delta virion. J Virol 1993;67(1):366–72.
13. Wang KS, Choo QL, Weiner AJ, et al. Structure, sequence and expression of the hepatitis delta (delta) viral genome. Nature 1986;323(6088):508–14.
14. Usman Z, Velkov S, Protzer U, et al. HDVdb: a comprehensive hepatitis D virus database. Viruses 2020;12(5). https://doi.org/10.3390/v12050538.
15. Abbas Z, Afzal R. Life cycle and pathogenesis of hepatitis D virus: a review. World J Hepatol 2013;5(12):666–75.
16. Macnaughton TB, Shi ST, Modahl LE, et al. Rolling circle replication of hepatitis delta virus RNA is carried out by two different cellular RNA polymerases. J Virol 2002;76(8):3920–7.
17. Greco-Stewart V, Pelchat M. Interaction of host cellular proteins with components of the hepatitis delta virus. Viruses 2010;2(1):189–212.
18. Glenn JS, Watson JA, Havel CM, et al. Identification of a prenylation site in delta virus large antigen. Science 1992;256(5061):1331–3.
19. Hwang SB, Lai MM. Isoprenylation mediates direct protein-protein interactions between hepatitis large delta antigen and hepatitis B virus surface antigen. J Virol 1993;67(12):7659–62.
20. Kamal H, Westman G, Falconer K, et al. Long-term study of hepatitis delta virus infection at secondary care centers: the impact of viremia on liver-related outcomes. Hepatology 2020;72(4):1177–90.
21. Brichler S, le Gal F, Butt A, et al. Commercial real-time reverse transcriptase PCR assays can underestimate or fail to quantify hepatitis delta virus viremia. Clin Gastroenterol Hepatol 2013;11(6):734–40.
22. Lampertico P, Agarwal K, Berg T, et al. EASL 2017 Clinical Practice Guidelines on the management of hepatitis B virus infection. J Hepatol 2017;67(2):370–98.
23. Yamashiro T, Nagayama K, Enomoto N, et al. Quantitation of the level of hepatitis delta virus RNA in serum, by real-time polymerase chain reaction–and its possible correlation with the clinical stage of liver disease. J Infect Dis 2004; 189(7):1151–7.
24. Le Gal F, Gordien E, Affolabi D, et al. Quantification of hepatitis delta virus RNA in serum by consensus real-time PCR indicates different patterns of virological response to interferon therapy in chronically infected patients. J Clin Microbiol 2005;43(5):2363–9.
25. Mederacke I, Bremer B, Heidrich B, et al. Establishment of a novel quantitative hepatitis D virus (HDV) RNA assay using the Cobas TaqMan platform to study HDV RNA kinetics. J Clin Microbiol 2010;48(6):2022–9.
26. Schaper M, Rodriguez-Frias F, Jardi R, et al. Quantitative longitudinal evaluations of hepatitis delta virus RNA and hepatitis B virus DNA shows a dynamic, complex replicative profile in chronic hepatitis B and D. J Hepatol 2010;52(5):658–64.
27. Le Gal F, Dziri S, Gerber A, et al. Performance characteristics of a new consensus commercial kit for hepatitis D virus RNA viral load quantification. J Clin Microbiol 2017;55(2):431–41.

28. Jena A, Konrad-Zuse-Strasse AG, Hofmann U, et al. Improved Management of Hepatitis D: Standardized Quantification of HDV RNA Publication Monitoring of HDV RNA Improved Management of Hepatitis D: Standardized Quantification of HDV RNA. Available at: www.analytik-jena.com. Accessed March 3, 2023.
29. Olivero A, Rosso C, Ciancio A, et al. Clinical application of droplet digital PCR for hepatitis delta virus quantification. Biomedicines 2022;10(4):792.
30. Pflüger LS, Nörz D, Volz T, et al. Clinical establishment of a laboratory developed quantitative HDV PCR assay on the cobas6800 high-throughput system. JHEP Reports 2021;3(6):100356.
31. Chudy M, Hanschmann KM, Bozdayi M, et al. EXPERT COMMITTEE ON BIOLOGICAL STANDARDIZATION Geneva, 21 to 25 October 2013 Collaborative Study to Establish a World Health Organization International Standard for Hepatitis D Virus RNA for Nucleic Acid Amplification Technique (NAT)-Based Assays.; 2013. Available at: http://www.who.int/about/licensing/copyright_form/en/index. html Accessed March 3, 2023.
32. le Gal F, Brichler S, Sahli R, et al. First international external quality assessment for hepatitis delta virus RNA quantification in plasma. Hepatology 2016;64(5): 1483–94.
33. Radjef N, Gordien E, Ivaniushina V, et al. Molecular phylogenetic analyses indicate a wide and ancient radiation of African hepatitis delta virus, suggesting a deltavirus genus of at least seven major clades. J Virol 2004;78(5):2537–44.
34. Su CW, Huang YH, Huo TI, et al. Genotypes and viremia of hepatitis B and D viruses are associated with outcomes of chronic hepatitis D patients. Gastroenterology 2006;130(6):1625–35.
35. Roulot D, Brichler S, Layese R, et al. Origin, HDV genotype and persistent viremia determine outcome and treatment response in patients with chronic hepatitis delta. J Hepatol 2020;73(5):1046–62.
36. Lempp FA, Ni Y, Urban S. Hepatitis delta virus: insights into a peculiar pathogen and novel treatment options. Nat Rev Gastroenterol Hepatol 2016;13(10):580–9.
37. Spaan M, Carey I, Bruce M, et al. Hepatitis delta genotype 5 is associated with favourable disease outcome and better response to treatment compared to genotype 1. J Hepatol 2020;72(6):1097–104.
38. Sarin SK, Kumar M, Lau GK, et al. Asian-Pacific clinical practice guidelines on the management of hepatitis B: a 2015 update. Hepatol Int 2016;10(1):1–98.
39. Lee AU, Lee C. Hepatitis D review: challenges for the resource-poor setting. Viruses 2021;13(10):1912.
40. Terrault NA, Lok ASF, McMahon BJ, et al. Update on prevention, diagnosis, and treatment of chronic hepatitis B: AASLD 2018 hepatitis B guidance. Clin Liver Dis 2018;12(1):33–4.
41. Palom A, Rando-Segura A, Vico J, et al. Implementation of anti-HDV reflex testing among HBsAg-positive individuals increases testing for hepatitis D. JHEP Reports 2022;4(10):100547.
42. Safaie P, Razeghi S, Rouster SD, et al. Hepatitis D diagnostics:Utilization and testing in the United States. Virus Res 2018;250:114–7.
43. Hutin Y, Nasrullah M, Easterbrook P, et al. Access to treatment for hepatitis B virus infection — worldwide, 2016. MMWR Morb Mortal Wkly Rep 2018;67(28):773–7.
44. Nguyen MH, Garcia RT, Trinh HN, et al. Histological disease in asian-Americans with chronic hepatitis B, high hepatitis B virus DNA and normal alanine aminotransferase levels. Am J Gastroenterol 2009;104(9):2206–13.
45. Marchio A, Cerapio JP, Ruiz E, et al. Early-onset liver cancer in South America associates with low hepatitis B virus DNA burden. Sci Rep 2018;8(1):12031.

46. Jeng WJ, Lok AS. Should treatment indications for chronic hepatitis B Be expanded? Clin Gastroenterol Hepatol 2021;19(10):2006–14.

47. McNaughton AL, Lemoine M, van Rensburg C, et al. Extending treatment eligibility for chronic hepatitis B virus infection. Nat Rev Gastroenterol Hepatol 2021;18(3):146–7.

48. Robinson A, Wong R, Gish RG. Chronic hepatitis B virus and hepatitis D virus. Clin Liver Dis 2023;27(1):17–25.

49. Wedemeyer H, Yurdaydìn C, Dalekos GN, et al. Peginterferon plus adefovir versus either drug alone for hepatitis delta. N Engl J Med 2011;364(4):322–31.

50. Heidrich B, Yurdaydın C, Kabaçam G, et al. Late HDV RNA relapse after peginterferon alpha-based therapy of chronic hepatitis delta. Hepatology 2014;60(1): 87–97.

51. Yurdaydin C, Abbas Z, Buti M, et al. Treating chronic hepatitis delta: the need for surrogate markers of treatment efficacy. J Hepatol 2019;70(5):1008–15.

52. Wedemeyer H, Yurdaydin C, Hardtke S, et al. Peginterferon alfa-2a plus tenofovir disoproxil fumarate for hepatitis D (HIDIT-II): a randomised, placebo controlled, phase 2 trial. Lancet Infect Dis 2019;19(3):275–86.

53. Lok AS, Negro F, Asselah T, et al. Endpoints and new options for treatment of chronic hepatitis D. Hepatology 2021;74(6):3479–85.

54. Metin O, Zeybel M, Yurdaydin C. Treatment endpoints for chronic hepatitis D. Liver Int 2022. https://doi.org/10.1111/liv.15447.

55. Niro GA, Smedile A, Fontana R, et al. HBsAg kinetics in chronic hepatitis D during interferon therapy: on-treatment prediction of response. Aliment Pharmacol Ther 2016;44(6):620–8.

56. Bazinet M, Pântea V, Cebotarescu V, et al. Safety and efficacy of REP 2139 and pegylated interferon alfa-2a for treatment-naive patients with chronic hepatitis B virus and hepatitis D virus co-infection (REP 301 and REP 301-LTF): a nonrandomised, open-label, phase 2 trial. Lancet Gastroenterol Hepatol 2017; 2(12):877–89.

57. Bazinet M, Pântea V, Cebotarescu V, et al. Persistent control of hepatitis B virus and hepatitis delta virus infection following REP 2139-Ca and pegylated interferon therapy in chronic hepatitis B virus/hepatitis delta virus coinfection. Hepatol Commun 2021;5(2):189–202.

58. Sandmann L, Yurdaydin C, Deterding K, et al. HBcrAg levels are associated with virological response to treatment with interferon in patients with hepatitis delta. Hepatol Commun 2022;6(3):480–95.

59. Heidrich B, Serrano B C, Idilman R, et al. HBeAg-positive hepatitis delta: virological patterns and clinical long-term outcome. Liver Int 2012;32(9):1415–25.

60. Lempp FA, Roggenbach I, Nkongolo S, et al. A rapid point-of-care test for the serodiagnosis of hepatitis delta virus infection. Viruses 2021;13(12):2371.

Triple Threat: HDV, HBV, HIV Coinfection

Debra W. Yen, MD[a], Vicente Soriano, MD, PhD[b],
Pablo Barreiro, MD, PhD[c], Kenneth E. Sherman, MD, PhD[a],*

KEYWORDS

- HIV • Hepatitis delta • HDV • Viral hepatitis • Coinfection • Liver disease

KEY POINTS

- Understanding the HDV life cycle and mechanisms of replication provides insights into novel treatment targets. For example, bulevirtide blocks entry of HBV and HDV into hepatocytes by targeting NTCP.
- About 350,000 to 700,000 people worldwide have HIV/HBV/HDV coinfection. In PLWH, HDV is associated with higher rates of cirrhosis, liver decompensation, HCC, and death.
- All HBsAg-positive patients with HIV should be screened for HDV with HDV Ab, and serum HDV RNA should be checked to confirm active infection if HDV ab is positive.
- New HDV therapeutic options undergoing clinical trials include bulevirtide, lonafarnib, and REP-2139, although liver transplantation remains an option for PLWH with end-stage liver disease or HCC.

INTRODUCTION

First discovered in the late 1970s, hepatitis delta virus (HDV) has emerged as an important driver of decompensated liver disease and hepatocellular carcinoma (HCC) worldwide. HDV requires hepatitis B virus (HBV) for transmission and occurs as either a coinfection with HBV or a superinfection in the setting of chronic HBV. The global prevalence is difficult to estimate, but HDV likely affects around 15 to 25 million people worldwide. Due to shared transmission routes, namely sexual and parenteral, people living with HIV (PLWH) often are coinfected by HBV, HDV, and hepatitis C virus (HCV). Despite the severe disease course and rapid progression of liver disease with HDV, it remains underdiagnosed, including in the HIV population. Fortunately, novel therapies are forthcoming although studies of these

[a] Division of Digestive Diseases, University of Cincinnati College of Medicine, Cincinnati, OH 45267, USA; [b] Health Sciences School & Medical Center, Universidad Internacional La Rioja (UNIR), Madrid, Spain; [c] Public Health Regional Laboratory, Hospital Isabel Zendal, Universidad Rey Juan Carlos, Madrid, Spain
* Corresponding author.
E-mail address: Kenneth.Sherman@UC.edu

Clin Liver Dis 27 (2023) 955–972
https://doi.org/10.1016/j.cld.2023.05.010
1089-3261/23/© 2023 Elsevier Inc. All rights reserved.
liver.theclinics.com

medications in PLWH are still lacking. In this article, we will review HDV virology and immunology, epidemiology and clinical course in the setting of HIV, challenges with screening and diagnosis, and existing and developing treatment options for HDV.

HEPATITIS DELTA VIRUS VIROLOGY AND IMMUNOLOGY IN THE SETTING OF HIV
HIV, Hepatitis Delta Virus, and Hepatitis B Virus—Similarities and Differences

HDV, HBV, and HIV are distinct viral entities, which are often linked due to shared routes of transmission. Each virus can influence the replication, immunopathogenesis, and natural history of the other through both direct and indirect mechanisms. **Table 1** summarizes the similarities and differences between these agents.

While HDV is the smallest mammalian virus in terms of genome size at 1700 nucleotides, HBV and HIV genomes are larger at 3200 and 9200 nucleotides, respectively.[1] HIV and HDV are both RNA viruses, as opposed to HBV which is a DNA virus.

HDV requires an envelope of hepatitis B surface antigens (HBsAg), and both HBV and HDV bind to heparan sulfate proteoglycans to interact with the hepatic sodium taurocholate cotransporting polypeptide (NTCP) receptor through the pre-S1 domain of large HBsAg (L-HBsAg) for hepatocyte entry.[3,4] Both viruses then replicate independently in the nucleus of the cell. HBV-DNA is remodeled into covalently closed circular DNA (cccDNA), which acts as a genomic reservoir, and replication occurs with host RNA polymerase and viral reverse transcriptase. Conversely, HDV exclusively utilizes host RNA polymerase for replication rather than coding for its own replication enzymes. Two isoforms of hepatitis D antigen (HDAg) are translated: small HDAg, which is responsible for HDV mRNA transcription and replication, and large HDAg (L-HDAg), which allows for HDV assembly through envelopment by HBV surface proteins.[5] Some of L-HDAg is prenylated by cellular farnesyltransferase, which allows for recognition of S-HBsAg and encapsulation into the HBV envelope.

Innate and Adaptive Immune Response

HDV activates interferon (IFN) response pathways, which results in upregulation of IFN-β and IFN-λ.[6] IFN predominantly suppresses cell division–mediated HDV spread.[7] HDV-induced IFNs might also suppress HBV replication and augment HBV antigen

Table 1
Comparison of HIV, HBV, and HDV

	HIV	HBV	HDV
Genome size[1]	9200 nucleotides	3200 nucleotides	1700 nucleotides
Genus classification	Lentivirus	Orthohepadnavirus	Deltaviridae
RNA or DNA	RNA	DNA	RNA
Route of transmission	Sexual, parental, vertical	Sexual, parental, vertical	Sexual, parental, vertical
Binding site	CD4 receptor	NTCP receptor	NTCP receptor
Site of replication	Cytoplasm	Nucleus	Nucleus
Viral proteins	Structural proteins, envelope proteins, viral enzymes such as reverse transcriptase, regulatory proteins for replication[2]	HBsAg (small, medium, and large), HBcAg, precore/HBeAg, HBx, polymerase	S-HDAg, L-HDAg

Abbreviations: L-HDAg, large hepatitis D antigen; S-HDAg, small hepatitis D antigen.

presentation, which partially explains the low HBV viral load often found in HBV-HDV coinfection.[8,9] However, HDV may have evolved to adapt to the IFN response by hiding through compartmentalization to the nucleus for replication, as well as directly counteracting IFN signaling pathways.[10] These pathways are already impaired in PLWH with decreased innate immune function in dendritic and natural killer cells that are involved with clearance of viral infected cells. The mechanisms related to this are an area of intense research but are probably related to disturbances in T-regulatory cell mechanisms which lead to a persistent viral infection state.

Anti-HDV antibodies lack neutralizing activity and thus do not play a major role in viral control or clearance.[11] Although the cellular adaptive immune response is a driver of viral elimination in HBV and HCV, the role of CD4+ and CD8+ T cells in HDV is still unclear. More recent studies have found HDV-specific CD4+ and CD8+ T cells present during chronic HDV infection and lack of correlation between clinical parameters and the strength of HDV-specific T-cell response.[12–15] Nonetheless, an association between HDV-specific CD4+ T-cell response and low HBV viral load has been found.[13] In addition, like other chronic infections such as HIV, HBV, and HCV, the mechanisms of HDV-specific CD8+ T-cell failure that contribute to HDV persistence include mutational viral escape and T-cell exhaustion.[4,6]

Viral Interactions

HDV is known to suppress HBV replication in HBV-HDV coinfected patients, with HBV DNA levels typically below 2000 IU/mL.[16] Likewise, HDV dominates in HBV/HDV/HCV triple infection and results in low levels of HBV and HCV viremia, which is independent of HIV status.[17–20] Besides the possible contribution of HDV-induced IFN response and cellular T-cell response to HBV suppression as mentioned previously, other proposed explanations for low HBV viremia include the repression of HBV enhancers by HDV antigens[21] and higher frequencies of deletions in the basal core promoter/precore region in HBV genomes in HDV-positive patients.[22]

With HIV coinfection, studies have been mixed on whether HDV replication is increased in patients with HIV.[23,24] It does appear that persistence of serum HDAg is seen in PLWH, possibly in the setting of an HIV-induced reduction of CD4+ T-cell count.[25] Notably, HBV is suppressed to a lesser extent in the setting of HIV compared to that in patients without HIV, suggesting that HIV counters the inhibitory effect of HDV on HBV replication.[24]

HEPATITIS DELTA VIRUS EPIDEMIOLOGY AND NATURAL HISTORY IN HIV PATIENTS

Both HIV and HDV share transmission routes, with new infections acquired from sexual, parenteral, or vertical exposures.[26,27] HDV particles in the blood and other body fluids of carriers can cause new infections after contact with mucosal epithelia or blood vessels from others.[27] From the inoculation site, HDV particles travel to the liver where they find the surface NTCP receptor at hepatocytes. The odds of HDV infection becoming a chronic infection depend on whether HBV infection was already chronic or occurred simultaneously with HDV infection. In cases of coinfection, acute hepatitis is observed, and chronicity of HBV and HDV occurs at similar rates as HBV infection alone. If HDV superinfection on top of chronic HBsAg positivity occurs, a flaring hepatitis is observed, and HDV persistence happens now in most of these patients.

Following the introduction of HIV and viral hepatitis screening tests, transfusion-transmitted viral infections have drastically declined.[26,27] Nowadays, sexual transmission and injection drug use are by far the most common routes of contagion for both HIV and HDV.[26,27] However, in regions where any of these viruses are endemic and access to mother-to-child preventive measures are limited, perinatal transmission still occurs.[26,27] For HDV, the most common situation is vertically acquired hepatitis B and, years later, HDV superinfection during childhood or early sexually active adulthood.[27]

The World Health Organization (WHO) has global estimates for hepatitis B and C viral infections,[28] but it does not have figures of prevalence or mortality for HDV. Despite being a neglected disease, however, hepatitis delta is included as part of the Global Health Sector Strategy on Viral Hepatitis in 2016. They called for the elimination of all viral hepatitis by 2030, meaning at least 65% reduction in mortality and 90% decline in incidence.[29] Approaches envisioned by WHO to face the challenge of HDV control have recently been released.[30] Expanding HBV vaccination and HDV testing are key elements of this roadmap. Nevertheless, specific interventions in target populations such as PLWH are scarcely addressed.

Overlapping Epidemics of HIV and Hepatitis Delta Virus

Global trends in the rate of major bloodborne chronic viral infections, namely HIV and viral hepatitis B, C, and D, have evolved during the last few decades, following the introduction of protective vaccines and/or antiviral therapies.[26,30–32] Current estimates and the intersection of these viral infections are graphically recorded in **Fig. 1**.

For HIV/AIDS, the current estimate of PLWH is around 38 million.[33] Nearly 1.5 million people worldwide are newly infected with HIV annually. Nowadays, the HIV pandemic can be split into three major forms. The first HIV epidemic form mostly affects Sub-Saharan Africa and is the largest, with estimates of 25 million PLWH. Heterosexual transmission is the predominant mechanism of contagion. Women are slightly more affected than men at roughly 55%. Although mother-to-child transmission has drastically declined, but HIV infections in children and adolescents continue to occur. The second HIV pandemic form mostly affects North America and Europe but is also seen in Japan and Australia, with estimates of 3 million PLWH. Persons who inject drugs (PWID) and men having sex with men (MSM) are by far the most affected high-risk populations. The third HIV pandemic form mostly occurs in Latin America and Asia. It evolves heterogeneously between the two prior forms, affecting sexually active individuals with a variable and larger weight of MSM and PWID (**Fig. 2A**).

For hepatitis delta, following wide discussions in the scientific literature,[34,35] Miao and Pan have concluded that the global prevalence of HDV infection must be around 0.7%, roughly affecting 13% of HBsAg+ patients[36] (**Table 2**).

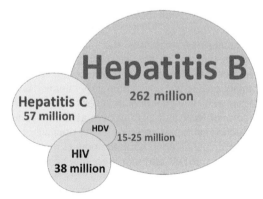

Fig. 1. Intersection of global viral hepatitis and HIV.

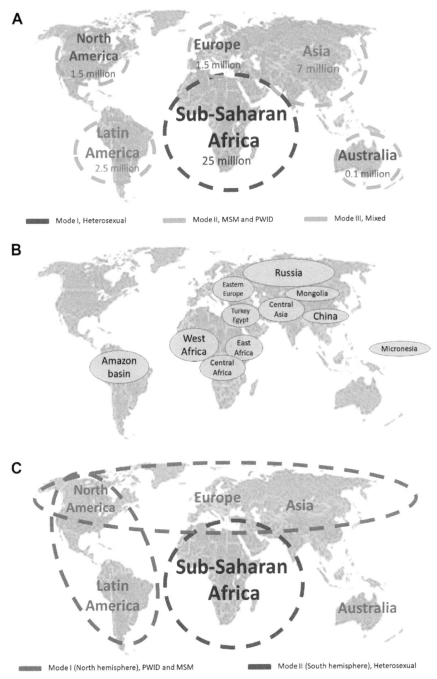

Fig. 2. (*A*) Major epidemiological forms of the HIV-1 pandemic. (*B*) Global geographic distribution of HDV infection. Major endemic regions. (*C*) Major global patterns of HIV-HDV coinfection.

Table 2
Prevalence of HDV infection-systematic reviews and meta-analysis

	Studies Analyzed	Anti-HDV + Among HBsAg +	Global Anti-HDV +	Estimated Absolute Numbers
Chen et al,[34] 2019	182	14.6%	0.98%	62–72 million
Stockdale et al,[35] 2020	282	4.5%	0.16%	12 million
Miao & Pan,[36] 2020	634	13%	0.70%	50 million

Given that only a fraction of anti-HDV-positive persons replicate the virus, the absolute number of HDV viremic individuals is thought to be between 15 and 25 million people worldwide.

By order, Asia, Africa, South America, Middle East, Eastern Europe, and the Western Pacific islands are the regions with the largest HDV populations[26,29,37] (**Fig. 2**B). Notably, China, India, and Nigeria are the major reservoirs of HBV infection and harbor at least one-third of total HDV infections. There are no reliable data from Russia and China, where HDV rates are high and underestimated.[37] Mongolia, a country in between, has one of the highest rates of HDV infection worldwide (30% of HBsAg+). In the Western Pacific, high rates of HDV have been reported in Micronesia, whereas Polynesia and Melanesia depict low HDV rates.

The widespread use of antiretroviral therapy has reduced HIV transmission significantly in most regions. However, 1.5 million new HIV infections still occur annually worldwide.[26] The introduction of treatment as early as HIV diagnosis is made and the prescription of antiretrovirals as pre-exposure prophylaxis in HIV-uninfected individuals engaged in high-risk behaviors have largely impacted MSM.[38,39] For other risk groups, such as PWID, individual and social challenges frequently preclude them from benefitting from medical services, which includes periodic testing, HBV vaccination, and access to medication.[38] These unfavorable factors largely increase the risk of HDV acquisition.[1,40]

In a recent survey conducted in Europe, 15% of nearly 2800 HIV-infected individuals with positive HBsAg had HDV antibodies.[41] While the rate was only 5% among MSM, which resembles the rate seen in the general HIV-negative population with positive HBsAg, it rose to 50% among PWID.[41] These numbers are similar to those reported in prior surveys conducted more than 1 decade ago.[42] Thus, PWID represent the largest HDV reservoir among PLWH in Europe and North America.[1,40–42] In the rest of the world, sexual risk groups make a greater contribution to the HDV reservoir.[30]

Producing estimates of the global population with HIV and HDV coinfection is difficult, while considering HIV and HDV overlapping geographic distribution, shared transmission routes, HBsAg+ prevalence and survival rates. Given that HDV only occurs among HBsAg+ individuals, we can start with estimates of HIV-HBV coinfection. If we assume that the rate of HBsAg among PLWH ranges from 5% to 10% and that there are 38 million PLWH worldwide, the population with HIV-HBV coinfection should range from 2 to 4 million. Then, if we apply the 15% rate of anti-HDV seen among European HBsAg+ PLWH, the estimated global number of HIV-HDV coinfected persons should range between 350,000 and 700,000 people. **Table 3** records estimates for viral hepatitis in PLWH based on the most updated figures.[39–41,43,44]

Double and triple viral hepatitis infections may occur in PLWH, including HBV plus HCV or HBV plus HDV plus HCV.[45] Classically, these patients exhibit the worst outcomes. Viral interference phenomena may occur with hepatic displacement of one virus when replication of another hepatitis virus takes over.[46] In this situation, antiviral treatment of all replicating viruses should be encouraged.

Table 3
Estimated number of individuals with viral hepatitis worldwide and coinfection with HIV

	All	PLWH
Total	8 billion	38 million
Hepatitis B[31]	262 million	5%–10% (2–4 million)
Hepatitis C[32,43]	57 million	5%–6% (2.3 million)
Hepatitis delta[36,41]	15–25 million	15% of HBsAg+ (350,000–700,000)

Abbreviation: PLWH, persons living with HIV.

Hepatitis Delta Virus Molecular Epidemiology in the HIV Setting

There are at least eight HDV genotypes (1–8).[47] Genotype 1 is prevalent worldwide. Genotype 2 is mostly reported from the Yakutia region of Russia, Taiwan, and Japan. Genotype 3 is common in the Amazon Basin and is associated with more severe forms of liver disease, earlier onset of HCC, and outbreaks of fatal acute liver failure. Genotype 4 is reported in the Far East, including the Miyako Islands in Japan and Taiwan.[48] Genotypes 5–8 are reported in Africa[49] and in Europe among African immigrants.[50]

Two major patterns of HIV and HDV coinfection have been recognized that exhibit distinct HIV-1 variants and HDV genotypes (**Fig. 2**C). In North America and Europe, HIV-1 subtype B and HDV genotype 1 are the predominant coinfections, with men more frequently affected than women. MSM and PWID are the largest groups.[47] A second pattern of HIV-HDV coinfection occurs in Sub-Saharan Africa where multiple HIV-1 non-B subtypes circulate, and co-infection with HDV genotypes 5–8 predominates along with HDV-1. Heterosexual transmission of HIV and HDV is the most common one, with women more affected than men.[47,49] As a result of migrant flows, this second pattern of HIV-HDV coinfection is increasingly being recognized in Europe and North America.[40,50]

Progression to Cirrhosis in People Living with HIV with Hepatitis Delta

Earlier studies have described a severe course of liver disease in chronic hepatitis D patients, who demonstrate faster progression toward liver cirrhosis with subsequent high liver-related morbidity and mortality.[51,52] However, many of those studies included risk groups such as PWID or patients with multiple comorbidities, including HIV or diabetes. During the last decade, the epidemiological landscape of hepatitis delta has changed with decreasing domestic cases and an increasing proportion of younger individuals immigrating from endemic regions to low-endemic regions.[50,53] Recent insights into the spectrum of HDV disease have highlighted an indolent course in a substantial proportion of persons with hepatitis delta.[54] However, at diagnosis, up to 30% may already show cirrhosis. Older age, liver cirrhosis, and HIV coinfection are the main predictors of worse clinical outcomes for HDV.[54]

In PLWH, chronic hepatitis delta has been associated with a disproportionate rate of cirrhosis[55] and poor clinical outcomes.[56] In a case-control study, 26 HIV-HDV coinfected patients experienced significantly higher rates of hepatitis flares, liver cirrhosis, liver decompensation, and death over a median follow-up period of 55 months than matched HIV monoinfected controls.[57] However, caution should be exercised when utilizing noninvasive fibrosis markers (transient elastography and serum markers) in patients with HIV/HBV/HDV coinfection, as there are no well-established thresholds.[58]

LIVER CANCER DUE TO HEPATITIS DELTA VIRUS IN HIV PATIENTS

Chronic HDV infection is associated with a higher risk of hepatic decompensation, HCC, and all-cause mortality among chronic HBV-infected persons.[51,52,59] In highly endemic regions for HDV, such as in Mongolia and Central Africa, liver cancer is very prevalent.[60,61] In one cohort study of 299 chronic hepatitis D patients in Italy (13 of whom had HIV coinfection), the annual incidence of HCC was 2.8% per year over a mean follow-up period of 19 years.[51] In another cohort study of 200 chronic hepatitis B patients with compensated cirrhosis, HDV infection was associated with a 3-fold increased risk of HCC over a median of 6.6 years.[52] The incidence of HCC was not compared by HIV status in either study.

Several reports have suggested that greater rates of HCC may be seen in PLWH with hepatitis delta along with unique clinical features, including multifocal lesions and younger age at diagnosis.[57,62–65] Two large studies have examined the risk of liver decompensation and HCC in PLWH with hepatitis delta. In one Spanish study,[66] 1147 PLWH (mean age, 42 years; 81% males; 46% PWID; 85% on antiretroviral therapy [ART]) were followed up for a mean of 8 years. Overall, 15 patients died of liver-related complications, and 26 developed hepatic decompensation events. The major predictors of hepatic outcomes were HDV coinfection and baseline liver fibrosis. Of note, 3 out of 17 PLWH with hepatitis delta developed HCC during the study period.

The second study reported data from the Swiss cohort.[67] Overall, 15% of 818 HBsAg+ individuals had antibodies to HDV infection, of whom 63% had active HDV replication defined as detectable and measurable serum HDV RNA. During a median follow-up period of 8 years, PLWH with hepatitis delta were 8 times more likely to die from liver-related causes and 9 times more likely to develop HCC.

The path toward the development of HCC in PLWH and hepatitis delta may be accelerated due to the conjunction of distinct pathogenic insults. The first is the intrinsic harmful effect of HDV causing more inflammation, fibrosis, and cirrhosis than any other hepatitis virus. The second is the persistent underlying direct carcinogenic effect of HBV. Third, HIV immunodeficiency has been associated with liver damage, and high HIV-RNA has been specifically linked to a direct carcinogenic effect.[68] Finally, comorbidities including toxic and metabolic effects of antiretroviral drugs as well as high rates of alcohol and/or tobacco consumption may contribute to the enhanced risk of HCC among PLWH with hepatitis delta (**Fig. 3**).

SCREENING AND DIAGNOSIS IN PEOPLE LIVING WITH HIV
Hepatitis Delta Virus Screening

Guidelines on the criteria for HDV screening differ by regional society, although all guidelines agree that patients with HIV who are HBsAg positive should be tested for

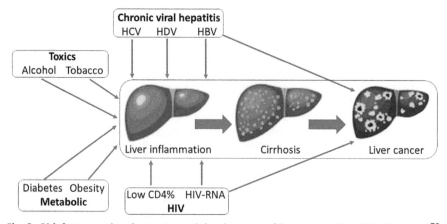

Fig. 3. Risk factors and pathways toward development of liver cancer. (*Modified from* Ref.[76])

HDV. The European Association for the Study of Liver Diseases and Asian-Pacific Association for the Study of the Liver recommend universal HDV testing for all patients with chronic HBV infection.[69,70] However, the American Association for the Study of Liver Diseases recommends testing only in select high-risk groups. In addition to PLWH, these include PWIDs, men who have sex with men, immigrants from highly HDV endemic areas, and HBsAg-positive patients with low or undetectable HDV DNA but high alanine aminotransferase (ALT) levels.[71]

Hepatitis Delta Virus Diagnosis

Diagnostic testing for HDV starts with total anti-HDV antibodies (HDV-Ab), which includes immunoglobulin M (IgM) and immunoglobulin G (IgG). Anti-HDV IgM typically is detectable about 2 to 4 weeks after symptom onset and becomes negative within 2 months after acute infection[72] although it may persist in chronic infection and serve as a marker of progressive disease.[73,74] Anti-HDV IgG appears 3 to 9 weeks after symptom onset and can persist for a long duration after viral clearance, thus causing anti-HDV IgG positivity to be unable to differentiate between current and prior HDV infection.[72,75] In patients who are HDV-Ab positive, HDV RNA is checked to confirm active infection. HDV RNA can be qualitatively or quantitatively detected by reverse transcriptase PCR although sensitivity between different HDV RNA detection methods vary greatly, and standardization is lacking.[75] In addition, HDV RNA levels can fluctuate over time and do not correlate with severity of liver disease.[16,76] Nonetheless, reduction in HDV RNA is being used as an alternative, a more realistic endpoint to HBsAg loss for HDV treatment. Unlike older methods that were limited in detection by genotype, newer tests are pan-genotypic and may be more reliable for the monitoring of virologic response to HDV treatment.[77]

Despite guideline recommendations, HDV remains underdiagnosed. A recent study evaluating two large United States cohorts found that among patients with chronic HBV, only 6.7% received testing in a Quest cohort and 19.7% in a Veteran's Administration (VA) cohort.[78] In PLWH, HDV underdiagnosis has been proposed to be less frequent due to the ability to perform HDV testing in patients regularly attending HIV clinics.[79] However, in a US Midwestern center, HDV testing was found to be lower in HBV-infected patients with HIV than that in those without HIV.[80] Correspondingly, an Italian study also found that HDV was underdiagnosed in HIV-HBV coinfected patients.[81] Implementation of anti-HDV reflex testing to HBsAg positivity has been shown to be a feasible strategy in increasing HDV detection.[82]

Hepatitis Delta Virus in Occult Hepatitis B Virus

In patients with HIV in whom serological responses to viral hepatitis may be impaired, the prevalence of occult HBV is 16%, which is 20 times higher than that in the general population.[83] Given cases of HDV survival for months after liver transplantation without HBV replication[84] and the discovery of HDV propagation through cell division in the absence of HBV coinfection,[85] the possibility of HDV infection in occult HBV has been considered. Aguilera and colleagues evaluated for HDV-Ab and HDV RNA in HBsAg-negative patients with markers of past HBV infection.[86] Of the patients with reactive HDV-Ab, all were negative for HDV RNA including all patients with HIV, which argues against HDV infection in HBsAg-negative patients. Conversely, in an Amerindian community from Argentina, Delfino and colleagues found 2 patients with occult HBV (isolated anti-HBV core positivity and detectable HBV DNA) that were positive for HDV RNA and interestingly both negative for HDV-Ab.[87] The difficulty in establishing HDV infection in the absence of HBsAg positivity may be attributable to imperfect diagnostic tests for low-level HDV-Ab and HDV viremia, as well as inadequate recognition of HDV-Ab in the context of highly divergent HDAg nucleotide sequences.[88,89]

UNIQUE TREATMENT CONSIDERATIONS

In patients with HIV-HBV coinfection, tenofovir is the preferred backbone for antiretroviral therapy given its high efficacy for long-term HBV treatment. There have been mixed results in whether tenofovir is associated with HDV suppression in PLWH. A cohort from Spain had demonstrated significant reduction in HDV RNA and liver stiffness with tenofovir exposure of 58 months.[90] In French and Swiss cohorts of triple-infected patients on tenofovir disoproxil fumarate (TDF) followed up over 3 to 5 years, however, most patients did not experience a significant reduction in HDV viral load or change in clinical outcomes such as liver fibrosis.[91,92]

The development of an HBV cure remains unsuccessful due to the inability to clear the HBV genome reservoir, HBV cccDNA. In contrast, the HDV replication cycle lacks chromosomal integration or a genomic reservoir, so attaining viral extinction by halting HDV replication for a finite duration of time may be achievable as has been done with HCV.[93] However, HDV evades targets of traditional antiviral therapies due to its use of host polymerase for replication instead of encoding its own.[94] Historically, IFN-α has been used for treatment of HDV, but it is poorly tolerated and has low rates of long-term effectiveness. Only 20% to 25% of patients achieved sustained virological response at 24 weeks after a 48-week treatment course, and out of all responders, half experienced late virological relapse.[95,96]

Newer Therapeutic Options

Newer therapeutic options on the horizon include bulevirtide, lonafarnib, REP-2139, and pegylated interferon-lambda (PEG-IFNλ). Bulevirtide, which is administered subcutaneously, is a lipopeptide that mimics the preS1 domain of L-HBsAg and inhibits the NTCP receptor, thus blocking entry of HBV and HDV. It received conditional approval from the European Medicines Agency in 2020 for treatment of compensated chronic HDV. In phase 2 trials, bulevirtide reduced HDV RNA levels at 24 weeks in TDF-treated patients,[97] as well as at 48 weeks with and without pegylated-interferon alpha (PEG-IFNα).[98] Bulevirtide was well-tolerated, with an asymptomatic dose-related increase in bile acids observed. A phase 3 trial (MYR301) that studies the safety and efficacy of bulevirtide monotherapy up to 144 weeks is underway.[99]

To date, the only report of bulevirtide use in persons with HIV/HBV/HDV coinfection enrolled 21 patients in an early access program in Europe.[100] Fourteen received bulevirtide 2 mg daily via subcutaneous injection, and 7 received this dose in combination with PEG-IFNα 2a. Combined response measures (>2 log reduction in HDV RNA and ALT <40) were seen at 3 months in 39% of those treated with bulevirtide only, while those on combination therapy had a 67% response rate. At 12 months by intention-to-treat analysis, 57% had a composite response in bulevirtide alone compared with 29% among those receiving a combination therapy. The intention-to-treat response was limited by the dropout of 8 patients, which was thought to be unrelated to bulevirtide use.

Lonafarnib is an oral farnesyl-transferase inhibitor that prevents prenylation of L-HDAg and interferes with HDV virion assembly and release. Lonafarnib and protease inhibitors are both substrates and potent CYP3A4 inhibitors, and ritonavir has been used to sustain higher postabsorption levels of lonafarnib and avoid gastrointestinal side effects.[101] Phase 2 studies showed that lonafarnib boosted by ritonavir significantly decreased HDV RNA levels at 24 weeks, with increased efficacy seen with the addition of PEG-IFNα.[102] The phase 3 D-LIVR study evaluating lonafarnib-ritonavir with and without PEG-IFNα at 48 weeks is ongoing. Although these studies summarily exclude patients with HIV, the use of ritonavir as a booster of lonafarnib can increase the number of potential CYP3A-related drug-drug interactions, particularly in PLWH who may require multiple other medications. Thus, it is likely that significant interactions may be observed with both protease inhibitors and nonnucleoside reverse transcriptase inhibitors.

REP-2139, a nuclear acid polymer, blocks the release of HBV subviral particles and clears circulating HBsAg. REP-2139 combined with PEG-IFNα in a small study showed that close to 60% of patients had undetectable HDV RNA, with clearance of HBsAg in 40%.[103] These virologic responses demonstrated durability up to 3.5 years off-treatment.[104] Lastly, PEG-IFNλ has better tolerability than PEG-IFNα, and 50% of patients had reduction in HDV viral load with 180-mcg subcutaneous injections weekly for 48 weeks.[105]

For PLWH, antiretroviral therapy is highly efficacious and well-tolerated, and unlike the multi-pill regimen in the past, regimens can now often be condensed into a single multidrug pill. In an effort to further improve adherence, not only have monthly intramuscular injectable formulations of antiretrovirals been developed,[106] but ultra-long-acting antivirals with sustained drug concentrations for 1 year in animal studies are also being investigated. Hypothetically, this same concept can be applied to HDV treatment with a once yearly injectable that could potentially even act as a cure.[79] However, the possibility of a cure in the form of HDV viral elimination despite HBV persistence, in addition to the required duration of HDV therapy to achieve this endpoint, is still being explored.

Liver Transplantation for Hepatitis Delta Virus

For patients with HDV with end-stage liver disease or HCC, liver transplantation is an option that may result in HBV and/or HDV cure with a protocol of intramuscular HBV immunoglobulin and nucleos(t)ide analogs for HBV prophylaxis.[107] Specifically, one study from Turkey showed no HDV recurrence in 128 transplanted patients with mean follow-up of 30 months,[108] while a second study from Turkey found 13% HDV recurrence rate in 104 patients with a mean follow-up duration of 82 months.[109] In addition, survival outcomes are promising, with a nationwide analysis in the United States demonstrating identical 5-year overall and graft survival at 78% to 79% between HBV monoinfected and HDV coinfected patients.[110]

Data regarding liver transplantation in HIV/HBV/HDV coinfected patients remain limited, yet existing studies suggest positive outcomes. In HIV-HBV liver transplant recipients, graft and patient survival are excellent and similar to HIV-negative patients as long as HIV replication is well suppressed.[111,112] In terms of patients with HDV, one study with 5 HIV/HBV/HDV coinfected patients who underwent liver transplantation found that HDV RNA remained negative at a maximum follow-up of 38 months.[113] Per European AIDS Clinical Society guidelines, liver transplantation from HBsAg-negative donors should be strongly considered in PLWH with HDV who are liver transplant candidates.[58]

SUMMARY

HDV occurs in about 15% of HIV-HBV coinfected patients and leads to faster rates of development of cirrhosis, liver decompensation, and liver-related death. In addition, disproportionate rates of HCC are seen in PLWH with HDV. Besides the need for improved HBV vaccination as a preventative strategy, HDV is largely underdiagnosed and thus unrecognized, even in patients with HIV. Clinicians should be aware that HDV screening with antibody testing is recommended for all patients with HIV who are HBsAg positive, and HDV RNA should be tested in patients with positive HDV ab. More effective therapies for HDV are in the pipeline, and although clinical trials exclude PLWH, bulevirtide appears to be efficacious in the real-world setting in patients with HIV. Lonafarnib is also a promising option; however, further examination of potential drug-drug interactions, particularly in PLWH, should be undertaken.

CLINICS CARE POINTS

- All patients with HIV who are HBsAg positive should be screened for HDV, and clinicians should not be misled by patients who are already on tenofovir who may have coincidental HBV suppression.
- Although HDV leads to faster development of cirrhosis, noninvasive assessment of liver fibrosis should be interpreted with caution in HIV/HBV/HDV coinfection due to the lack of established thresholds.
- In patients with HIV/HDV who require liver transplantation, donors who are HBsAg negative should be considered to increase the likelihood of HBV and HDV cure after transplantation.

REFERENCES

1. Soriano V, Sherman K, Barreiro P. Hepatitis delta and HIV infection. AIDS (Lond) 2017;31(7):875–84.
2. German advisory committee blood (arbeitskreis blut), subgroup 'assessment of pathogens transmissible by blood'. Human immunodeficiency virus (HIV). Transfus Med Hemother 2016;43(3):203–22.
3. Verrier ER, Colpitts CC, Bach C, et al. A targeted functional RNA interference screen uncovers glypican 5 as an entry factor for hepatitis B and D viruses. Hepatology 2016;63(1):35–48.
4. Urban S, Neumann-Haefelin C, Lampertico P. Hepatitis D virus in 2021: virology, immunology and new treatment approaches for a difficult-to-treat disease. Gut 2021;70(9):1782–94.
5. Lucifora J, Delphin M. Current knowledge on hepatitis delta virus replication. Antivir Res 2020;179:104812.
6. Oberhardt V, Hofmann M, Thimme R, et al. Adaptive immune responses, immune escape and immune-mediated pathogenesis during HDV infection. Viruses 2022;14(2):198.
7. Zhang Z, Ni Y, Urban S. SAT-202-Endogenous and exogenous IFN responses suppress HDV persistence during proliferation of hepatocytes in vitro. J Hepatol 2019;70(1):e718–9.
8. Alfaiate D, Lucifora J, Abeywickrama-Samarakoon N, et al. HDV RNA replication is associated with HBV repression and interferon-stimulated genes induction in super-infected hepatocytes. Antivir Res 2016;136:19–31.
9. Tham CYL, Kah J, Tan AT, et al. Hepatitis delta virus acts as an immunogenic adjuvant in hepatitis B virus-infected hepatocytes. Cell reports. Medicine 2020;1(4):100060.
10. Zhang Z, Urban S. Interplay between hepatitis D virus and the interferon response. Viruses 2020;12(11):1334.

11. Grabowski J, Wedemeyer H. Hepatitis delta: immunopathogenesis and clinical challenges. Dig Dis 2010;28(1):133–8.
12. Grabowski J, Yurdaydìn C, Zachou K, et al. Hepatitis D virus-specific cytokine responses in patients with chronic hepatitis delta before and during interferon alfa-treatment. Liver Int 2011;31(9):1395–405.
13. Landahl J, Bockmann JH, Scheurich C, et al. Detection of a broad range of low-level major histocompatibility complex class II–restricted, hepatitis delta virus (HDV)–Specific T-cell responses regardless of clinical status. J Infect Dis 2019;219(4):568–77.
14. Kefalakes H, Koh C, Sidney J, et al. Hepatitis D virus-specific CD8+ T cells have a memory-like phenotype associated with viral immune escape in patients with chronic hepatitis D virus infection. Gastroenterology 2019;156(6):1805–19.e9.
15. Karimzadeh H, Kiraithe MM, Oberhardt V, et al. Mutations in hepatitis D virus allow it to escape detection by CD8+ T cells and evolve at the population level. Gastroenterology 2019;156(6):1820–33.
16. Zachou K, Yurdaydin C, Drebber U, et al. Quantitative HBsAg and HDV-RNA levels in chronic delta hepatitis. Liver Int 2010;30(3):430–7.
17. Arribas JR, González-García JJ, Lorenzo A, et al. Single (B or C), dual (BC or BD) and triple (BCD) viral hepatitis in HIV-infected patients in Madrid, Spain. AIDS 2005;19(13):1361–5.
18. Mathurin P, Thibault V, Kadidja K, et al. Replication status and histological features of patients with triple (B, C, D) and dual (B, C) hepatic infections. J Viral Hepat 2000;7(1):15–22.
19. Jardi R, Rodriguez F, Buti M, et al. Role of hepatitis B, C, and D viruses in dual and triple infection: influence of viral genotypes and hepatitis B precore and basal core promoter mutations on viral replicative interference. Hepatology 2001;34(2):404–10.
20. Boyd A, Lacombe K, Miailhes P, et al. Longitudinal evaluation of viral interactions in treated HIV-hepatitis B co-infected patients with additional hepatitis C and D virus. J Viral Hepat 2010;17(1):65–76.
21. Williams V, Brichler S, Radjef N, et al. Hepatitis delta virus proteins repress hepatitis B virus enhancers and activate the alpha/beta interferon-inducible MxA gene. J Gen Virol 2009;90(Pt 11):2759–67.
22. Pollicino T, Raffa G, Santantonio T, et al. Replicative and transcriptional activities of hepatitis B virus in patients coinfected with hepatitis B and hepatitis delta viruses. J Virol 2011;85(1):432–9.
23. Buti M, Esteban R, Español MT, et al. Influence of human immunodeficiency virus infection on cell-mediated immunity in chronic D hepatitis. J Infect Dis 1991; 163(6):1351–3.
24. Pol S, Wesenfelde L, Dubois F, et al. Influence of human immunodeficiency virus infection on hepatitis δ virus superinfection in chronic HBsAg carriers. J Viral Hepat 1994;1(2):131–7.
25. Roingeard P, Dubois F, Marcellin P, et al. Persistent delta antigenaemia in chronic delta hepatitis and its relation with human immunodeficiency virus infection. J Med Virol 1992;38(3):191–4.
26. DeCock KM, Jaffe HW, Curran JW. Reflections on 40 Years of AIDS. Emerg Infect Dis 2021;27(6):1553–60.
27. Kushner T. Delta hepatitis epidemiology and the global burden of disease. J Viral Hepat 2023. https://doi.org/10.1111/jvh.13797.
28. World Health Organization. Global hepatitis report. Geneva: World Health Organization; 2017.

29. World Health Organization. Global health sector strategy on viral hepatitis 2016-2021. Geneva: World Health Organization; 2016.

30. Hayashi T, Takeshita Y, Hutin YJ-, et al. The global hepatitis delta virus (HDV) epidemic: what gaps to address in order to mount a public health response? Arch Publ Health 2021;79(1):1–180.

31. Ippolito H, Abbasi-Kangevari M, Abdoli A, et al. Global, regional, and national burden of hepatitis B, 1990–2019: a systematic analysis for the Global Burden of Disease Study 2019. The lancet. Gastroenterology & hepatology 2022;7(9): 796–829.

32. Tacke F, Craxi A, Tanaka J, et al. Global change in hepatitis C virus prevalence and cascade of care between 2015 and 2020: a modelling study. The lancet. Gastroenterology & hepatology 2022;7(5):396–415.

33. UNAIDS. HIV/AIDS report 2022.

34. Chen H, Shen D, Ji D, et al. Prevalence and burden of hepatitis D virus infection in the global population: a systematic review and meta-analysis. Gut 2019;68(3): 512–21.

35. Stockdale AJ, Kreuels B, Henrion MYR, et al. The global prevalence of hepatitis D virus infection: systematic review and meta-analysis. J Hepatol 2020;73(3): 523–32.

36. Miao Z, Pan Q. Revisiting the estimation of hepatitis D global prevalence. J Hepatol 2020;73(5):1279–80.

37. Wedemeyer H, Negro F. Devil hepatitis D: an orphan disease or largely under-diagnosed? Gut 2019;68(3):381–2.

38. Centers for Disease Control and Prevention. US Public Health Service: pre-exposure prophylaxis for the prevention of HIV infection in the United States—2021 update: a clinical practice guideline.

39. Gandhi RT, Bedimo R, Hoy JF, et al. Antiretroviral drugs for treatment and prevention of HIV infection in adults: 2022 recommendations of the international antiviral society–USA panel. JAMA, J Am Med Assoc 2023;329(1):63–84.

40. Ferrante ND, LoRe V. Epidee. Curr HIV AIDS Rep 2020;17(4):405–14.

41. Beguelin C, Atkinson A, Boyd A, et al. Hepatitis delta infection among persons living with HIV in Europe. Liver Int 2023. https://doi.org/10.1111/liv.15519.

42. Soriano V, Grint D, dArminio Monforte A, et al. Hepatitis delta in HIV-infected individuals in Europe. AIDS 2011;25(16):1987.

43. Platt L, Easterbrook P, Gower E, et al. Prevalence and burden of HCV co-infection in people living with HIV: a global systematic review and meta-analysis. Lancet Infect Dis 2016;16(7):797–808.

44. Kenfack-Momo R, Kenmoe S, Takuissu GR, et al. Epidemiology of hepatitis B virus and/or hepatitis C virus infections among people living with human immuno-deficiency virus in Africa: a systematic review and meta-analysis. PLoS One 2022;17(5):e0269250.

45. Chen S, Ren F, Huang X, et al. Underestimated prevalence of HIV, hepatitis B virus (HBV), and hepatitis D virus (HDV) triple infection globally: systematic review and meta-analysis. JMIR public health and surveillance 2022;8(11): e37016.

46. Maida I, Rios MJ, Perez-Saleme L, et al. Profile of patients triply infected with HIV and the hepatitis B and C viruses in the HAART era. AIDS Res Hum Retrovir 2008;24(5):679–83.

47. Le Gal F, Gault E, Ripault M, et al. Eighth major clade for hepatitis delta virus. Emerg Infect Dis 2006;12(9):1447–50.

48. Han M, Littlejohn M, Yuen L, et al. Molecular epidemiology of hepatitis delta virus in the Western Pacific region. J Clin Virol 2014;61(1):34–9.
49. Andernach IE, Leiss LV, Tarnagda ZS, et al. Characterization of hepatitis delta virus in sub-saharan Africa. J Clin Microbiol 2014;52(5):1629–36.
50. Aguilera A, Trastoy R, Barreiro P, et al. Decline and changing profile of hepatitis delta among injection drug users in Spain. Antivir Ther 2018;23(1):87–90.
51. Romeo R, Del Ninno E, Rumi M, et al. A 28-year study of the course of hepatitis Δ infection: a risk factor for cirrhosis and hepatocellular carcinoma. Gastroenterology 2009;136(5):1629–38.
52. Fattovich G, Giustina G, Christensen E, et al. Influence of hepatitis delta virus infection on morbidity and mortality in compensated cirrhosis type B. Gut 2000;46(3):420–6.
53. Ramos-Rincon J, Pinargote H, Ramos-Belinchón C, et al. Hepatitis delta in patients hospitalized in Spain (1997–2018). AIDS (Lond) 2021;35(14):2311–8.
54. Kamal H, Aleman S. Natural history of untreated HDV patients: always a progressive disease? Liver Int 2022. https://doi.org/10.1111/liv.15467.
55. Castellares C, Barreiro P, Martín-Carbonero L, et al. Liver cirrhosis in HIV-infected patients: prevalence, aetiology and clinical outcome. J Viral Hepat 2008;15(3):165–72.
56. Lee C, Tsai H, Lee SS, et al. Higher rate of hepatitis events in patients with human immunodeficiency virus, hepatitis B, and hepatitis D genotype II infection: a cohort study in a medical center in southern Taiwan. J Microbiol Immunol Infect 2013;48(1):20–7.
57. Sheng W, Hung C, Kao J, et al. Impact of hepatitis D virus infection on the long-term outcomes of patients with hepatitis B virus and HIV coinfection in the era of highly active antiretroviral therapy: a matched cohort study. Clin Infect Dis 2007; 44(7):988–95.
58. European AIDS Clinical Society (EACS) Guidelines version 11.1. 2022.
59. Alfaiate D, Clément S, Gomes D, et al. Chronic hepatitis D and hepatocellular carcinoma: a systematic review and meta-analysis of observational studies. J Hepatol 2020;73(3):533–9.
60. Candia J, Bayarsaikhan E, Tandon M, et al. The genomic landscape of Mongolian hepatocellular carcinoma. Nat Commun 2020;11(1):4383.
61. Amougou MA, Noah DN, Moundipa PF, et al. A prominent role of Hepatitis D Virus in liver cancers documented in Central Africa. BMC Infect Dis 2016; 16(1):647.
62. Garcia-Samaniego J, Rodriguez M, Berenguer J, et al. Hepatocellular carcinoma in HIV-infected patients with chronic hepatitis C. Am J Gastroenterol 2001;96(1):179–83.
63. Puoti M, Bruno R, Soriano V, et al. Hepatocellular carcinoma in HIV-infected patients: epidemiological features, clinical presentation and outcome. AIDS 2004; 18(17):2285–93.
64. Bruno R, Puoti M, Sacchi P, et al. Management of hepatocellular carcinoma in HIV- infected patients. J Hepatol 2006;44(Supplement 1):146.
65. Bräu N, Fox RK, Xiao P, et al. Presentation and outcome of hepatocellular carcinoma in HIV-infected patients: a U.S.–Canadian multicenter study. J Hepatol 2007;47(4):527–37.
66. Fernández-Montero JV, Vispo E, Barreiro P, et al. Hepatitis delta is a major determinant of liver decompensation events and death in HIV-infected patients. Clin Infect Dis 2014;58(11):1549–53.

67. Béguelin C, Moradpour D, Sahli R, et al. Hepatitis delta-associated mortality in HIV/HBV-coinfected patients. J Hepatol 2016;66(2):297–303.

68. Torgersen J, Kallan MJ, Carbonari DM, et al. HIV RNA, CD4+ percentage, and risk of hepatocellular carcinoma by cirrhosis status. JNCI : J Natl Cancer Inst 2020;112(7):747–55.

69. Lampertico P, Agarwal K, Berg T, et al. EASL 2017 Clinical Practice Guidelines on the management of hepatitis B virus infection. J Hepatol 2017;67(2):370–98.

70. Sarin SK, Kumar M, Lau GK, et al. Asian-Pacific clinical practice guidelines on the management of hepatitis B: a 2015 update. Hepatol Int 2016;10(1):1–98.

71. Terrault NA, Lok ASF, McMahon BJ, et al. Update on prevention, diagnosis, and treatment of chronic hepatitis B: AASLD 2018 hepatitis B guidance. Hepatology 2018;67(4):1560.

72. Aragona M, Caredda F, Lavarini C, et al. Serological response to hepatitis delta virus in hepatitis D. Lancet 1987;329(8531):478–80.

73. Farci P, Gerin JL, Aragona M, et al. Diagnostic and prognostic significance of the IgM antibody to the hepatitis delta virus. JAMA 1986;255(11):1443–6.

74. Mederacke I, Yurdaydin C, Dalekos GN, et al. Anti-HDV immunoglobulin M testing in hepatitis delta revisited: correlations with disease activity and response to pegylated interferon-α2a treatment. Antivir Ther 2012;17(2):305–12.

75. Chen L, Pang X, Goyal H, et al. Hepatitis D: challenges in the estimation of true prevalence and laboratory diagnosis. Gut Pathog 2021;13(1):1–66.

76. Schaper M, Rodriguez-Frias F, Jardi R, et al. Quantitative longitudinal evaluations of hepatitis delta virus RNA and hepatitis B virus DNA shows a dynamic, complex replicative profile in chronic hepatitis B and D. J Hepatol 2010;52(5): 658–64.

77. LeGal F, Dziri S, Gerber A, et al. Performance characteristics of a new consensus commercial kit for hepatitis D virus RNA viral load quantification. J Clin Microbiol 2017;55(2):431–41.

78. Wong RJ, Kaufman HW, Niles JK, et al. Low performance of hepatitis delta virus testing among 2 national cohorts of chronic hepatitis B patients in the United States. Am J Gastroenterol 2022;117(12):2067–70.

79. Soriano V, de Mendoza C, Treviño A, et al. Treatment of hepatitis delta and HIV infection. Liver Int 2022. https://doi.org/10.1111/liv.15345.

80. Safaie P, Razeghi S, Rouster SD, et al. Hepatitis D diagnostics:Utilization and testing in the United States. Virus Res 2018;250:114–7.

81. Brancaccio G, Shanyinde M, Puoti M, et al. Hepatitis delta coinfection in persons with HIV: misdiagnosis and disease burden in Italy. 2022.

82. Palom A, Rando-Segura A, Vico J, et al. Implementation of anti-HDV reflex testing among HBsAg-positive individuals increases testing for hepatitis D. JHEP Rep 2022;4(10):100547.

83. Ji D, Pang X, Shen D, et al. Global prevalence of occult hepatitis B: a systematic review and meta-analysis. J Viral Hepat 2022;29(5):317–29.

84. Mederacke I, Filmann N, Yurdaydin C, et al. Rapid early HDV RNA decline in the peripheral blood but prolonged intrahepatic hepatitis delta antigen persistence after liver transplantation. J Hepatol 2011;56(1):115–22.

85. Giersch K, Bhadra OD, Volz T, et al. Hepatitis delta virus persists during liver regeneration and is amplified through cell division both in vitro and in vivo. Gut 2019;68(1):150–7.

86. Aguilera A, Rodríguez-Calviño J, de Mendoza C, et al. Short article: hepatitis delta in patients with resolved hepatitis B virus infection. Eur J Gastroenterol Hepatol 2018;30(9):1063.

87. Delfino CM, Eirin ME, Berini C, et al. HDAg-L variants in covert hepatitis D and HBV occult infection among Amerindians of Argentina: new insights. J Clin Virol 2012;54(3):223–8.
88. Oubiña J, Delfino C, Mathet V. Hepatitis D virus infection in patients with hepatitis B virus occult infection. Eur J Gastroenterol Hepatol 2019;31(5):646.
89. Ponzetto A, Ciancio A, Figura N. Delta hepatitis in resolved hepatitis B. Eur J Gastroenterol Hepatol 2018;30(12):1528.
90. Soriano V, Vispo E, Sierra-Enguita R, et al. Efficacy of prolonged tenofovir therapy on hepatitis delta in HIV-infected patients. AIDS (Lond) 2014;28(16): 2389–94.
91. Boyd A, Miailhes P, Brichler S, et al. Effect of tenofovir with and without interferon on hepatitis D virus replication in HIV–hepatitis B virus–hepatitis D virus-infected patients. AIDS Res Hum Retrovir 2013;29(12):1535–40.
92. Béguelin C, Friolet N, Moradpour D, et al. Impact of tenofovir on hepatitis delta virus replication in the Swiss human immunodeficiency virus cohort study. Clin Infect Dis 2017;64(9):1275–8.
93. Soriano V, Mendoza Cd, Barreiro P, et al. Envisioning a hepatitis delta cure with new antivirals. Future Microbiol 2021;16(13):927–30.
94. Lok AS, Negro F, Asselah T, et al. Endpoints and new options for treatment of chronic hepatitis D. Hepatology (Baltimore, Md 2021;74(6):3479–85.
95. Abbas Z, Memon MS, Mithani H, et al. Treatment of chronic hepatitis D patients with pegylated interferon: a real-world experience. Antivir Ther 2014;19(5): 463–8.
96. Heidrich B, Yurdaydın C, Kabaçam G, et al. Late HDV RNA relapse after peginterferon alpha-based therapy of chronic hepatitis delta. Hepatology 2014;60(1): 87–97.
97. Wedemeyer H, Schöneweis K, Bogomolov P, et al. Safety and efficacy of bulevirtide in combination with tenofovir disoproxil fumarate in patients with hepatitis B virus and hepatitis D virus coinfection (MYR202): a multicentre, randomised, parallel-group, open-label, phase 2 trial. Lancet Infect Dis 2023;23(1):117–29.
98. Wedemeyer H, Schöneweis K, Bogomolov PO, et al. 48 weeks of high dose (10 mg) bulevirtide as monotherapy or with peginterferon alfa-2a in patients with chronic HBV/HDV co-infection. J Hepatol 2020;73:S52–3.
99. Wedemeyer H, Aleman S, Andreone P, et al. Bulevirtide monotherapy at low and high dose in patients with chronic hepatitis delta: 24-week interim data of the phase 3 MYR301 study. Dig Liver Dis 2022;54:S24–5.
100. de Ledinghen V, Gervais A, Hilleret M, et al. Bulevirtide +/- PEG-IFN in HIV/HBV/HDV Coinfected Patients in Real-Life Settings Abstract 589. Presented at: 30th Conference on Retroviruses and Opportunistic Infections. 2023.
101. Yurdaydin C, Keskin O, Kalkan Ç, et al. Optimizing lonafarnib treatment for the management of chronic delta hepatitis: the LOWR HDV-1 study. Hepatology 2018;67(4):1224–36.
102. Yurdaydin C, Keskin O, Yurdcu E, et al. A phase 2 dose-finding study of lonafarnib and ritonavir with or without interferon alpha for chronic delta hepatitis. Hepatology 2022;75(6):1551–65.
103. Bazinet M, Pântea V, Cebotarescu V, et al. Safety and efficacy of REP 2139 and pegylated interferon alfa-2a for treatment-naive patients with chronic hepatitis B virus and hepatitis D virus co-infection (REP 301 and REP 301-LTF): a non-randomised, open-label, phase 2 trial. lancet. Gastroenterology & hepatology 2017;2(12):877–89.

104. Bazinet M, Pântea V, Cebotarescu V, et al. Persistent control of hepatitis B virus and hepatitis delta virus infection following REP 2139-Ca and pegylated interferon therapy in chronic hepatitis B virus/hepatitis delta virus coinfection. Hepatology communications 2021;5(2):189–202.

105. Etzion O, Hamid S, Lurie Y, et al. Treatment of chronic hepatitis d with peginterferon lambda - the phase 2 LIMT-1 clinical trial. Hepatology 2023. https://doi.org/10.1097/HEP.0000000000000309.

106. Benítez-Gutiérrez L, Soriano V, Requena S, et al. Treatment and prevention of HIV infection with long-acting antiretrovirals. Expet Rev Clin Pharmacol 2018; 11(5):507–17.

107. Roche B, Samuel D. Liver transplantation in delta virus infection. Semin Liver Dis 2012;32(3):245–55.

108. Adil B, Fatih O, Volkan I, et al. Hepatitis B virus and hepatitis D virus recurrence in patients undergoing liver transplantation for hepatitis B virus and hepatitis B virus plus hepatitis D virus. Transplant Proc 2016;48(6):2119–23.

109. Serin A, Tokat Y. Recurrence of hepatitis D virus in liver transplant recipients with hepatitis B and D virus–related chronic liver disease. Transplant Proc 2019; 51(7):2457–60.

110. Kushner T, Da BL, Chan A, et al. Liver transplantation for hepatitis D virus in the United States: a UNOS study on outcomes in the meld era. Transplantation Direct 2022;8(1):e1253.

111. Stock PG, Terrault NA. Human immunodeficiency virus and liver transplantation: hepatitis C is the last hurdle. Hepatology 2015;61(5):1747–54.

112. Coffin CS, Stock PG, Dove LM, et al. Virologic and clinical outcomes of hepatitis B virus infection in HIV-HBV coinfected transplant recipients. Am J Transplant 2010;10(5):1268–75.

113. Tateo M, Roque-Afonso A, Antonini TM, et al. Long-term follow-up of liver transplanted HIV/hepatitis B virus coinfected patients: perfect control of hepatitis B virus replication and absence of mitochondrial toxicity. AIDS 2009;23(9):1069.

What Is the Real Epidemiology of Hepatitis D Virus and Why so Many Mixed Messages?

Zoë Post, MD[a], Nancy Reau, MD[b],*

KEYWORDS

- Hepatitis D virus • Epidemiology • HDV screening • HDV testing

KEY POINTS

- The prevalence of HDV is poorly understood and recent meta-analyses demonstrate vastly different prevalence estimates
- Estimates are performed based on biased chronic HBV populations, but HBV burden in itself is not well established and it is estimated that only 10% of HBsAg-positive individuals are diagnosed
- Prevalence rates vary greatly between different countries, risk groups as well as between different regions within the same countries
- Testing for HDV infections is suboptimal, as only a minority of at-risk patients are being tested and there is a lack of confirmatory PCR testing. In addition, there is no global guideline or consensus when it comes to the testing of HDV. Indeed, test availability for delta hepatitis are limited both in the US and internationally.
- Implementation of HBV vaccination programs has reduced the prevalence of HDV in younger populations and it is estimated that HBV vaccination rates of 80% could eradicate HDV

MANUSCRIPT BODY

The World Health Organization (WHO) aims to eradicate all viral hepatitis globally within the next 10 years. In order to fully eradicate these viruses, it is imperative to accurately identify the disease prevalence and adequately treat affected individuals. One of these hepatitis viruses is hepatitis D virus (HDV). The virus was initially discovered by Mario Rizetto in 1977, when he was looking at a hepatitis B virus (HBV) patient population with severe hepatitis.[1,2] Despite its discovery nearly 50 years ago, HDV

[a] Department of Digestive Diseases, Rush University Medical Center, 1725 West Harrison Street, Suite 206, Chicago, IL 60612, USA; [b] Section of Hepatology, Solid Organ Transplantation, Rush University Medical Center, 1725 West Harrison Street, Suite 319, Chicago, IL 60612, USA
* Corresponding author.
E-mail address: Nancy_Reau@Rush.edu

Clin Liver Dis 27 (2023) 973–984
https://doi.org/10.1016/j.cld.2023.05.011
1089-3261/23/© 2023 Elsevier Inc. All rights reserved.

liver.theclinics.com

remains a virus that has been largely neglected until recently. HDV is associated with more rapid progression to cirrhosis and the development of HCC, which prompted medical specialists to focus on the disease prevalence. Epidemiologic studies have been limited and there is significant difficulty in determining the global prevalence of HDV, as well as in specific subpopulations that are at higher risk for disease.[3] This review aims to provide an overview of the current literature on the prevalence of HDV and discuss the rationale for significant heterogeneity in data.

HDV is a satellite ribonucleic acid (RNA) virus and it is commonly referred to as a "defective" virus: in order to replicate, it requires host enzymes and the presence of hepatitis B surface antigen (HBsAg) to use this as a viral envelope and it shares the same hepatocyte receptor for entry into the cell.[4] There are 8 defined genotypes that can be found in different parts of the world. Genotype 1 is the most common globally, and is mostly encountered in Europe, North America, Australia, and the Middle East. Genotype 2 is commonly encountered in Asia and Russia. Genotype 3 is prevalent in South America, genotype 4 can be found in Japan and Taiwan, genotype 5 in Western Africa, and genotypes 6 through 8 are found in Middle Africa.[5] Knowing the specific HDV genotype is important, as it impacts disease severity and outcomes.

Nearly 300 million people worldwide are affected by chronic hepatitis B infection and therefore at risk for acquiring HDV.[6] Transmission of HDV is mainly through exposure to blood or blood products, including blood transfusions, needle-stick injury, intravenous drug use (IVDU), and through sexual intercourse. As opposed to HBV mono-infection, where the risk of transmission from mother to fetus is high, especially with higher levels of HBV DNA, transmission of HDV from mother to fetus is uncommon. HDV suppresses HBV by interfering with HBV messenger RNA synthesis and stability, and the production of IFN-beta and IFN-delta, which both inhibit HBV replication as well as increase resistance to innate immune responses.[7–11] By suppressing HBV, HDV limits transmission for both HDV and HBV, as it decreases the high HBV viral loads that are required for transmission.

Active infection with HDV can present as one of the 2 ways, depending on the individual's HBV infection status: (1) it can be co-transmitted with HBV, known as co-infection or (2) patients can acquire HDV after having HBV infection, known as super-infection.[12,13] These 2 pathways of obtaining HDV lead to vastly different disease phenotypes. Despite its dependence on another virus for replication, it is associated with the most severe forms of hepatitis in human beings. In co-transmission, patients can have an acute hepatitis with extensive hepatic necrosis that can present as fulminant hepatitis, but they often clear the infection spontaneously.[1,4] They become HDV antibody positive but have a negative HDV RNA level. The rate of HDV infection was found to be higher in patients with fulminant hepatitis as compared to less symptomatic acute hepatitis (26.7% vs 11.7% respectively).[14] On the contrary is a superinfection, in which patients with HBV (defined as HBsAg-positive state) who acquire HDV have accelerated progression of their liver disease, including more rapid development of cirrhosis, liver failure, and need for liver transplant, as well as a three times higher risk of developing hepatocellular carcinoma (HCC),[14,15] likely from persistent HDV within the body[16] in addition to the risk of advanced liver disease. Superinfection can present insidiously, with a rise in aspartate aminotransferase (AST) and alanine transaminase (ALT) being the only sign. Miao and colleagues found that nearly 40% of patients with HDV infection develop cirrhosis in approximately 1.5 years time, with an additional 30% that progress to cirrhosis within 3 years.[14] A French study demonstrated that the prevalence of cirrhosis increased from 28.1% to nearly 50% at 3-year follow-up, and nearly 10% of patients had developed HCC.[17]

It is estimated that 1 in 5 to 6 cases of cirrhosis or HCC among people with HBV are attributable to HDV.[5] Asymptomatic HBsAg carriers are at smaller risk for having HDV due to their mild disease phenotype and therefore have a lower prevalence as compared to patients with HBV cirrhosis that are much more likely to have HDV, as HDV leads to the progression of disease. This is evidenced by patients with HDV/HBV cirrhosis often times being younger due to the faster progression of disease.

There is an ongoing debate on the true prevalence of HDV. Multiple recent studies have attempted to estimate the global prevalence of HDV based on meta-analyses of available data. However, the estimated rates vary significantly between the studies. For example, Stockdale and colleagues calculated that the global prevalence of HDV is 0.16% based on a meta-analysis of 282 studies, comprising 376 population samples from 95 different countries.[5] A total number of 120,293 HBsAg-positive patients were included, and among these the HDV prevalence was estimated to be 4.5%, ranging from 3.0% in Europe to 6.0% in African regions. Two other studies estimated a much higher prevalence of HDV. For example, Miao and colleagues performed a meta-analysis on 634 studies including a total of 271,629 HBsAg-positive patients from 83 different countries and regions.[14] Based on their calculations, the prevalence of HDV in HBsAg-positive patients is 13.02%, and when extrapolated to the general population the prevalence would be 0.8%. Similarly, Chen and colleagues performed a meta-analysis on 182 studies including a total of 40,127,988 individuals from 61 countries and regions and estimated an HDV prevalence of 0.98% in the global population and a prevalence of 14.57% in the HBsAg-positive population.[18] These 3 studies highlight the heterogeneity of HDV prevalence in the literature as they report vastly different global preferences depending on studies included in the meta-analyses.

The prevalence of HDV varies greatly between countries, but overall Africa and Asia have the highest rates of HDV as well as the largest number of chronic HBV-infected individuals.[19] In the study by Stockdale and colleagues, Mongolia was found to have the highest HDV prevalence of 36.9%, followed by the Republic of Moldova and countries in Western and Middle Africa. There were also multiple isolated communities, such as indigenous Amazonian Amerindian tribes in Bolivia, Brazil and Colombia that showed high rates of HDV.[5] The highest prevalence in the study by Miao and colleagues was found in Asia (44%–56%) and Africa (22%–38%) in terms of HDV burden in the HBsAg-positive population, whereas in the general population the highest prevalence of HDV was found in Tunisia (15.33%), Mongolia (8.31%) and Niger (5.04%).[15] The third meta-analysis noted the highest prevalence of HDV in the general population of Mongolia with rates up to 8%, as well as high prevalence in African countries such as Niger and Gabon.[18] Unfortunately, these meta-analyses are significantly limited by biased sampling of high-risk individuals and low sample sizes from the majority of countries included.

An association has been established between higher HDV rates and lower income countries; the prevalence of HDV was low in high socio-economic countries, at 0.42%, whereas low socio-economic countries had an average prevalence of 3.41%, which is more than 8 times higher.[18] Interestingly, the high-middle socioeconomic countries had lower prevalence rates as compared to high socio-economic countries (0.07% and 0.42% respectively). The low-income countries account for half of the world population, 60% of the global HBV burden, but up to 75% of global HDV burden and are therefore the most important population to target.[14,20]

Within the United States, HDV prevalence ranges between 3% and 8%.[21–25] A National Health and Nutrition Examination Survey (NHANES) from 2011 until 2016 estimated the prevalence of HDV among 113 HBsAg-positive individuals to be 42%

(43 out of 113).[25] Looking at their subgroups, it appears that most of these individuals are foreign born (HBsAg-positive status: 80 vs 33; HBV/HDV-positive status: 34 vs 9) and the majority reported an Asian ethnicity (HBsAg-positive status: 70 vs 43; HBV/HDV-positive status: 29 vs 14 individuals). Interestingly, a similar yet much larger NHANES study including 52,209 HBsAg-positive patients undergoing HDV testing a decade earlier, between 1999 and 2012, had determined that only 0.02% of individuals with HBsAg or HBV DNA were positive for anti-HDV (10 out of 52,209).[26] In their sample, the majority of patients were either non-Hispanic white (40%), Mexican American (23%) or non-Hispanic Black (23%), whereas only 6% were deemed "other race," including Asian. Of note, Njei's study had an HDV testing rate of nearly 73% in their selected HBsAg-positive population, which is much higher than estimated national averages, as we will discuss later. These two studies illustrate how vastly different prevalence numbers can be estimated based on the "general" population selected for these calculations. It therefore appears that even within a country with many resources for epidemiologic studies, the prevalence of HDV remains uncertain.

We also have to keep in mind that intra-country variations exist in terms of HDV prevalence, especially in large countries, which could be secondary to differences in health care access.[20] For example, in Turkey, where infection rates have significantly improved over time and only 2.8% of HBsAg-positive individuals were found to have anti-HDV, rates were up to 61.4% in the Elazir Region and 18.4% in Van.[27–29] A similar observation is made in Iran, where rates in the North-West are significantly lower than in Eastern regions, with prevalence rates of 1.7% to 2.1% and 21.8% to 65.5% respectively in HBsAg-positive individuals.[30–33] In Africa, prevalence was found to be 25.6% in Central Africa, 7.3% in Western Africa and 0.05% in the general population of Eastern and Southern Africa, although data from these regions is extremely limited.[34] Furthermore, in Asia similar differences can be found, with higher HDV prevalence found in the center of the continent. For example, 50% to 60% of HBsAg-positive patient in Mongolia have anti-HDV.[35,36] In Kazakhstan, 7.9% of HBsAg-positive individuals had anti-HDV, as compared to 82% of HBsAg-positive patients with cirrhosis in Uzbekistan, 15% in Tajikistan and 42% in Kyrgyzstan.[37,38] In Pakistan, 30% to 50% of HBsAg-positive patients have anti-HDV, whereas in India, the anti-HDV prevalence was 5% in HBsAg-positive patients.[39] These significant regional differences in HDV prevalence further complicate unraveling the true prevalence of HDV in a specific country. In addition, it also shows that it is not possible to take prevalence data from one region and superimpose it onto another region within the same country, even if HBsAg prevalence is similar between the 2 regions.

The number one risk factor for acquiring HDV in developed countries is IVDU, followed by immigration from an endemic region.[40] In less developed countries, additional risk factors are mostly related to compromised hygienic practices, such as tattoo placement with non-sterile needles, use of unsterile tools in hospitals, unprotected sexual intercourse, and transmission within households.[41] Establishing the prevalence in high-risk groups such as IVDU or individuals engaging in high-risk sexual behavior is challenging due to the paucity of data. Existing data show that patients with IVDU were found to have significantly higher rates of HDV, with odds ratios (OR) ranging from 15 to 19.[5,14] In addition, patients undergoing hemodialysis (HD) were also found to be at increased risk for acquiring HDV.[5] Commercial sex workers and men who have sex with men (MSM), collectively referred to as individuals with high-risk sexual behavior, were also found to be at increased risk (OR 18.7 and 16.0 respectively).[5] Furthermore, patients with HCV or human immunodeficiency virus (HIV) also have higher odds of having HDV, with OR of 3.05 and 2.99 respectively.[5,14] Even within a high-risk group such as IVDU, attempts at minimizing transmission through needle exchange programs and offering HBV vaccinations have shown to be impactful, as evidenced by decreased frequency of HDV transmission over time in this population. In Spain, the anti-HDV prevalence in this population decreased from 30% before 2000 to 4.2% in 2018, which is attributed to needle exchange programs that are available in many Western countries, as well as higher rates of HBV vaccinations in this patient population.[42] As with the other hepatitis viruses, gender does not affect the risk for acquiring HDV, as evidenced by no significant differences in HDV infection rates being found between males and females.[14]

In determining the accurate population to test, it has come to light that viruses other than HBV can act as helper viruses for the transmission of HDV, such as HCV and HIV.[43,44] Perez-Vargas et al demonstrated that HDV particles were propagated by HCV in a mouse model, whereas Fernandez-Montero et al identified 17 anti-HDV-positive patients in their HIV-positive population of 1147 patients, although they did not specify whether these patients were HBsAg positive or negative. The hypothesis that other viruses can aid in HDV transmission requires further testing, but could imply that there is an overlooked patient population, those who are HIV or HCV positive and HBV negative, that is not included in epidemiologic studies.

In the past 2 decades, HBV vaccination programs have been implemented which offer individuals protection against HDV as well. By 2015, nearly 100 countries had implemented neonatal HBV vaccinations and 180 countries offered the hepatitis B vaccination series as part of their routine immunization schedule.[45] Various countries have published data on reduced HDV prevalence due to HBV vaccinations: In Spain, the HDV prevalence decreased by nearly 90%, from 30% in 1990 to 4% in 2018.[42] Similar changes were observed in Italy, where HDV prevalence rates decreased from 24% in 1990 to 8.5% in 2006.[46] The favorable impact of HBV vaccination programs is also evidenced by lower HDV rates among the younger population taking part in the vaccination program: an Italian study showed that the majority of anti-HDV in the HBsAg-positive population is found in individuals over the age of 50, whereas only 3% were found to be younger than 30.[47] Improvements were also noted outside of Europe: implementation of an HBV vaccination program in an indigenous population of the Peruvian Amazon proved to eliminate HDV in children.[48] A meta-analysis using global data showed a significantly lower prevalence of HDV in the era in which HBV vaccines were recommended (after 1997) versus before 1997, with a definite association between HBV vaccine rates and HDV prevalence.[18] Using a mathematical model, it is estimated that if more than 80% of a population is vaccinated against HBV, it could eradicate both HBV and HDV infections.[18,49] The authors did not specify the time it would take to eradicate the viruses. Despite these hopeful numbers in mainly high-income countries in Europe, HBV vaccination rates remain low in low-income countries. For example, in Africa, only 11 out of 54 countries implemented HBV vaccinations at birth.[50] HDV prevalence estimates should therefore take into account the significant decrease in HDV prevalence in high-income countries due to high HBV vaccination rates, whereas low-income countries do not exhibit these changes. In addition, the data from high-income countries mainly shows low HDV prevalence rates among the younger populations, that is, those who benefited from the implementation of HBV vaccination programs. The older generation with higher HDV prevalence is slowly disappearing, which would further lower the HDV prevalence rates in these countries as time passes.

The most important reason for challenges in determining the prevalence of HDV is the lack of appropriate testing. A major factor that contributes to the lack of testing in the United States and elsewhere is the lack of knowledge about HDV. As one can imagine, if a clinician is not thinking about the possibility of HDV co-infection/superinfection in their HBsAg-positive patient, appropriate testing will not be ordered. It is therefore imperative to increase awareness on HDV among clinicians and other healthcare professionals. Another important factor to consider in this realm is the availability of tests. Most HDV tests are not universally available and can be quite expensive. Only as of recently have these tests been made available in some commercial laboratories (review by Emmanuel Gordien). A major lab in the US, LabCorp, does not have delta total antibody or quantitative HDV RNA.

Screening tests for HDV include measuring total antibodies against HDV (anti-HDV) followed by validation through enzyme immunoassay testing. Total anti-HDV is a marker of exposure rather than active infection, and could represent a resolved infection. Moreover, the sensitivity and specificity for antibody testing in genotypes 5 through 8 is lower as compared to other genotypes,[51] which could result in under detection of HDV in this subpopulation of patients. Most prevalence estimation studies are based on the presence of HDV antibody, but not active disease, which is determined based on the presence of HDV RNA using reverse transcription polymerase chain reaction (RT-PCR).[52] This limits the identification of individuals with active infection, as a significant proportion of individuals with HDV antibody do not have active viral replication.[22,53] More accurate estimates could be established by looking at active disease, like we currently do for HBV by looking at HBsAg positivity, and for HCV, which is based on detectable HCV RNA levels. In addition, increasing the use of standardized confirmatory RT-PCR testing could help epidemiologic studies in determining the migration of specific genotypes to other continents. Unfortunately, information on HDV RNA is often lacking due to poor access to confirmatory RT-PCR tests, not only in low-income countries in Asia and Africa, but also in the US where Kushner and colleagues demonstrated that only 8.2% of HDV-Ab positive patients at the VA underwent confirmatory RT-PCR testing.[21]

There is no global guideline or consensus on who should undergo HDV testing. Even among the major liver societies, their guidelines on testing differ from one another. A number of guidelines, including in Europe and Asia, recommend that *every* individual with chronic HBV (ie, positive HBsAg) should get tested at least once for HDV.[52,54] The issue with merely recommending one-time testing for HDV is that it results in the false assumption that the individual will remain HDV negative for the rest of their life. A superinfection can occur at any time in HBsAg-positive individuals, even after a negative HDV test, and risk behavior should therefore be taken into account in these guidelines. Other guidelines, including in the United States, recommended only testing individuals with chronic HBV *at risk* for having HDV.[55] Risk factors include immigration from a country with high HDV prevalence, current or past IVDU, men who have sexual intercourse with men, individuals with multiple sexual parts, individuals with a history of a sexually transmitted disease (STD), and individuals with HCV or HIV. Risk-based testing has failed for HBV, HCV, and HIV, yet it is not clear why risked based testing for HDV is advised. We are currently at all adult screening for HBV, HCV, and HIV, thus HDV testing for all HBV-infected individuals may follow. In addition, an individual is considered "at risk" for HDV when laboratory testing shows an elevated alanine aminotransferase (ALT) or aspartate aminotransferase (AST) with a low or undetectable HBV deoxyribonucleic acid (DNA) level (<2000 IU/mL) (**Box 1**). However, the guideline does state that if there is any uncertainty on whether to test for HDV, screening would be recommended.

Within the United States, where testing is recommended in at risk patients, the actual testing rates vary greatly: in a study at the Veterans Affairs medical system including over 25,000 patients, merely 8.5% of HBsAg-positive patients were tested

Box 1
Individuals at risk for HDV infection
Immigration from a country with high HDV prevalence
Current or past IVDU
High risk sexual behavior (MSM, commercial sex workers)
Multiple sexual partners
History of STD
HCV positive
HIV positive
Elevated AST or ALT with low/undetectable HBV DNA levels (<2000 IU/mL)
Abbreviations: ALT, alanine aminotransferase; AST, aspartate aminotransferase; DNA, deoxyribonucleic acid; HCV, hepatitis C virus; HDV, hepatitis D virus; HIV, human immunodeficiency virus; IVDU, intravenous drug use; MSM, men who have sex with men; STD, sexually transmitted disease.

for HDV by antibody testing, of which 3.5% tested positive of HDV-Ab.[21] Only 8.2% of individuals with a positive HDV-Ab test underwent confirmatory testing with PCR. Of those meeting criteria per national guidelines, that is, elevated ALT with low HBV DNA levels, only 20% were appropriately screened for HDV. They found that cirrhosis was a predictor of positive HDV test result, which is also evidenced by higher prevalence of HDV in this patient population.[14] On the other hand, at an academic center the testing rate was 42%, with approximately 8% of patients having a positive HDV test.[22] Over 90% of HDV-positive patients underwent confirmatory RT-PCR testing. More than half of patients had undetectable HDV RNA levels. Again, and as expected, cirrhosis was a positive predictor for a positive HDV test. Despite the European recommendation to test *every* individual with HBV, the rates of testing are inappropriately low, with less than half of chronic HBV patients undergoing screening.[56] Given that co-infection is clinically indistinguishable from an acute HBV mono-infection, it is suspected that clinicians do not suspect HBV/HDV co-infections. The rates of testing are even lower in less developed countries, likely due to insufficient awareness on HDV, its consequences and access to affordable tests.[5]

As previously discussed, in high-income countries the prevalence of HDV is significantly declining due to the implementation and adherence to HBV vaccination programs. However, increase in the immigration of individuals from high endemic areas to these high-income countries leads to the re-introduction HDV to these populations. The decline in HDV infections has plateaued in the last 10 years in European countries,[57] which is attributed to immigration from endemic regions is resulting in higher HDV rates in non-endemic countries. Studies in Greece and Germany demonstrated that more than half of their HDV-positive population are immigrants.[15,58] A French study demonstrated that 77% of immigrants had active HDV infection.[17]

This is also evidenced by the detection of HDV genotypes that were previously limited to Africa in continents outside of Africa, such as Europe.[1] Despite substantial adherence to HBV vaccination programs in European countries, HDV infection rates are not decreasing.[1] In addition, immigrants were found to have lower HBV vaccination rates, suggesting that they have limited access to medical care in their country of residence and may therefore be excluded from HDV prevalence testing, especially if they are considered illegal immigrants.[34]

In order to intensify testing in at-risk populations in the United States, we need to determine how best to approach the highest risk population in Western countries, that is, individuals with IVDU. This is often the population that has the least exposure to health care facilities and might therefore be difficult to track down. In this key population, prevention rather than detection might be the best strategy, for example, by offering needle exchange programs to limit transmission of HDV and offering HBV vaccinations, as proven successful in Spain.[1,42] In low socioeconomic countries, HDV prevalence can be improved by intensifying the implementation of HBV vaccination programs. It is estimated that world-wide, less than 40% of children receive HBV vaccines at birth.[59] In addition, HDV prevalence rates can be lowered by improving the process of blood product screening and the use of sterile medical equipment.[60]

Until recently, no effective treatment options were available for patients with HDV. This may have contributed to low testing rates for HDV as clinicians were unable to change the outcome for their patients. However, with recent drug developments, attempts can be made at eradicating HDV and this would hopefully incentivize clinicians to increase their testing frequency. These novel drug therapies will be discussed separately (review by Tarik Asselah). Given the significant progression of underlying liver disease in patients with HDV, it is imperative that testing is being performed to identify these patients. Increasing the detection of HDV will allow us to better study risk factors for rapid disease progression and response to treatment.

As evidenced in this review article, the disease burden of HDV is poorly understood. There are multiple reasons why mixed messages are portrayed in the literature when it comes to the prevalence of HDV: (1) there is an overestimation of HDV infection rates in the general population due to limited sample sizes from many countries that are not representative of the general population in those countries as evidenced by significant regional variations in prevalence, (2) estimates are performed based on chronic HBV populations, but HBV burden in itself is not well established and it is estimated that only 10% of HBsAg-positive individuals are getting diagnosed,[19,61] (3) there is a significant lack of testing in at-risk populations as evidenced by the merely 20% of patients with risk factors that were appropriately tested, (4) prevalence testing is based on HDV antibody testing and not HDV RNA, which is needed to distinguish between active infection vs prior exposure, (5) many older studies used ELISA testing to determine prevalence, which was found to be a less reliable test, and (6) implementation of HBV vaccination programs in both developed and less developed countries has affected the prevalence of HDV, but is often not accounted for in meta-analyses.

Unfortunately, the true prevalence of HDV is yet to be discovered. Acceptable attempts have been made at establishing the global prevalence of HDV, but due to the lack of high-quality data and inappropriately low testing rates, it is impossible to determine the true prevalence of HDV. By improving testing rates in all countries, more accurate attempts at estimating the global prevalence can be made.

CLINICS CARE POINTS

- The prevalence of HDV is poorly understood and prevalence rates vary greatly between different countries, regions and risk groups
- HDV testing rates are inappropriately low world-wide due to poor access to HDV testing (HDV-Ab and PCR testing) and insufficient awareness on HDV
- Successful HBV vaccination programs and needle-exchange programs for IVDU can significantly lower HDV prevalence

DISCLOSURE

Z. Post: There are no financial conflicts of interest to disclose. N. Reau: There are no financial conflicts of interest to disclose.

REFERENCES

1. Hughes SA, Wedemeyer H, Harrison PM. Hepatitis delta virus. Lancet 2011;378: 73–85.
2. Rizzetto M, Hamid S, Negro F. The changing context of hepatitis. D. J Hepatol 2021;74(5):1200–11.
3. Kushner T. Delta hepatitis epidemiology and the global burden of disease. J Viral Hepat 2023. https://doi.org/10.1111/jvh.13797. Epub ahead of print.
4. Botelho-Souza LF, Vasconcelos MPA, Dos Santos AO, et al. Hepatitis delta: virological and clinical aspects. Virol J 2017;14:177.
5. Stockdale AJ, Kreuels B, Henrion MYR, et al. The global prevalence of hepatitis D virus infection: systematic review and meta-analysis. J Hepatol 2020;73(3): 523–32.
6. Hepatitis B. In: World Health Organization Fact Sheets. Updated: 24 June 2022. Available at: https://www.who.int/news-room/fact-sheets/detail/hepatitis-b. Accessed 26 February 2023.
7. Sellier PO, Maylin S, Brichler S, et al. Hepatitis B Virus-Hepatitis D Virus mother-to-child co-transmission: a retrospective study in a developed country. Liver Int 2018;38(4):611–8.
8. Chilaka VN, Konje JC. Viral hepatitis in pregnancy. Eur J Obstet Gynecol Reprod Biol 2021;256:287–96.
9. Sureau C, Negro F. The hepatitis delta virus: replication and pathogenesis. J Hepatol 2016;64:102–16.
10. Suslov A, Heim MH, Wieland S. New insights into HDV- induced innate immunity: MDA5 senses HDV replication. J Hepatol 2018;69:5–7.
11. Zhang Z, Filzmayer C, Ni Y, et al. Hepatitis D virus replication is sensed by MDA5 and induces IFN-β/λ responses in hepatocytes. J Hepatol 2018;69:25–35.
12. Gilman C, Heller T, Koh C. Chronic hepatitis delta: a state-of-the-art review and new therapies. World J Gastroenterol 2019;25(32):4580–97.
13. Negro F. Hepatitis D virus coinfection and superinfection. Cold Spring Harb Perspect Med 2014;4:a021550.
14. Miao Z, Zhang S, Ou X, et al. Estimating the global prevalence, disease progression, and clinical outcome of hepatitis delta virus infection. J Infect Dis 2020; 221(10):1677–87.
15. Manesis EK, Vourli G, Dalekos G, et al. Prevalence and clinical course of hepatitis delta infection in Greece: a 13-year prospective study. J Hepatol 2013;59: 949–56.
16. Fattovich G, Giustina G, Christensen E, et al. Influence of hepatitis delta virus infection on morbidity and mortality in compensated cirrhosis type B. The European Concerted Action on Viral Hepatitis (Eurohep). Gut 2000;46:420–6.
17. Roulot D, Brichler S, Layese R, et al. Origin, HDV genotype and persistent viremia determine outcome and treatment response in patients with chronic hepatitis Delta. J Hepatol 2020;S0168-8278(20):30441–4.
18. Chen HY, Shen DT, Ji DZ, et al. Prevalence and burden of hepatitis D virus infection in the global population: a systematic review and meta-analysis. Gut 2019; 68(3):512–21.

19. Polaris Observatory. In: CDA Foundation. Available at: https://cdafound.org/polaris/. Accessed: 26 February 2023.

20. Polaris Observatory Collaborators. Global prevalence, treatment, and prevention of hepatitis B virus infection in 2016: a modelling study. Lancet Gastroenterol Hepatol 2018;3(6):383–403.

21. Kushner T, Serper M, Kaplan DE. Delta hepatitis within the Veterans Affairs medical system in the United States: prevalence, risk factors, and outcomes. J Hepatol 2015;63(3):586–92.

22. Gish RG, Yi DH, Kane S, et al. Coinfection with hepatitis B and D: epidemiology, prevalence and disease in patients in Northern California. J Gastroenterol Hepatol 2013;28(9):1521–5.

23. Safaie P, Razeghi S, Rouster SD, et al. Hepatitis D diagnostics: utilization and testing in the United States. Virus Res 2018;250:114–7.

24. Kucirka LM, Farzadegan H, Feld JJ, et al. Prevalence, correlates, and viral dynamics of hepatitis delta among injection drug users. J Infect Dis 2010;202(6):845–52.

25. Patel EU, Thio CL, Boon D, et al. Prevalence of hepatitis B and hepatitis D virus infections in the United States, 2011-2016. Clin Infect Dis 2019;69(4):709–12.

26. Njei B, Do A, Lim JK. Prevalence of hepatitis delta infection in the United States: national health and nutrition examination survey, 1999-2012. Hepatology 2016;64:681–2.

27. Tozun N, Ozdogan O, Cakaloglu Y, et al. Seroprevalence of hepatitis B and C virus infections and risk factors in Turkey: a fieldwork TURHEP study. Clin Microbiol Infect 2015;21:1020–6.

28. Bahcecioglu IH, Aygun C, Gozel N, et al. Prevalence of hepatitis delta virus (HDV) infection in chronic hepatitis B patients in eastern Turkey: still a serious problem to consider. J Viral Hepat 2011;18:518–24.

29. Dulger AC, Suvak B, Gonullu H, et al. High prevalence of chronic hepatitis D virus infection in Eastern Turkey: urbanization of the disease. Arch Med Sci 2016;12:415–20.

30. Pouri AA, Ghojazadeh M, Baiaz B, et al. Prevalence of hepatitis D virus among HBsAg-positive individuals, 2015- 2016: azar cohort study. Health Promot Perspect 2020;10:38–42.

31. Sayad B, Naderi Y, Alavian SM, et al. Hepatitis D virus infection in Kermanshah, west of Iran: seroprevalence and viremic infections. Gastroenterol Hepatol Bed Bench 2018;11:145–52.

32. Bakhshipour A, Mashhadi M, Mohammadi M, et al. Seroprevalence and risk factors of hepatitis delta virus in chronic hepatitis B virus infection in Zahedan. Acta Med Iran 2013;51:260–4.

33. Sharifan P, Amoueian S. Histological and serological epidemiology of hepatitis Delta virus coinfection among patients with chronic active hepatitis B virus in Razavi Khorasan Province, Northeastern Iran. Iran J Publ Health 2018;47:1906–12.

34. Stockdale aJ, Chaponda M, Beloukas a, et al. Prevalence of hepatitis D virus infection in sub-Saharan Africa: a systematic review and meta-analysis. Lancet Glob Health 2017;5:e992–1003.

35. Tsatsralt-Od B. Viral hepatitis in Mongolia: past, present, and future. Euroasian J Hepato-Gastroenterol 2016;6:56–8.

36. Chen X, Oidovsambuu O, Liu P, et al. A novel quantitative microarray antibody capture assay identifies an extremely high hepatitis delta virus prevalence among hepatitis B virus- infected Mongolians. Hepatology 2017;66:1739–49.

37. Khodjaeva M, Ibadullaeva N, Khikmatullaeva A, et al. The medical impact of hepatitis D virus infection in Uzbekistan. Liver Int 2019;39:2077–81.
38. Khan A, Kurbanov F, Tanaka Y, et al. Epidemiological and clinical evaluation of hepatitis B, hepatitis C, and delta hepatitis viruses in Tajikistan. J Med Virol 2008;80:268–76.
39. Acharya SK, Madan K, Dattagupta S, et al. Viral hepatitis in India. Natl Med J India 2006;19:203–17.
40. Da BL, Rahman F, Lai WC, et al. Risk factors for delta hepatitis in a North American cohort: who should Be screened? Am J Gastroenterol 2021;116(1):206–9.
41. Daw MA, Daw AM, Sifennasr NEM, et al. The epidemiology of hepatitis D virus in North Africa: a systematic review and meta-analysis. Sci World J 2018;2018: 9312650.
42. Aguilera A, Trastoy R, Barreiro P, et al. Decline and changing profile of hepatitis delta among injection drug users in Spain. Antivir Ther 2018;23(1):87–90.
43. Perez-Vargas J, Amirache F, Boson B, et al. Enveloped viruses distinct from HBV induce dissemination of hepatitis D virus in vivo. Nat Commun 2019;10:2098.
44. Fernández-Montero JV, Vispo E, Barreiro P, et al. Hepatitis delta is a major determinant of liver decompensation events and death in HIV-infected patients. Clin Infect Dis 2014;58:1549–53.
45. Soriano V, Young B, Reau N. Report from the international conference on viral hepatitis 2017. AIDS Rev 2018;20:58–70.
46. Sagnelli E, Sagnelli C, Pisaturo M, et al. Epidemiology of acute and chronic hepatitis B and delta over the last 5 decades in Italy. World J Gastroenterol 2014; 20(24):7635–43.
47. Stroffolini T, Sagnelli E, Sagnelli C, et al. Hepatitis delta infection in Italian patients: towards the end of the story? Infection 2017;45:277–81.
48. Cabezas C, Trujillo O, Balbuena J, et al. Reduction of HBV and HDV infection in two indigenous peoples of Peruvian Amazon after the vaccination against hepatitis B. Salud Publica Mex 2020;62:237–45.
49. Goyal A, Murray JM. The impact of vaccination and anti-viral therapy on hepatitis B and hepatitis D epidemiology. PLoS One 2014;9:e110143.
50. Breakwell L, Tevi-Benissan C, Childs L, et al. The status of hepatitis B control in the African region. Pan Afr Med J 2017;27(Suppl 3):24.
51. Le Gal F, Brichler S, Sahli R, et al. First international external quality assessment for hepatitis delta virus RNA quantification in plasma. Hepatology 2016;64: 1483–94.
52. European Association for the Study of the Liver. EASL 2017 Clinical Practice Guidelines on the management of hepatitis B virus infection. J Hepatol 2017; 67(2):370–98.
53. Béguelin C, Moradpour D, Sahli R, et al. Hepatitis delta-associated mortality in HIV/HBV-coinfected patients. J Hepatol 2017;66:297–303.
54. Sarin SK, Kumar M, Lau GK, et al. Asian-Pacific clinical practice guidelines on the management of hepatitis B: a 2015 update. Hepatol Int 2016;10(1):1–98.
55. Terrault NA, Lok ASF, McMahon BJ, et al. Update on prevention, diagnosis, and treatment of chronic hepatitis B: AASLD 2018 hepatitis B guidance. Clin Liver Dis 2018;12(1):33–4.
56. El Bouzidi K, Elamin W, Kranzer K, et al. Hepatitis delta virus testing, epidemiology and management: a multicentre cross-sectional study of patients in London. J Clin Virol 2015;66:33–7.

57. Wedemeyer H1, Manns MP. Epidemiology, pathogenesis and management of hepatitis D: update and challenges ahead. Nat Rev Gastroenterol Hepatol 2010;7:31–40.
58. lempp Fa, ni Y, Urban S. Hepatitis delta virus: insights into a peculiar pathogen and novel treatment options. Nat Rev Gastroenterol Hepatol 2016;13:580–9.
59. Lemoine M, Thursz MR. Battlefield against hepatitis B infection and HCC in Africa. J Hepatol 2017;66:645–54.
60. Schweitzer A, Horn J, Mikolajczyk RT, et al. Estimations of worldwide prevalence of chronic hepatitis B virus infection: a systematic review of data published between 1965 and 2013. Lancet 2015;386:1546–55.
61. Basnayake SK, Easterbrook PJ. Wide variation in estimates of global prevalence and burden of chronic hepatitis B and C infection cited in published literature. J Viral Hepat 2016;23:545–59.

What is the Path Forward to Treat Hepatitis Delta Virus?
Old Treatments and New Options

Tarik Asselah, MD, PhD*

KEYWORDS

- Chronic hepatitis D • HDV therapy • Pegylated interferon • Bulevirtide • Lonafarnib
- Replicor • HBV cure

KEY POINTS

- Hepatitis Delta Virus (HDV) is a small RNA virus that requires Hepatitis B Surface Antigen (HBsAg) for its envelope, for entry into hepatocytes and secretion.
- Reinforcement of HBV vaccine coverage, increasing screening, linkage to care, access to therapy are essential to reduce HDV infection.
- Current treatment of chronic hepatitis delta (CHD) is Pegylated-interferon for 48 weeks with mild efficacy and poor tolerability.
- Entry inhibitor, Bulevirtide (Hepcludex), has been conditionally approved in Europe in 2020, with around half of patients achieving a more than 2 log decline and ALT normalization at one year of therapy.
- Drugs under development include different modes of actions: entry inhibitors, prenylation inhibitors, and nucleic acid polymers, and also those aiming for an HBV cure.

INTRODUCTION

Hepatitis D virus (HDV) infection increases the risk of cirrhosis and hepato-cellular carcinoma when compared to hepatitis B virus (HBV) mono-infection. There is an urgent need to develop new drugs for chronic hepatitis D (CHD). Pegylated interferon alpha (PEG-IFNα) (direct-antivirals and immune modulators) has been used and recommended by scientific guidelines, although not approved, with moderate efficacy and poor tolerability. There are several drugs in development which target the host: bulevirtide (BLV), lonafarnib (LNF), nucleic acid polymer and others. HDV use the cell enzymes for its own replication, and the HBsAg as envelope. Because of the limited enzyme

Financial support: no financial support.
University of Paris-Cité, Hôpital Beaujon, Service d'hépatologie AP-HP & INSERM UMR1149, Clichy, France
* Corresponding author. Service d'hépatologie, Hôpital Beaujon, 100 Boulevard du Général Leclerc, 92110 Clichy, France.
E-mail address: tarik.asselah@aphp.fr

targets, it appears difficult to develop direct acting antivirals. In this article, we review current and future treatments for chronic hepatitis D.

OLD TREATMENTS
Interferon alfa (IFN-α)

Historically, the use of IFN-α for the treatment for chronic delta hepatitis has been based on the limited number of small series reporting moderate efficacy and poor tolerability. The exact mode of action of IFN remains unclear, however IFN acts as an anti-viral and immune modulator.

In an early pilot study published in 1990, 12 patients with chronic delta hepatitis were treated with interferon alfa-2b (IFN-α), initiated at 5 million units per day subcutaneously (sc) for at least 4 months, being reduced by half if side effects occurred.[1] IFN-α resulted in decreased of serum alanine aminotransferase (ALT) levels, hepatitis delta virus (HDV) RNA and hepatitis delta antigen. On the cessation of therapy, most patients experienced a relapse over 6 months, but ALT levels could be normalized once more by restarting IFN-α therapy. Finally, IFN-α decreased hepatic inflammation by the inhibition of HDV replication, although relapse occurred when IFN-α was stopped. Therefore, it appears that long-term therapy is required for long-term control of the disease.

A landmark study aimed to evaluate the efficacy of treatment with IFN-α, 42 patients with CHD who were randomly assigned to receive either 9 million or 3 million units of IFN-α-2a (three times a week for 48 weeks) or no treatment.[2]

By the end of the treatment, serum ALT had become normal in 10 of 14 patients receiving 9 million units, as compared with 4 of 14 treated with 3 million units and 1 of 13 untreated controls. Seven patients among 14 treated with the higher dose of IFN had a complete response (normal ALT levels and no detectable serum HDV RNA, as compared with 3 of those who received the lower dose, and none of the controls. Furthermore, treatment with a high dose of IFN was associated with improvement in histology features (reduced periportal necrosis and portal and lobular inflammation), whereas in the untreated controls there was considerable histologic deterioration. In 5 of the 10 patients treated with 9 million units of IFN whose ALT became normal, the biochemical responses persisted for up to 4 years (mean, 39 months), but the effects of treatment on viral replication were not sustained. In contrast, none of those who received 3 million units and none of the untreated controls had a sustained biochemical or virologic response. Finally, in about half the patients with CHD treated with high doses of IFN alfa-2a, the serum ALT level becomes normal, serum HDV RNA becomes undetectable, and there is histologic improvement. However, a relapse is common after treatment cessation.

The same group evaluated the long-term outcomes of patients with CHD after an extended course of PEG-IFNα.[3] The 36 patients with CHD who participated in the previous randomized controlled trial of a 48-week course of high (9 million units) or low (3 million units) doses of IFN-α or no treatment were followed for an additional 2 to 14 years. Long-term survival was significantly longer in the high-dose group than in untreated controls or in the low-dose group but did not differ between patients treated with 3 million units and controls. Among surviving patients at 12 years of follow-up, a biochemical response was present in 7 of 12 treated with 9 million units, in 2 of 4 who received 3 million units, and in none of 3 controls. Long-term ALT normalization correlated with improved hepatic function and loss of IgM antibody to hepatitis delta antigen (anti-HD). Patients in the high-dose group had a sustained decrease in HDV replication, leading to clearance of HDV RNA and, eventually, HBV)in some patients, as well as a dramatic improvement in liver histology with respect to activity grade and fibrosis stage. They documented an absence of fibrosis in the final biopsy of 4 patients with a long-term biochemical response and an initial diagnosis of active cirrhosis. Finally, high doses of IFN-α-2a significantly improved the long-term clinical outcome and survival of patients with CHD, even though the majority had active cirrhosis before starting therapy.

Pegylated interferon alpha

Several scientific societies recommend, for patients with HDV infection on active replication, the use of PEG-IFN-α for a minimum of 48 weeks, or more if tolerability is favorable.[4–6] These recommendations relies also, as for IFN-α, on small series of patients. It is well known that PEG-IFN-α is more convenient for patients (1 time weekly vs daily), with a favorable pharmaco-kinetic. Endpoint for efficacy, similarly to historical treatment for hepatitis C virus (HCV), has been usually defined by undetectable HDV-RNA levels at 24 weeks post-treatment. In these studies evaluating PEG-IFN-α, efficacy was reported between 23% and 57% of patients.[7–10]

We have to emphasize that HDV-RNA serum levels should be regularly monitored in patients with a virological response, since relapse is common. A study reported that in patients treated with PEG-IFN-α for 48 weeks, although 40% achieved undetectable HDV-RNA levels at 24 weeks post-treatment, only 12% had maintained such levels after a 4.5 years follow-up study.[11] Therefore, the term sustained virological response (used for therapy of HCV infection) should not be used for HDV infection. The term durable response appears to be more appropriate (when HDV RNA remains undetectable).

In a small series of 12 patients with CHD, who received more than 6 months of PEG-IFN-α treatment, with further follow-up, an extended course of PEG-IFN-α therapy resulted in sustained clearance of HDV RNA and favorable clinical outcomes in more than half of patients and loss of HBsAg in a third.[8]

It is well known that PEG-IFN-α treatment is associated with significant side effects: flu-like symptoms (headaches, myalgias, arthralgias), pancytopenia (anemia, leukopenia, thrombocytopenia), depression and risk of suicide, and high serum aminotransferase values. This treatment is contra-indicated for patients with decompensated cirrhosis, major psychiatric illness, and autoimmune diseases. Finally, long-term durable antiviral efficacy of IFN remains limited (around 10%–20%) with a poor tolerability. **Box 1** describes available and investigational drugs for HDV infection.

Bulevirtide

Sodium taurocholate cotransporting polypeptide (NTCP) has been identified as a receptor for human hepatitis B virus, and therefore for also for HDV.[12] BLV (Hepcludex) is a myristoylated synthetic peptide of 47 amino acids derived from the S1 domain of HBsAg that inhibits viral entry by interfering with viral binding to the NTCP, thus avoiding the novel infection of hepatocytes.[13] Phase 2 clinical trials showed that BLV (2 mg/d; sc) was well tolerated and effective in reducing ALT and HDV RNA serum levels, however the majority of patients had a relapse after the cessation of therapy.[14,15]

BLV was given conditional marketing authorization by European Medical Agency (EMA) in 2020.[16] BLV was approved at a dose of 2 mg sc per day for the treatment of chronic HDV infection in adult patients with compensated liver disease and positive HDV viremia. Treatment is not indicated in patients with decompensated cirrhosis (because of the lack of data). The optimal treatment duration has not been determined and according to EMA "treatment should be continued if a clinical benefit is observed with BLV administration". However, this clinical benefit is not defined. Treatment

---

Box 1
Considerations for Current and investigantioanl drugs for HDV infection

- Treatment should be considered in all patients with compensated CHD and detectable HDV RNA.
- Durable virological response (HDV RNA undetectable) appears to be a surrogate marker of long-term benefit.
- BLV, entry inhibitor, received marketing authorization by the European Medical Agency in 2020, with around half of the patients achieving control of the disease (HDV RNA decline and normal ALT) at one year of therapy.
- Lonafarnib, an orally active farnesyltransferase inhibitor, is being evaluated in a large phase III study with more than 400 patients.
- A success in the HBV cure program (with HBs loss) will hopefully lead to HDV cure.

---

discontinuation could be considered in the rare case of HBsAg seroconversion for at least 6 months. BLV monotherapy may be considered as a long-term therapy, that is, maintenance therapy (as analogs for HBV infection).

BLV has also demonstrated similar early virological efficacy and favorable safety in real world-setting.[17,18]

Currently, BLV efficacy and safety are being assessed in at least three ongoing phase 2 and phase 3 clinical trials exploring different doses employed alone or in combination with PEG-IFN-α-2a (NCT02888106, NCT03852719, and NCT03852433). BLV is also being evaluated in several real life cohorts, among whom a French observational cohort (ANRS HDEP01 BuleDelta, NCT04166266) which is currently recruiting 400 patients for monitoring 48 weeks post-treatment. There remain open questions regarding BLV treatment: What is the optimal duration of treatment? Are there futility rules (when to stop treatment, specially in non responders ?) ? Should BLV be combined with PEG-IFN for selected patients ?

Lonafarnib

LNF inhibits the prenylation of HDV replication inside hepatocytes and blocks assembly through interaction with the large hepatitis delta antigen (L-HDAg).[19] Early studies demonstrated LNF efficacy in patients with CHD.[20,21]

The LNF with ritonavir for HDV-2 (LOWR-2) study's aim was to identify optimal combination regimens of LNF + ritonavir (RTV) $\pm$ PEG-IFNα for up to 24 weeks (NCT02430194).[22] Fifty-five patients with CHD were consecutively enrolled in an open-label, single-center, phase 2 dose-finding study. There were three main treatment groups: high-dose LNF (LNF $\geq$ 75 mg twice daily [bid] + RTV) (n = 19, 12 weeks); all-oral low-dose LNF (LNF 25 or 50 mg po bid + RTV) (n = 24, 24 weeks), and combination low-dose LNF with PEG-IFNα (LNF 25 or 50 mg po bid + RTV + PEG-IFNα) (n = 12, 24 weeks). The primary endpoint, $\geq$2 log$_{10}$ decline or < lower limit of quantification of HDV-RNA from baseline at end of treatment, was reached in 46% (6 of 13) and 89% (8 of 9) of patients receiving the all-oral regimen of LNF 50 mg bid + RTV, and combination regimens of LNF (25 or 50 mg bid) + RTV + PEG-IFNα, respectively. Furthermore, several patients experienced well-tolerated transient posttreatment ALT increases, resulting in HDV-RNA negativity and ALT normalization. The proportions of grade 2 and 3 gastrointestinal adverse events in the high-dose versus low-dose groups were 49% (37 of 76) and only 22% (18 of 81), respectively. Finally, LNF boosted with low-dose RTV, is a promising all-oral therapy, and maximal efficacy is achieved with PEG-IFNα addition.

In the LOWR-HDV 3, different doses of LNF (50, 75 or 100 mg/ritonavir 100 mg) were evaluated, once daily for 12 or 24 weeks.[21] LNF 50 mg/ritonavir was found superior compared to higher LNF doses. The LOWR-HDV 4 study is a dose-escalation/ maintenance up to LNF 100 mg BID/ritonavir 100 mg for 24-week study.[23]

To summarize, these studies demonstrated the antiviral effect of LNF, a dose-dependent anti-viral efficacy. RTV boosting allowed use of lower LNF doses, reducing side effects, mainly gastro-intestinal (nausea, vomiting, and diarrhea). In these early studies, the antiviral efficacy of LNF appears to be synergistic with PEG-IFNα.

An international, multi-center, phase 3 study of around 300 patients treated with LNF (with a total of 400 patients including controls) to evaluate an all-oral arm of LNF boosted with ritonavir and a combination arm of LNF boosted with ritonavir combined with PEG-IFNα, with each arm to be compared to a placebo arm (background HBV nucleos(t)ide only), in patients with CHD, is ongoing (The D-LIVR (Delta Liver Improvement and Virologic Response in HDV)) (NCT03719313).

Replicor, Rep2139

REP 2139-Ca is a nucleic acid polymer. It has been shown that nucleic acid polymers clear serum HBsAg both in duck HBV-infected ducks and in human patients and to act synergistically with PEG-IFN alpha 2a or thymosin alpha-1.[24,25]

The mode of action of REP 2139-Ca in removing serum HBsAg and its synergistic effect with PEG-IFN 2a is supposed to restore immunity and to induce the antiviral effect against HBV and HDV infection.[26] An increase in serum ALT was observed in many patients treated with REP 2139-Ca, and safety should be important to confirm in patients with cirrhosis. More clinical trials (increasing the number of patients) are needed to confirm efficacy and safety.

Pegylated-interferon lambda

PEG-IFNλ is a secreted cytokine which is close to the IL-10 cytokines family. PEG-IFNλ acts through ISG signaling pathways to induce antiviral activities.[27,28] The restricted expression of IFNλ receptor in a tissue-specific manner (mainly lung, liver and gut), leads to less systemic immune adverse events when compared to those caused by PEG-IFNα.[29]

An open-label study evaluated the safety and efficacy of PEG-IFNλ (120 or 180 mcg, administered once weekly by sc injections for 48 weeks) followed by 24 weeks of post-treatment follow-up in patients with CHD.[30] Thirty tree patients were allocated to PEG-IFNλ 180 mcg (n = 14) or 120 mcg (n = 19). Intention to treat rates of virologic response to Lambda 180 mcg and 120 mcg, 24 weeks following treatment cessation were 5 of 14(36%) and 3 of 19 (16%), respectively. Post-treatment response rate of 50% was seen in low BL viral load ($\leq$4 log10) on 180 mcg. Common on-treatment AEs included flu-like symptoms and elevated transaminase levels. Eight (24%) cases of hyperbilirubinemia with or without liver enzyme elevation, leading to drug discontinuation were mainly observed in the cohort from Pakistan. The clinical course was uneventful, and all responded favorably to dose reduction or discontinuation. In conclusion, PEG-IFNλ in patients with CHD may result in virologic response during and following treatment cessation.

An ongoing phase 3 clinical trial (LIMT-2, NCT05070364) has recruited patients in 13 countries for 48 weeks of treatment consisting of weekly sc injections of 180 µg of PEG-IFNλ. Also, a phase 2 study (NCT03600714) evaluated the safety and efficacy of combined treatment with lonafarnib, ritonavir, and IFNλ with promising results.

The hepatitis B virus cure strategy

The extraordinary revolution with direct-acting antivirals against HCV infection,[31] has led to important expectation for a cure to HBV.[32] A functional cure for HBV infection is defined as an HBs loss (with or without HBs antibodies).[33] Of course, a cure of HBV is associated with a cure of HDV. HBV drug development is promising with different molecules and different mode of actions including entry inhibitors; polymerase inhibitors; RNA silencers, capsid assembly modulators; and release inhibitors.[34–46] Several trials with the goal of an HBV cure will also include arms with patients with HDV infection.

How to improve screening?

There is a need to improve screening and linkage to care. The hepatitis D double reflex testing defined by anti-HDV testing of all hepatitis B surface antigen (HBsAg)-positive individuals and HDV RNA testing of all anti-HDV positive individuals could be a strategy to improve screening.[47] This strategy would need availabilities of diagnostic tests (HDV antibodies and RT-PCR) but also availabilities of therapeutics with efficacy and favorable tolerability. There is a lack worldwide of reliable and/or affordable tests for anti-HDV and HDV RNA. HDV RNA assays are needed to identify active HDV infection among those who test positive for anti-HDV, to monitor those with chronic hepatitis D, and to assess treatment response. These assays must be sensitive, specific, and provide reliable quantification regardless of HDV genotype and genetic diversity. They must be standardized, externally validated, and easily accessible.[48]

Who to treat ?

Because of the severity of chronic hepatitis D with high risk of cirrhosis and hepatocellular carcinoma,[49,50] treatment should be considered in all patients with chronic hepatitis D and active HDV replication (HDV RNA detectable). There is a debate whether all patients should be currently treated. There are recent data reporting patients with chronic hepatitis D and mild disease.[51] For patients, with mild disease, that is, with normal serum ALT, low HDV replication, and mild fibrosis, there may be no emergency to start treat, and treatment could be delayed with close monitoring (each 3–6 months). We may consider to better understand natural history, there might be patients with HDV infection (and no hepatitis) and a favorable outcome; and patients with CHD (hepatitis) with a risk of cirrhosis and HCC. Follow-up pf well phenotype prospective cohorts of patients will help to better describe natural history (similarly to HBV infection).

PEG-IFN is contra-indicated in patients with decompensated cirrhosis, and there are no data regarding BLV in these patients with Child-Pugh B or C. Several drugs and strategies are ongoing. Combining direct-acting antivirals and immune modulators might be an interesting perspective.

How to treat ?

PEG-IFN-α for patients with CHD, compensated liver disease and active replication, for a minimum of 48 weeks or more if tolerability is favorable, is recommended by several scientific societies. BLV has received a marketing authorization by EMA in 2020. BLV appears to be well tolerated with an antiviral efficacy that increases with the duration of treatment. Thus, BLV may be suitable for prolonged administration as a maintenance therapy. It should be noted that the best results, at least during the first year, have been obtained when BLV is combined with PEG-IFN. Whether combination with PEG-IFN will remain superior at long-term remains to be evaluated.

There is a need to define which patients may benefit more from the combination therapy and those who may benefit from the monotherapy. There is also a need to define futility rules and predict non response to stop therapy.

What are the endpoints for therapy?

In patients with CHD, persistent viremia has been associated with poor outcome, with mortality and morbidity, with decompensated cirrhosis and HCC.[52,53] At the opposite, durable virological response (HDV RNA undetectability during several years) has been associated with fibrosis regression[3] and favorable outcome.[11] Therefore a durable virological response may be considered as a surrogate marker of clinical efficacy (good prognosis).

Of course, the ideal endpoint of CHD treatment would be HBsAg loss, alike to the proposed definition for functional HBV cure.[33] However, since HBs loss is rarely obtained, a secondary important endpoint to achieve (surrogate marker of long-term benefit) would be a durable virological response (HDV RNA undetectable on the long-term).

The Food and Drug Administration (FDA) proposed that "drugs that are intended to be used as chronic suppressive therapy, a greater than or equal to 2-$\log_{10}$ decline in HDV-viral load and ALT normalization on-treatment could be considered an acceptable surrogate endpoint reasonably likely to predict clinical benefit".[54]

These endpoints need to be shown to be associated with clinical benefit, such as histologic improvement or decreased risk of cirrhosis, decompensation or HCC.[55] Furthermore, other endpoints and biomarkers, such as HDV RNA, should be definitely further investigated.

SHOULD WE USE ANALOGUES FOR HEPATITIS B VIRUS TREATMENT ?

Analogues have no effect for CHD, and therefore are not approved or recommended for the treatment.[8] HDV usually can reduce HBV replication. If a therapy is started to treat chronic hepatitis D, there is a risk of reactivations of the HBV following control of HDV. Therefore, tenofovir, entecavir or tenofovir alafenamide, have been added to HDV therapy to prevent possible reactivations of the HBV following control of HDV.

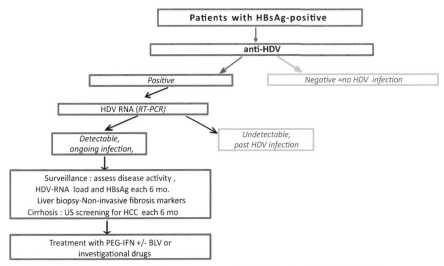

Fig. 1. An algorithm regarding the management of patients with HDV infection.

SUMMARY

The exact prevalence of HDV worldwide is unknown since diagnostic tests (serology and PCR) are not widely available. Not only HDV RNA testing is not widely available, but the sensitivity of many assays has not been evaluated and validated. HBV vaccination is the best preventive strategy to decrease HBV and HDV infections worldwide. HDV, when compared to HBV mono-infection, increases the risk of cirrhosis and HCC. PEG-IFN has been used so far, as off-label therapy, with moderate efficacy (around 10%–20%) and poor tolerability. BLV received marketing authorization by the EMA in 2020; preliminary data after 1 year of therapy indicate control of disease in more than half of the patients. An algorithm regarding the management of patients with HDV infection is proposed in **Fig. 1**. Other new drugs are investigated with the hope of a cure for CHD.

CLINICS CARE POINTS

- Developing rapid Point-of-Care Test for the serodiagnosis of HDV will be important to increase screening and diagnosis.

AUTHORS' CONTRIBUTIONS

T. Asselah prepared the article, contributed to the drafting of the article, the critical revision of the article, and its final approval.

CONFLICTS OF INTEREST

T. Asselah has acted as a speaker and/or advisor board and/or investigator for Antios, Eiger Biopharmaceutical, Enyo, Janssen, Gilead, GSK, Roche, and Vir Biotechnology.

REFERENCES

1. Di Bisceglie AM, Martin P, Lisker-Melman M, et al. Therapy of chronic delta hepatitis with interferon alfa-2b. J Hepatol 1990;11(Suppl 1):S151–4.
2. Farci P, Mandas A, Coiana A, et al. Treatment of chronic hepatitis D with interferon alfa-2a. N Engl J Med 1994;330(2):88–94.
3. Farci P, Roskams T, Chessa L, et al. Long-term benefit of interferon alpha therapy of chronic hepatitis D: regression of advanced hepatic fibrosis. Gastroenterology 2004;126:1740–9.
4. European Association for the Study of the Liver. Clinical practice guidelines Manag. Hepatitis B virus infection. J Hepatol 2017;67:370–98.
5. Terrault NA, Lok ASF, McMahon BJ, et al. Update on prevention, diagnosis, and treatment of chronic hepatitis B: AASLD 2018 hepatitis B guidance. Hepatology 2018;67:1560–99.
6. Sarin SK, Kumar M, Lau GK, et al. Asian- Pacific clinical practice guidelines on the management of hepatitis B: a 2015 update. Hepatol. Int. 2016;10:1–98.
7. Castelnau C, Le Gal F, Ripault M-P, et al. Efficacy of peginterferon alpha-2b in chronic hepatitis delta: relevance of quantitative RT- PCR for follow-up. Hepatology 2006;44:728–35.
8. Heidrich B, Yurdaydin C, Kabacam G, et al. HIDIT-1 Study Group, Late HDV RNA relapse after peginterferon alpha-based therapy of chronic hepatitis delta. Hepatology 2014;60:87–97.

9. Wedemeyer H, Yurdaydin C, Hardtke S, et al. HIDIT-II study team. Peginterferon alfa-2a plus tenofovir disoproxil fumarate for hepatitis D (HIDIT-II): a randomised, placebo controlled, phase 2 trial. Lancet Infect Dis 2019;19:275–86.

10. Loureiro D, Castelnau C, Tout I, et al. New therapies for hepatitis delta virus infection. Liver Int 2021;41(S1):30–7.

11. Heller T, Rotman Y, Koh C, et al. Long-term therapy of chronic delta hepatitis with peginterferon alfa. Aliment Pharmacol Ther 2014;40:93–104.

12. Yan H, Zhong G, Xu G, et al. Sodium taurocholate cotransporting polypeptide is a functional receptor for human hepatitis B and D virus. Elife 2012;1:e00049.

13. Ni Y, Lempp FA, Mehrle S, et al. Hepatitis B and D viruses exploit sodium taurocholate co-transporting polypeptide for species-specific entry into hepatocytes. Gastroenterology 2014;146:1070–83.

14. Wedemeyer H, Bogomolov P, Blank A, et al. Final results of a mul-ticenter, open-label phase 2b clinical trial to assess safety and efficacy of Myrcludex B in combination with tenofovir in patients with chronic HBV/HDV co-infection. J Hepatol 2018;68:S3.

15. Bogomolov P, Alexandrov A, Voronkova N, et al. Treatment of chronic hepatitis D with the entry inhibitor myrcludex B: first results of a phase Ib/IIa study. J Hepatol 2016;65:490–8.

16. European Medicines Agency https://www.ema.europa.eu/en/medicines/human/EPAR/hepcludex, Accessed April 15, 2021.

17. Lampertico P, Roulot D, Wedemeyer H. Bulevirtide with or without pegIFNα for patients with compensated chronic hepatitis delta: from clinical trials to real-world studies. J Hepatol 2022;77:1422–30.

18. Asselah T, Loureiro D, Le Gal F, et al. Early virological response in six patients with hepatitis D virus infection and compensated cirrhosis treated with Bulevirtide in real-life. Liver Int 2021;41(7):1509–17.

19. Glenn JS, Watson JA, Havel CM, et al. Identification of a prenylation site in delta virus large antigen. Science 1992;256:1331–3.

20. Koh C, Canini L, Dahari H, et al. Oral prenylation inhibition with lonafarnib in chronic hepatitis D infection: a proof-of-concept randomised, double-blind, placebo-controlled phase 2A trial. Lancet Infect Dis 2015;15:1167–74.

21. Yurdaydin C, Keskin O, Kalkan C, et al. Optimizing lonafarnib treatment for the management of chronic delta hepatitis: the LOWR HDV-1 study. Hepatology 2018;67:1224–36.

22. Yurdaydin C, Keskin O, Yurdcu E, et al. A phase 2 dose-finding study of lonafarnib and ritonavir with or without interferon alpha for chronic delta hepatitis. Hepatology 2022;75(6):1551–65.

23. Wedemeyer H, Port K, Deterding K, et al. PS-039 – a phase 2 dose- escalation study of lonafarnib plus ritonavir in patients with chronic hepatitis D: final results from the lonafarnib with ritonavir in HDV-4 (LOWR HDV-4) study. J Hepatol 2017;66(S24).

24. Quinet J, Jamard C, Burtin M, et al. Nucleic acid polymer REP 2139 and nucleos(T)ide analogues act synergistically against chronic hepadnaviral infection in vivo in Pekin ducks. Hepatology 2018;67:2127–40.

25. Bazinet M, Pantea V, Cebotarescu V, et al. Safety and efficacy of REP 2139 and pegylated interferon alfa-2a for treatment-naive patients with chronic hepatitis B virus and hepatitis D virus co- infection (REP 301 and REP 301-LTF): a non-randomised, open- label, phase 2 trial. Lancet Gastroenterol Hepatol 2017;2:877–89.

26. Bazinet M, Pantea V, Cebotarescu V, et al. Persistent control of hepatitis B virus and hepatitis delta virus infection following REP 2139-Ca and pegylated interferon therapy in chronic hep- atitis B virus/hepatitis delta virus coinfection. Hepatol Commun 2021;5:189–2022.

27. Kotenko SV, Gallagher G, Baurin VV, et al. IFN-lambdas mediate antiviral protection through a distinct class II cytokine receptor complex. Nat Immunol 2003;4:69–77.

28. Sheppard P, Kindsvogel W, Xu W, et al. IL-28, IL-29 and their class II cytokine receptor IL-28R. Nat Immunol 2003;4:63–8.

29. Lasfar A, Zloza A, Cohen-Solal KA. IFN-lambda therapy: current status and future perspectives. Drug Discov Today 2016;21:167–71.

30. Etzion O, Hamid S, Lurie Y, et al. Treatment of chronic hepatitis d with peginterferon lambda - the phase 2 LIMT-1 clinical trial. Hepatology 2023. https://doi.org/10.1097/HEP.0000000000000309. NCT02765802).

31. Asselah T, Marcellin P, Schinazi RF. Treatment of hepatitis C virus infection with direct-acting antiviral agents: 100% cure? Liver Int 2018;38(Suppl 1):7–13.

32. Asselah T, Loureiro D, Boyer N, et al. Targets and future direct-acting antiviral approaches to achieve hepatitis B virus cure. Lancet Gastroenterol Hepatol 2019;4:883–92.

33. Tout I, Loureiro D, Mansouri A, et al. Hepatitis B surface antigen seroclearance: immune mechanisms, clinical impact, importance for drug development. J Hepatol 2020;73:409–22.

34. Janssen HLA, Hou J, Asselah T, et al. Randomised phase 2 study (JADE) of the HBV capsid assembly modulator JNJ-56136379 with or without a nucleos(t)ide analogue in patients with chronic hepatitis B infection. Gut 2023;2022–328041.

35. Gish RG, Asselah T, Squires K, et al. Active site polymerase inhibitor nucleotides (ASPINs): Potential agents for chronic HBV cure regimens. Antivir Chem Chemother 2022;30. 20402066221138705.

36. Daffis S, Balsitisc S, Chamberlain J, et al. Toll-like receptor 8 agonist GS-9688 induces sustained efficacy in the woodchuck model of chronic hepatitis B. Hepatology 2021;73:53–67.

37. Luk A, Jiang Q, Glavini K, et al. A single and multiple ascending dose study of toll-like receptor 7 agonist (RO7020531) in Chinese healthy volunteers. Clin Transl Sci 2020;13:985–93.

38. Bertoletti A, Tan AT. HBV as a target for CAR or TCR T cell therapy. Curr Opin Immunol 2020;66:35–41.

39. Gane E, Verdon DJ, Brooks AE, et al. Anti-PD-1blockade with nivolumab with and without therapeutic vaccination for virally sup- pressed chronic hepatitis B: a pilot study. J Hepatol 2019;71:900–7.

40. Schinazi RF, Ehteshami M, Bassit L, et al. Towards HBV cura- tive therapies. Liver Int 2018;38(Suppl 1):102–14.

41. Hoogeveen RH, Boonstra A. Checkpoint inhibitors and therapeutic vaccines for the treatment of chronic HBV infection. Front Immunol 2020;401:1–9.

42. Gane E, Locarnini S, Lim TH, et al. Short interfering RNA JNJ-3989 combination therapy in chronic hepatitis B shows potent reduction of all viral markers but no correlate was identified for HBsAg reduc- tion and baseline factors. J Hepatol 2021;75:S289.

43. Squires KE, Mayers DL, Bluemling GR, et al. ATI-2173, a novel liver-targeted non-chain-terminating nucleotide for hepatitis B virus cure regimens. Antimicrob Agents Chemother 2020;64(9). 008366-e920.

44. Yuen MF, Lim SG, Plesniak R, et al. Efficacy and safety of bepiro- virsen in chronic hepatitis B infection. N Engl J Med 2022;387:1957–68.
45. Gane E, Lim YS, Cloutier D, et al. Safety and antiviral activity of VIR- 2218, an X-targeting RNAi therapeutic, in participants with chronic hepatitis B infection: week 48 follow-up results. J Hepatol 2021;75:S287.
46. Yuen MF, Lim YS, Cloutier D, et al. Preliminary results from a phase 2 study evaluating VIR-2218 alone and in combination with pegylated interferon alfa-2a in participants with chronic hepatitis B infection. Hepatology 2021;74:63A.
47. Polaris Observatory Collaborators. Hepatitis D double reflex testing of all hepatitis B carriers in low HBV and high HBV/high HDV prevalence countries. J Hepatol 2023. S0168-8278(23)00206-214.
48. Le Gal F, Brichler S, Sahli R, et al. First international external quality assessment for hepatitis delta virus RNA quantification in plasma. Hepatology 2016;64(5): 1483–94.
49. Fattovich G, Giustina G, Christensen E, et al. Influence of hepatitis delta virus infection on morbidity and mortality in compensated cirrhosis type B. Gut 2000; 46:420–6.
50. Alfaiate D, Clément S, Gomes D, et al. Chronic hepatitis D and hepatocellular carcinoma: a systematic review and meta-analysis of observational studies. J Hepatol 2020;73:533–9.
51. Kamal H, Westman G, Falconer K, et al. Long-term study of hepatitis delta virus infection at secondary care centers: the impact of viremia on liver-Related outcomes. Hepatology 2020;72:1177–90.
52. Roulot D, Brichler S, Layese R, et al. Origin, HDV genotype and persistent viremia determine outcome and treatment response in patients with chronic hepatitis delta. J Hepatol 2020;73(5):1046–62.
53. Palom A, Rodríguez-Tajes S, Navascués CA, et al. Long-term clinical outcomes in patients with chronic hepatitis delta: the role of persistent viraemia. Aliment Pharmacol Ther 2020;51:158–66.
54. Food and Drug Administration (FDA). Chronic hepatitis D virus infection: developing drugs for treatment. Guidance for Industry 2019;84. FR 58724:58724–6.
55. Lok AS, Negro F, Asselah T, et al. Endpoints and new options for treatment of chronic hepatitis D. Hepatology 2021;74(6):3479–85.

Back to "B"

Test All for Hepatitis B Virus

Link to Care and Treatment if Quantitative DNA Positive, Vaccinate if Susceptible

Katerina Roma, DO[a,*], Zahra Dossaji, DO[a], Lubaba Haque, DO[a],
Tooba Laeeq, MD[a], Robert G. Gish, MD[b,1], Carol Brosgart, MD[c,2]

KEYWORDS

- Hepatitis B virus • Triple panel testing • Linkage to care • Emerging therapies
- HBV treatment

KEY POINTS

- Test all adults with a "triple panel": HBsAg, anti-HBc antibody, anti-HBs antibody.
- Vaccinate all adults who are triple panel negative.
- If HBsAg-positive, follow up with qDNA and anti-HDV testing.
- Treat all HBV-DNA-positive patients including those with cirrhosis. Treat until HBsAg loss +12 months consolidation.
- Surveillance for HCC and treatment of concomitant liver disease (ie, MAFLD, MASH, HDV, HCV).

INTRODUCTION

The hepatitis B virus (HBV) affects an estimated 262 million individuals worldwide and is responsible for approximately 900,000 deaths annually, mostly from complications of cirrhosis and hepatocellular carcinoma (HCC).[1] In 2018, it was estimated that 1.47 million foreign-born people in the United States had chronic HBV infection.[2] This has increased from estimated 1.32 million in 2009.[3] We currently are not projected to meet the World Health Organization (WHO) goal to eliminate HBV as a health threat by 2030. By improving awareness, diagnosis, and treatment of those

[a] Internal Medicine, Kirk Kerkorian School of Medicine at the University of Nevada, 1701 West Charleston Boulevard - Suite 230, Las Vegas, NV 89102, USA; [b] Hepatitis B Foundation, Doylestown, PA, USA; [c] Medicine, Biostatistics, and Epidemiology, University of California San Francisco, San Francisco, CA, USA
[1] Present address: 6022 La Jolla Mesa Drive, San Diego, CA 92037.
[2] Present address: 3133 Lewiston Avenue, Berkeley, CA 94705.
* Corresponding author.
E-mail address: Katerinaromado@gmail.com

Clin Liver Dis 27 (2023) 997–1022
https://doi.org/10.1016/j.cld.2023.05.009
1089-3261/23/© 2023 Elsevier Inc. All rights reserved.
liver.theclinics.com

with HBV, we can reduce stigma and discrimination due to HBV infection, improve quality of life, decrease extrahepatic manifestations of HBV, reduce infectivity, and decrease incidences of cirrhosis, HCC and other cancers, liver transplant, and death due to HBV.

Unfortunately, only 1% to 10% achieve functional cure with antiviral treatment.[4] HBV cure remains difficult to achieve because of the persistence of covalently closed circular DNA (cccDNA), HBV-DNA integration into the host genome, and impaired immune response.[5] It was previously believed that chronic hepatitis infection progressed through immune-tolerant, immune-reactive, and inactive carrier; however, these terms have become obsolete, as shown in **Table 1**.

In terms of HBV testing, southern blotting is regarded as the gold standard for quantitative cccDNA detection; however, given its complexity, it is not deemed suitable for screening. Polymerase chain reaction (PCR)-based methods, invader assays, in situ hybridization, and surrogate markers have proven to be more sensitive for cccDNA detection.[6] Although advances in serology and viral nucleic acid testing over the last decades significantly reduced the risk of transfusion-transmitted HBV, there is still a residual risk to recipients from those blood donors with extremely low viral DNA levels.[7]

Despite the advancement in technology, occult hepatitis B infection (OBI) has been a medical concern during the last decade.[8,9] This is due to the fact that the standard lower limit of detection (LLOD) for HBV-DNA is 5 IU/mL or 30 copies/mL.[9] Luckily, target amplification assays, such as the real-time PCR assay or the transcription-based mediated amplification assay, make it possible to detect quantities of less than 5 IU/mL of HBV-DNA and are rapidly approaching the level of a single HBV genome.[9] Another emerging concern is HBV reactivation associated with immune-suppressive and biological therapies. This is touted to be an important cause of morbidity and mortality in patients with chronic HBV (CHB) infection.[10] HBV reactivation generally occurs in overt or occult HBV infection with chemotherapy or immuno-suppressive therapy.[11]

In the setting of progression of the disease with untreated chronic HBV infection, OBI, high rates of HBV reactivation, and increased transmission via solid organ transplant and transfusions, it has become imperative to test all patients for HBV and to treat all who are HBV-DNA positive. Testing only those with known or admitted risk factors, including country of origin, has failed dismally and does not identify all patients with chronic HBV. This chapter further sheds light on the emerging concerns, ongoing efforts to curb the spread, linkage to care, treating all who are HBV-DNA positive, and introduce a 5-line guideline for HBV (**Box 1**).

Table 1
Terminologies for chronic HBV infection

Old Terminology	New Terminology	Characteristics
Immune-tolerant phase	HBeAg-positive chronic infection	HBeAg+, normal Liver enzymes, high HBV-DNA
Immune-reactive phase	HBeAg-positive chronic infection	HBeAg+, abnormal enzymes, high HBV-DNA
Inactive carrier phase	HBeAg-negative chronic infection	HBeAg−, normal liver enzymes, HBV-DNA < 2000 IU/mL

Abbreviations: HBeAg, hepatitis B e antigen; HBV, hepatitis B virus; HBV-DNA, hepatitis B virus-DNA; LFTs, liver function tests.

> **Box 1**
> **The 5-line guidelines for HBV in adults**
>
> - Test all adults with HBV triple panel: HBsAg, anti-HBc antibody, anti-HBs antibody.
> - Vaccinate all adults who are triple panel negative.
> - If HBsAg-positive, follow-up with qDNA and anti-HDV testing.
> - Treat all HBV-DNA-positive patients including those with cirrhosis (treat until HBsAg loss +12 months consolidation).
> - Surveillance for HCC and treatment of concomitant liver disease (ie, MAFLD, MASH, HDV, HCV).
>
> *Abbreviations:* HBsAg, hepatitis B surface antigen; HBV, hepatitis B virus; HCC, hepatocellular carcinoma; HDV, hepatitis delta virus; MAFLD, metabolic-associated fatty liver disease; MASH, metabolic-associated steatohepatitis; qDNA, quantitative DNA.

DISCUSSION
Test All Patients with a "Triple Hepatitis B Virus Panel": Hepatitis B Surface Antigen, Total Antibody to Hepatitis B Core Antigen, Hepatitis B Surface Antibody

There are many factors that underly the importance of testing all individuals for HBV infection. Traditionally, only those with a high risk for acquiring the infection were tested. This risk-based screening involved those from high and intermediate endemic areas, men who have sex with men, injection drug users, people with multiple sexual partners, those with a history of sexually transmitted infections, correctional facility inmates, pregnant women, and more.[12] Given the many modes of transmission, limited questioning by practitioners regarding risk for HBV (creating bias against individuals with high risk), stigmatization reducing the number of patients who might answer the risk questions, continued high prevalence of the disease both globally and domestically within the United States, and the mortality associated with untreated infection, it has become clear that testing all individuals for HBV is paramount. Furthermore, many believe that they were vaccinated as children; however, infant immunization did not begin in the United States until 1991.[13] Other indications for testing all adults include the potential to reverse liver disease progression with early detection, early counseling to help manage disease burden, and the possibility of detecting HCC at a treatable stage. The most recent morbidity and mortality weekly report (MMWR) published by the Centers for Disease Control and Prevention (CDC) recommends that HBV testing should be routinely performed.[14]

There is also a growing concern about a global comorbidity, the prevalence of nonalcoholic fatty liver disease (NAFLD), now called metabolic (dysfunction)-associated fatty liver disease (MAFLD) in over 60 countries, nonalcoholic steatohepatitis (NASH), now called metabolic-associated steatohepatitis (MASH), as they are becoming the most frequent causes of chronic liver disease and cirrhosis.[15] The old terminology NAFLD is a diagnosis of exclusion, thus difficult to diagnose and has caused stigmatization. International panel experts state that NAFLD does not reflect current knowledge and that MAFLD is more an appropriate term.[15] MAFLD is prevalent in about 25% of the population in western countries and 30% in the Asia Pacific region.[16] MAFLD is due to insulin resistance and related metabolic dysfunction with or without secondary cause. These secondary cause(s) include alcohol consumption, viral hepatitis (such as HBV and hepatitis C virus [HCV]), pregnancy, medication-induced, and/or genetic disorder. If there is significant steatohepatitis, at a histological level, then MAFLD can be named MASH.[15,17] MAFLD and MASH prevalence is increasing due to the growth of sedentary lifestyles, diabetes, and obesity. In addition, fatty liver can increase the risk of HCC up to 27%.[18] Because it can be exacerbated by viral hepatitis (HBV and HCV), it is becoming more important to test all for HBV with a triple panel. Indeed, HBV now like HIV and HCV has the recommendation for routine testing for adults, by the CDC.[14]

Triple-panel testing, which includes hepatitis B surface antigen (HBsAg), anti-HBc, and anti-HBs, is the best way to test individuals for HBV infection exposure and vaccine-induced immunity or the need for vaccination. Positivity for HBsAg indicates an active HBV infection, and positive anti-HBc indicates exposure to HBV. This should automatically prompt providers to test these patients for hepatitis delta virus (HDV) co-infection, as well as a quantitative HBV-DNA level (**Fig. 1**). HDV is only present in those with coexistent HBV infection. If HBsAg and HBV-DNA is positive, then this indicates a chronic infection and that the host could not mount the appropriate immune response to cease and control viral replication.[19] Notably, in HBV, HBsAg is usually present for up to 6 months after acute infection[20]; therefore, it is not considered a chronic infection, unless HBsAg is present beyond the 6 months after an acute infection.

For those who are HBV-DNA positive, reversing liver disease progression is often done with the help of oral antiviral treatment, such as entecavir, tenofovir disoproxil fumarate (TDF), or tenofovir alafenamide fumarate (TAF). Interferon is rarely used today. Adequate treatment can significantly suppress HBV replication and prevent progression of the disease to HCC, liver cirrhosis, or liver failure.[21] Early counseling of patients who test positive for infection can prevent complications of the infection.

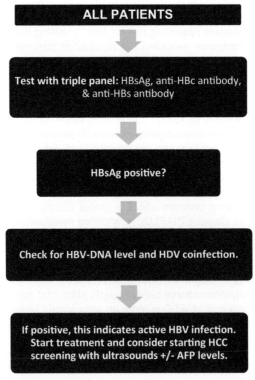

Fig. 1. Summary of recommendations for testing and treatment of HBV. FP, alpha-fetoprotein; HBsAg, hepatitis B surface antigen; HBV, hepatitis B virus; HBV-DNA, hepatitis B virus-DNA; HCC, hepatocellular carcinoma; HDV, hepatitis delta virus.

Oftentimes, routine interventions include vaccinating these individuals with the hepatitis A vaccine, routine screening for coinfections (HDV, HIV, and/or HCV), encouraging decreased alcohol consumption, and minimizing the progression to MAFLD, by managing HTN, diabetes, and hyperlipidemia.[21] HCC is often associated with chronic, untreated HBV infection and is amplified by abundant alcohol use. It is crucial that anyone who is HBsAg-positive to get surveyed routinely for HCC if they meet risk groups. The AASLD recommends monitoring with an ultrasound with or without quantitative alpha-fetoprotein (AFP) measurement every 6 months.[21] This further reinforces the idea of why testing everyone in the general population is imperative.

OBI (occult hepatitis B infection), also known as persistent HBV infection, is described as serum-negative HBsAg despite having serum-positive HBV-DNA (**Table 2**). This is due to the presence of cccDNA and integrated viral DNA in hepatocytes.[20] Those with OBI also tend to have antibodies positive for anti-HBc, but rarely anti-HBs.[19] In addition, hepatitis B core antigen (HBcAg) is often positive, indicating active viral replication. This infection is often difficult to detect because it is often only established in specific conditions and settings[22] and because the gold standard involves detection of HBV genomes in liver DNA samples.[23] The diagnosis also depends on the sensitivity of testing used to detect HBsAg and HBV-DNA; the LLOD often varies from laboratory to laboratory, so this is often varying without standardization especially with HBV DNA.[23] The HBV vaccine booster is not recommended in these patients. It is recommended to also keep a watchful eye on those with OBI as reactivation of the virus is possible, especially if they have comorbidities such as solid or hematologic malignancies, autoimmune diseases, or organ transplantation.[20] And, if they are undergoing the associated therapies for malignancies, autoimmune diseases, and organ transplantation, it is crucial to educate these patients on the possibility of reactivation and be aware of the signs and symptoms of reactivation (eg, nausea, vomiting, abdominal pain, jaundice). Reactivation due to immunosuppressants is dependent on doses, duration, and administration routes (**Table 3**).

OBI prevalence varies from country to country. However, it is to be noted that high-risk groups, such as people who inject drugs or those with HIV coinfections, have a higher prevalence.[23] If patients are seropositive for anti-HBs antibody, anti-HBc antibody with or without the presence of an HBsAg, and low levels of HBV-DNA, this typically indicates immune control. The phrase "immune control" typically refers to seroclearance of the HBsAg in a patient with acquired HBV. Despite the clearance of HBsAg, these patients can have low levels of HBV-DNA in their bloodstream. Although HBsAg is not in the bloodstream, this phase is still considered infectious.[29] If anti-HBc antibodies are negative but anti-HB antibodies are positive, this indicates vaccine immunity (see **Table 2**). As demonstrated, testing for 3 markers conjunctively in a triple panel provides useful information in directing management therapies.

Reasons to Treat

Stigma reduction and improvement of quality of life
Health-related stigma surrounding HBV infection is prevalent in several communities (**Table 4**). In societal groups, stigma often manifests in the form of status loss within societal groups, resulting in stigma, discrimination, alienation, and ostracization. Misconceptions about the disease are driven by misunderstanding about disease transmission, fear of the virus itself, and association of the disease with sexual promiscuity and other risky behaviors.[30] Social stigma is a barrier both to HBV testing and to obtaining HBV treatment. In addition, stigma can come from the patient themselves (self-stigma). Many who are suffering from chronic HBV infection blame themselves, leading to isolation, depression, self-hatred, and avoidance of diagnosis and

Table 2
Hepatitis B and D serology markers[20,24]

HBV Status	HBsAg	HBcAg	Anti-HBs Antibody	Anti-HBc Antibody (IgM)	Anti-HBc Antibody (IgG)	HBeAg	Anti-HBe Antibody	HBV-DNA	HDAg	Anti-HDV Antibody (IgM)	Anti-HDV Antibody (IgG)	HDV-RNA
OBI	-	+	+/-	+/-	-	+/-	+/-	+/-	-	-	-	-
Vaccine immunity	-	-	+	-	-	-	-	-	-	-	-	-
Immune-controlled	-	-	+	-	+	-	+/-	+ (low)	-	-	-	-
Chronic infection	+	+	-	-	+	+/-	+/-	+	-	-	-	-
Acute HBV/HDV coinfection	+/-	+	+/-	+/-	+	+	+/-	+	+ (early)	+/-	+ (late, low)	+/-
Acute HBV/HDV superinfection	+	+	-	+/-	+	+	+/-	+	+ (early)	+	+ (late)	+
Chronic HDV	-	-	-	-	-	-	-	-	+	+	+	+

Abbreviations: HBcAg, hepatitis B core antigen; HBeAg, hepatitis B e antigen; HBsAg, hepatitis B surface antigen; HBV, hepatitis B virus; HBV-DNA, hepatitis B virus-DNA; HDV, hepatitis delta virus; IgG, immunoglobulin G; IgM, immunoglobulin M; OBI, occult HBV infection.

Table 3
Immunosuppressants and reactivation rates[25–28]

Medications	Reactivation Rates
Azathioprine Mercaptopurine Methotrexate Systemic corticosteroids (low dose, <1 wk) Intra-articular steroids	<1%
Infliximab Etanercept Adalimumab Ustekinumab Natalizumab Imatinib Nilotinib	1%–10%
Inhaled corticosteroids	3.2%
Rituximab Systemic corticosteroid (≥20 mg, ≥4 wk)	>10%

treatment. Reducing stereotypes and preconceived notions about HBV is imperative in ensuring that individuals get tested and acquire the proper treatment.

Patient-reported outcomes (PROs) measure and assesses the patient's perception of the status of their health condition without interpretation from a health professional. This encourages the patient to assess their disease severity, symptomatic presentation, and its impact on self-sufficiency and overall quality of life (QoL).[31] A commonly used PRO is the Chronic Liver Disease Questionnaire (CLDQ)-HBV.[32] Another questionnaire is called the Short Form-36 (SF-36).[33] In a recent article, Younossi and colleagues explored PROs with the CLDQ-HBV, SF-36, and a third questionnaire. It found that PROs appeared to be much improved with treatment when compared to without treatment as patients enjoyed a higher health-related QoL with lower HBV-DNA

Table 4
Reasons to treat HBV

Stigma reduction and improvement of quality of life	Increased awareness and treatment can reduce stigma (societal and self) and improve the quality of life
Infection reduction	Treatment can reduce the number of people who are infectious and therefore reduce the spread of the infection.
Cirrhosis and HCC prevention	Treatment can decrease the rapid progression of the disease and subsequent development of HCC.
Extrahepatic manifestation reduction	Treatment can reduce extrahepatic manifestations, which is linked to elevated HBsAg levels and immune complexes.
WHO HBV elimination	We currently are not projected to meet the WHO goal to eliminate HBV as a health threat by 2030.
Death	Treatment can reduce deaths due to HBV infection.

Abbreviations: HBsAg, hepatitis B surface antigen; HBV, hepatitis B virus; HCC, hepatocellular carcinoma; WHO, World Health Organization.

levels.[34] Therefore, it is important to identify those who are susceptible and treat all who are HBV-DNA positive.

Reducing spread of infection

HBV is actually considered 50 to 100 times more infectious than HIV.[35] There are several high-risk subgroups, including veterans, men who have sex with men, prisoners, people who inject drugs, patients with HCV and/or HIV coinfections, health care professionals, and homeless individuals.[36] Estimates for the percentage of incarcerated individuals with seropositivity for HBsAg ranges from 0.9% to 11.4%.[37] Other special, high-risk groups include pregnant women, newborns, and people with diabetes.[36] Transmission from mother to newborn remains one of the most important and preventable sources of HBV infection despite the availability of vaccination. Focused strategies on testing everyone with the triple panel can assist in identifying individuals that need to be treated and reduce the spread of infection.

Decreasing rates of liver cirrhosis, liver transplant, hepatocellular carcinoma, and death

Liver cirrhosis and HCC remain some of the most dreaded complications of HBV. Cirrhosis is a leading cause of morbidity and mortality, accounting for approximately 2.2% of deaths across the globe, with viral hepatitis being its leading cause.[38] With the increase in MAFLD and MASH, globally and domestically, it is growing as one of the risk factors for HBV-related cirrhosis.[18] HCC is known as the most common type of liver malignancy globally, composing about 75% of all liver cancers.[39] About 10% to 25% of HBV carriers have a lifetime risk of developing HCC[39]; and 29% of cirrhotic patients are HBV carriers.[38] Oftentimes, the prevalence of both HCC and liver cirrhosis is concurrent and represents an overall picture of poor prognosis.

Several randomized controlled trials have shown that antivirals, specifically nucleos(t)ide analogs (NAs), can achieve a significant decrease in HBV-DNA levels. Thus, these drugs can work to improve liver function and histology.[39] Given the positive change in hepatocellular architecture and functionality, as well as the consequent reduction in disease prevalence that is attainable with induction of antivirals, the treatment of HBV becomes even more important. Two people die every minute of HBV, and this has not changed in over 20 years and with greater than 20 editions of various medical professional liver and infectious disease association HBV treatment guidelines. Unfortunately, unlike the current HCV curative therapy, current treatment for HBV is long term or life long as most patients with chronic HBV do not clear the infection with available therapies.

Lowering the presence of extrahepatic manifestations

Extrahepatic manifestations are experienced in approximately 20% of those with HBV infection.[40] These manifestations can involve many different organ systems and categories, including renal, cardiovascular, musculoskeletal, dermatologic, and autoimmune, or they can be systemic. Common renal manifestations include glomerulopathies, such as membranous nephropathy and membranoproliferative glomerulonephritis (MPGN).[41] Cardiovascular, musculoskeletal, and autoimmune manifestations are often localized to the vasculature and include cryoglobulinemic vasculitis, polyarteritis nodosa (PAN), serum sickness-like syndrome, and nonrheumatoid arthritis.[41] Dermatologic manifestations include skin rashes and popular acrodermatitis.[42] Systemic manifestations include non-Hodgkin lymphoma.[43]

Extrahepatic syndromes have been linked to increased serum HBsAg levels and immune complexes that it creates. This can lead to more frequent doctor visits and hospitalizations, diagnostic tests, and life-long treatment, contributing to poor QoL. There are several studies that have shown treatment of HBV with antivirals can lead to complete resolution of the extrahepatic manifestation[40] due to the decrease in the HBsAg levels. This further highlights the need to treat all who are HBV-DNA positive.

Diminishing the death toll

Chronic HBV infection results in approximately 47% of all deaths in relation to viral hepatitis[44] with a majority of deaths secondary to HCC and progressive liver cirrhosis.[33] By treating those who are HBV-DNA positive, the rates of liver progression to cirrhosis and development of HCC can be halted.

Linkage to Care

Although the World Health Organization (WHO) committed to eliminating viral hepatitis (B and C) as a public health threat by 2030, hepatitis B models showed that no country is on track to achieve all HBV targets by 2030 or even by 2050.[45] HBV elimination strategies will need to focus on effective and implementable preventive and therapeutic strategies. These include upscaling HBV birth-dose vaccination, full HBV vaccine coverage of adults, vaccination of everyone who is susceptible, prevention of mother-to-child transmission, identification of all HBV-infected individuals (by changing the recommendations to test all routinely for HBV, not just those with known risk factors), and improving linkage to care for those who have chronic HBV.[46] What we can do today is treat all HBV-DNA positive to decrease infectivity and also HCC risk, starting with routine HBV screening as recommended by the recent *MMWR*.[14]

Public health interventions can increase HBV testing rates, diagnosis, treatment rates, and access to care. Many individuals worldwide are not aware of their HBV serological status. Even in those who are aware of their HBV status, access to clinical service coverage might be limited.[47] Access to screening and treatment is currently fraught with challenges in both the developed and developing world. For example, the shortage of liver specialists is exacerbated in low- and middle-income countries. In high-income countries with a large number of specialists, they are often located at the tertiary centers in major cities.[48] Another concern is treatment of HBV being limited to specialists, creating more barrier to access. There is not enough hepatologists and infectious disease physicians domestically or globally to treat all with HBV. There has been success in improving diagnosis and treatment of HIV and HCV in the community with the training of local primary care physicians, nurse practitioners, and physician assistants.[49,50] Therefore, awareness and education among primary care providers, nurse practitioners, and physician assistants regarding treatment of HBV will be crucial in terms of expanding care for HBV.

Widespread screening is needed to link the infected population to care and therefore decrease the possible consequences of untreated infection, including liver cancer, cirrhosis, and death.[51] A success story for widespread screening is the San Francisco Hep B Free Campaign. It used a unique health communication strategy to break the silence and normalize discussions about HBV[52] with foreign-born Asians and Pacific Islanders with chronic HBV. It promoted the use of the existing health care system for HBV screening and follow-up, raised $1,000,000 in resources, and established follow-up for 6.5% of patients with chronic HBV-infections.[53]

Based on the surveys about HBV programs, 17 countries (30%) had governments with the strongest political will to eliminate HBV, and 30 countries (51%) had top scores for financing their national HBV programs.[45] Evidently more effort is needed in this arena by countries to aid in developing an HBV-free world. Countries need to put substantial effort in funding HBV elimination programs to access and implement comprehensive strategies for vaccination of all susceptible adults and diagnosis and linkage to care for all with chronic HBV.[54] Domestic and global efforts should focus on improving awareness, decreasing discrimination and stigma, training primary care providers, financial resources, political will and commitment, vaccination drives, affordability of care, systematic screening, and referral programs.

Treat All Who Are Hepatitis B Virus-DNA-Positive

HBV infections are a major cause of chronic hepatitis, cirrhosis, and HCC worldwide. In up to 30% and 53% of patients, cirrhosis and HCC are due to HBV, respectively.[55] About 15% to 40% of patients with chronic HBV will develop liver cirrhosis, liver failure with a mortality rate of more than 820,000 deaths per year.[36,55–63] The persistence of chronic HBV infection and hepatitis is due to cccDNA64. cccDNA is a template to viral RNAs and virions64. Unfortunately, the cccDNA is not targeted by current treatments and a cure for chronic HBV will require elimination of cccDNA.[64,65] Therefore, the current treatment goals are to achieve HBV-DNA suppression to undetectable levels and HBsAg loss or HBsAg seroconversion (ie, functional cure).

A longitudinal study of patients with chronic HBV found that baseline HBV-DNA plus RNA was most positively correlated with cccDNA than HBsAg, HBV-RNA alone, HBV-DNA alone, HBV-RNA/DNA ratio, or HBcrAg in a HBeAg-positive patient. This correlation was not significant after 60 months of NA therapy. However, the decrease in HBV-DNA plus RNA was positively associated with cccDNA decline compared with HBV-RNA alone, HBV-DNA alone, and HBsAg in those receiving NA therapy. HBsAg levels and its association to cccDNA levels may not be as strong due to the fact that HBsAg is also produced by HBV-DNA that is integrated into the host genome. In addition, HBV-RNA and HBV-DNA alone may be insufficient in reflecting intrahepatic cccDNA due to NA treatment blocking reverse transcription of pregenomic RNA (pgRNA).[66]

The AASLD 2018 guidelines did not recommend treating everyone who is HBV-DNA-positive.[21] However, recent CDC guidelines recommend universal screening for HBV for adults aged 18 years and older with HBsAg, anti-HBc antibody, and anti-HBs antibody testing.[14] The current treatment recommendations are more complicated and based on whether the patient has chronic HBV infection versus hepatitis and if they are HBeAg-positive or -negative with elevated HBV-DNA and alanine aminotransferase (ALT) levels. For those who are pregnant, treatment is only indicated if the serum HBV-DNA is greater than 200,000 IU/mL.[21] These complicated guidelines, both for hepatologists and primary care practitioners, have made it difficult to treat patients with chronic HBV and obtain coverage through insurance companies. This has led to increased vertical and horizonal transmission to risk of HBV infection.

In addition, there is still a risk of HCC development in patients with detectible HBV-DNA or intrahepatic cccDNA.[67] The serum HBV-DNA levels have been positively correlated with the risk for HCC development in a dose-response relationship. This positive relationship was most prominent in those who were HBeAg-negative with normal ALT levels and no liver cirrhosis.[68] In addition, a multivariate analysis has confirmed that increasing levels of HBV-DNA and HBsAg has been linked to increased risk of HCC development.[69] A retrospective study in Korea found that there was still a risk for HCC development (14.3% at 5 years) for those who were outside current treatment guidelines.[70]

With current guidelines, we have been able to achieve ALT normalization, reduce HBV-DNA to undetectable levels, gain histological improvement, acquire HBeAg seroclearance, and reduce fibrosis, HCC, transplant need, and mortality. However, we have yet to achieve improvement in HBsAg seroclearance with current treatment guidelines. Functional cure (HBsAg seroclearance) is extremely rare (less than 1%

per year),[21] and we cannot achieve it without HBV-DNA negativity. Therefore, we recommend treating everyone who is HBV-DNA positive, releasing less stringent and confusing guidelines, and following up all patients who are or have been HBV-DNA positive with ongoing screening for HCC. This will allow treatment for all at risk of HCC development, cirrhosis, and death due to chronic HBV infection and reduce horizonal and vertical transmission rates. Here, we propose simplified 5-line guidelines for HBV in adults (see **Box 1**).

Current Treatments

The first line treatment for chronic HBV is with nucleos(t) ide (NAs) or interferons (INFs). In the United States, we have lamivudine, telbivudine, adefovir, entecavir, TDF, TAF, and conventional or pegylated interferon (pegINF) as treatment options. Generally, NAs are better tolerated and have better efficacy than the INFs. However, both NAs and INFs have their limitations (**Table 5**). For example, TAF has a more stable structure than TDF, leading to more effective delivery to the liver. This results in less renal or bone toxicity than TDF. In light of these limitations, TAF is usually a first-line treatment for those without renal impairment (creatinine clearance [CrCl] < 15 mL/min) or those receiving dialysis.[21] In addition, due to high rates of relapse after cessation of NAs, the American Association for The Study of Liver Diseases (AASLD) recommends stopping treatment only after HBsAg loss with or without seroconversion. Furthermore, discontinuation of therapy is not recommended for those with cirrhosis due to hepatitis flares with increased risk of liver failure and death.[71]

Because MAFLD/MASH is primarily due to metabolic dysfunction and insulin resistance, the most effective therapy for these comorbidities is weight reduction. A 10% weight reduction can lead to resolution of steatohepatitis or improvement of fibrosis.[72] From previous studies, vitamin E has shown potential benefit for nondiabetic noncirrhotic (≥F2) MAFLD. Pioglitazone also has shown potential benefit in a diabetic and

Table 5
Summary of current HBV therapies and their advantages and limitations

	Advantages	Limitations
Conventional INF and pegINF		Poor efficacy and tolerability.[71] Avoided in decompensated liver failure.[71] HBsAg loss after 5 y: <10% of patients.[73]
Entecavir	No bone or renal toxicity risk.[71]	Higher risk of resistance.[71] Avoid in women of childbearing age or in children.[71] Risk of severe lactic acidosis in those with MELD > 20.[74]
TDF	Stronger antiviral effect than adefovir and LAM-resistant HBV.[75] Reduced viral integrations and gene dysregulations compared to placebo.[76]	Increased renal and bone toxicity compared to TAF.[21]
TAF	Less renal and bone toxicity.[21] Better ALT suppression.[21]	Not recommended for CrCl <15 mL/min or those receiving dialysis.[21]

Abbreviations: ALT, alanine aminotransferase; CrCl, creatinine clearance; HBsAg, hepatitis B surface antigen; HBV, hepatitis B virus; LAM, lamivudine; MELD, model for end-stage liver disease; pegINF, pegylated interferon; TAF, tenofovir alafenamide fumarate; TDF, tenofovir disoproxil fumarate.

nondiabetic ($\geq$F2) MAFLD.[72] Unfortunately, statins, metformin, polyunsaturated fatty acids, ursodeoxycholic acid, and pentoxifylline have shown no clear benefit.[72] Statin is, however, recommended if the patient has a cardiovascular disease indication.[72]

Emerging Therapies

With current available treatments, more than 70% of treated patients achieve HBV-DNA suppression; however, HBsAg loss occurs only in a small subset of patients. This is because it is difficult to achieve HBsAg loss as current therapies have very little effect on HBsAg production and do not modify the immune response.[77,78] Thus, present treatment is a suppressive therapy with expectation of long-term treatment. Fortunately, there are over 30 new medications and 10 antivirals that are in development. With these new therapies, there is hope that a finite course of HBV treatment may be achieved with HBsAg loss and HBV-DNA suppression (**Table 6**).

A. Entry inhibitor. One way to reduce chronic HBV infection is to prevent entry of the virus into hepatocytes. Bulevirtide (BLV) is a competitive inhibitor for HBsAg envelope protein. When bound, it prevents entry of HBV into healthy cells.[71,79,80] When used with other antivirals, it has shown to improve HDV-RNA clearance.[81]
B. Inhibiting protein synthesis (siRNA, LNA, ASO). Small interfering RNA (siRNA) locked nucleic acid (LNA), and antisense oligonucleotide (ASO) targets specific gene products and cause degradation of mRNA. There are many siRNA therapies that are currently being studied. For example, a siRNA ARC520 has shown to silence transcription of HBsAg by targeting cccDNA-derived pgRNA in HBeAg-positive patients.[71,82] Another, siRNA, bepirovirsen, has shown significant reduction of HBsAg and HBV-DNA in treatment naïve patients with chronic HBV.[83]
C. Inactivating cccDNA (CRISPR/Cas9). CRISPR/Cas9 targets cccDNA and cause double-stranded breaks and deactivation of the targeted genes. Previous studies have shown combining siRNA with CRISPR/Cas9 improved reduction and even

Table 6
Emerging therapies

Mechanism	Drugs
Blocking entry	BLV
Blocking protein synthesis (siRNA, LNA, ASO)	ARC520 RG6004/RO7062931 GSK3389404 Bepirovirsen
Inactivating cccDNA (CRISPR/Cas9)	
Blocking core synthesis (CpAMs)	NVR3-778 Vebicorvir (ABI-H0731)
Blocking release and formation of virions (HBsAg).	REP-2139
Directly inhibit HBsAg with monoclonal antibody	Lenvervimab VIR-3434
Mediate T-cell response	GS-4774
TRL7 agonist	Vestaolimod (GS-9620)
TRL8 agonist	GS-9688
PD-1 inhibitors	Nivolumab

Abbreviations: ASO, antisense oligonucleotide; BLV, bulevirtide; ccDNA, closed covalent circular DNA; CpAMs, capsid assembly modulators; HBsAg, hepatitis B surface antigen; HBV, hepatitis B virus; LNA, locked nucleic acid; PD-1, programmed death-1; siRNA, small interfering RNAs.

disappearance of cccDNA.[84,85] However, there is a risk of cross-reactivity with human genetic material[85] when using CRISPR/Cas9 for patients with chronic HBV.

D. Inhibiting core synthesis (CpAMs). The capsid assembly modulators (CpAMs) target capsid assembly. It will result in aberrant assembly causing disassembly, creating aberrant capsids or empty capsids.[86] By affecting capsid assembly, it inhibits formation and release of new viruses, spread of the virus to uninfected cells, and prevents relaxed-circular DNA (rcDNA) transformation to cccDNA.[71,87] But several CpAMs have been discontinued due to liver toxicity (AB-506, AB-836, and ABI-H2173).[88]

Combination therapy of NVR3-778 (CpAM) and pegINF or entecavir was found to reduce HBV-DNA levels more so than with CpAM alone. However, it did not reduce HBsAg levels, and viral rebound was observed after treatment cessation.[71,89] When a CpAM vebicorvir (ABI-H0731) was combined with entecavir, TDF, or TAF, 100% of HBeAg-negative patients with chronic HBV achieved virological suppression of HBV-DNA plus pgRNA less than 20 IU/mL after 48 weeks of treatment.[90]

E. Inhibiting release and formation of virions (HBsAg). REP-2139 inhibits assembly and/or secretion of subviral particles (SVPs), reducing circulating HBsAg levels.[91] When REP-2139 was combined with TDF or pegINF in HBeAg-negative patients, it resulted in significantly reduced HBsAg levels (60%) and functional cure (35%) at follow-up after 48 weeks being treatment-free.[91]

F. HBsAg inhibition with monoclonal antibody. Lenvervimab is a monoclonal antibody that binds to HBsAg directly neutralizing the antigen and preventing entry into hepatocytes.[92] Another monoclonal antibody, VIR-3434, was studied with a siRNA. When combined, there was a significant reduction in HBsAg levels in all participants and HBsAg less than 10 IU/mL in most participants. The serum HBsAg levels were reduced more in combination therapy than either alone.[93]

G. Therapeutic vaccines. A vaccine, GS-4774, was developed to mediate T-cell response. Unfortunately, it only had a small effect on the HBsAg levels.[94] Another vaccine, INO-1800, which contains HBsAg and HBV core/capsid antigen encoding is currently being studied.[90]

H. Stimulation of innate immune response. There are many drugs in development that affect host's immune response to the HBV infection.

TLR7 or TLR8 agonist
Vesatolimod (GS-9620) is an oral TLR7 agonist that influences both innate and adaptive immune response as well as antiviral cytokine responses. Unfortunately, weekly administration only led to viral suppression but had no effect on HBsAg levels in treatment-naïve patients with chronic HBV.[71] Another is a TRL8 agonist, GS-9688, that stimulates myeloid cells (myeloid dendritic cells, monocytes, and Kupffer cells). Study of this new drug is currently underway.[90]

PD-1 (programmed death-1) inhibitors
An anti-PD-1, nivolumab, has been approved for gastrointestinal, renal, lung, skin, and urothelial cancers. When it was combined with GS-4774, a significant decline of HBsAg from baseline was experienced.[95] More studies are needed to determine the right dosage to avoid immune-mediated HBV flares and triggering of autoimmune conditions.[71,96]

Currently, HBV therapy is long term for most patients; however, with over 30 new medications and more than 10 antiviral drugs in development, we are hopeful for a future with agents that combine functional cure with a finite course of therapy. Recent studies suggest that we are headed toward combination therapy with up to 4 drugs to achieve greater than 50% HBsAg loss. Ongoing clinical trials for these new emerging therapies can be found in https://clinicaltrials.gov/ and Drug Watch webpage on the Hepatitis B Foundation website.

Vaccinate all who are susceptible

Vaccination is the most effective strategy to prevent individuals from contracting HBV and to reduce the global incidence of HBV.[97] In 1991, the WHO recommended that all countries implement a universal hepatitis B vaccination policy to prevent and control HBV infection on a global scale.[97] To date, vaccination remains the most effective way in preventing HBV, cirrhosis of the liver, and HCC worldwide. We recommend vaccination of all who do not have evidence of chronic HBV infection or HBV immunity.

The first available vaccines were created by harvesting the HBsAg from plasma of chronically infected individuals. The plasma-derived vaccines contained highly purified HBsAg particles that were inactivated via a combination of urea, pepsin, formaldehyde, and heat.[97] The second generation of vaccines used recombinant DNA technology to express the HBsAg in HBV-transfected yeasts. Since the advent of the recombinant hepatitis B vaccine in 1986, approximately one hundred million doses of the vaccine have been safely administered worldwide.[97] The hepatitis B vaccine is one of the most widely used vaccines globally, especially after it was incorporated as part of the routine vaccination schedule for infants and children.[97] Within 10 years of the initiation of the universal hepatitis B vaccination program, a 68% decrease in HBV infection prevalence among children was noted in the United States.[98]

A key strategy of control of the HBV epidemic is universal infant vaccination. In 2018, the Advisory Committee on Immunization Practices (ACIP) recommended Heplisav-B (HepB-CpG) vaccine as an option for adults aged 18 years and older who are unvaccinated, incompletely vaccinated, or those with specific risk factors. This is a 2-dose vaccine, given at least 4 weeks apart.[99] This is more convenient than the previous 3-dose vaccine series (Engerix-B, PreHevbrio, Recombivax HB), which is given over a 6-month period. It is not surprising to have a higher completion rate than the previous 3-dose vaccines (**Table 7**). The seroprotection rates were also higher for Heplisav-B vaccine than for the previous Engerix-B.[100–102]

Given that perinatal or early postnatal transmission is the primary method of HBV transmission globally, it is recommended that all infants should receive their first dose of the monovalent hepatitis B vaccine within 24 hours of delivery,[103] with an additional 2 doses of hepatitis B vaccine in the first year of life (**Table 8**). The pentavalent vaccine is a combination vaccine against HVB, DTP (diphtheria, tetanus toxoids and pertussis), and Hib (hemophilus influenzae type b).[98] Infants born to HBsAg-positive mothers should receive the hepatitis B vaccine and 0.5 mL of hepatitis B immunoglobulin (HBIG) within 12 hours of birth.[98] These infants should then be tested for HBsAg and anti-HBs between the ages of 9 and 12 months. If these infants did not receive the hepatitis B vaccination series within 24 hours after birth, they should be tested 1 to 2 months after completion of the series.[98] Infants born to a mother with an unknown HBsAg status should receive the hepatitis B vaccine within 12 hours of birth regardless of birth weight. The hepatitis B monovalent vaccine is only administered to infants before 6 weeks of age.

All pregnant women should be screened for HBV (**Table 9**). HBV vaccination can be safely administered in pregnancy, and all noninfected pregnant women who are not immune to the virus should be offered an accelerated vaccine series.[21] An accelerated vaccine schedule has been shown to be efficacious in pregnant women at high risk. Women who test positive for HBsAg should be tested for HBV-DNA. HBV flares in

Table 7
Children and adult hepatitis B vaccine schedule[98,104,105]

Patient Population	Vaccine	Dose 1	Dose 2	Dose 3	Follow-up Recommendations
Unvaccinated children	3-Dose vaccine series for infants <1 y	Now	1 mo after dose 1	6 mo after dose 1	No booster or follow-up recommended in immunocompetent children.
Unvaccinated adults Immunocompromised adults including those who are HIV-positive, have end-stage renal disease undergoing hemodialysis, have chronic liver disease or diabetes, or those receiving immunosuppressant therapy.	2-Dose vaccine series	Now	1 mo after dose 1		Heplisav-B (Not recommended in pregnancy)
	3-Dose vaccine series	Now	1 mo after dose 1	6 mo after dose 1	Engerix-B, PreHevbrio, or Recombivax HB (PreHevbrio not recommended in pregnancy). The CDC recommends a second series at 0, 1, and 6 mo in those who are nonresponders to the initial vaccine series.[21] The WHO recommends an additional dose of the vaccine at 2 mo or an adjuvanted vaccine with aluminum phosphate and monophosphorylate lipid A to achieve an appropriate immune response[103,97] Patients should be tested for their response to the vaccination 1–2 mo after the last dose of the vaccine.

(continued on next page)

Table 7
(continued)

Patient Population	Vaccine	Dose 1	Dose 2	Dose 3	Follow-up Recommendations
					Follow-up testing is recommended annually in those receiving hemodialysis. Booster dose recommended if anti-HBs titers fall below 10 mIU/mL.[21]
Exposure to known HBsAg + individual:					
Unvaccinated	HBIG and 3-dose vaccine series	Within 24 h of exposure	1 mo after dose 1	6 mo after dose 1	Undergo anti-HBs testing 1–2 mo after receiving the last vaccine dose.[104]
Partially unvaccinated adults (did not finish full vaccination series)	HBIG and complete vaccine series				Undergo anti-HBs testing 1–2 mo after receiving the last vaccine dose.[104]
Fully vaccinated with known exposure to HBsAg +	1 dose of HBV vaccine booster				
Exposure to unknown HBsAg status:					
Unvaccinated	3-dose vaccine series	Within 24 h of exposure	1 mo after dose 1	6 mo after dose 1	Undergo anti-HBs testing 1–2 mo after receiving the last vaccine dose.[104]
Partially unvaccinated adults (did not finish full vaccination series)	Complete vaccine series				Undergo anti-HBs testing 1–2 mo after receiving the last vaccine dose.[104]
Fully vaccinated with known exposure to HBsAg +	No treatment is needed				

Abbreviations: CDC, centers for disease control and prevention; HBIG, hepatitis B immunoglobulin; HBsAg, hepatitis B surface antigen; HBV, hepatitis B virus.

Table 8
International hepatitis B vaccination for all ages[106]

3-Dose Vaccine Series			
Age	Dose 1	Dose 2	Dose 3
Infants <1 y	Within 24 h of birth	1 mo after dose 1	6 mo after dose 1
Children >1 y and adults	Now	1 mo after dose 1	6 mo after dose 1

4-Dose Combination Vaccine (Pentavalent or Hexavalent Vaccine)			
Dose 1	Dose 2	Dose 3	Dose 4
Within 24 h of birth (HBV monovalent vaccine)	6 wk of age (combination vaccine)	10 wk of age (combination vaccine)	14 wk of age (combination vaccine)

pregnant women with chronic HBV were observed in up to 9% of patients and 4% of postpartum patients; thus, all women with chronic HBV should be closely monitored during pregnancy and early postpartum.

All unvaccinated children and adults who did not receive the vaccine in infancy or those that are anti-HBs-negative should receive the "catch up" vaccination schedule summarized in **Table 7**.[98] Sexual and household contacts of HBV-infected persons

Table 9
Suggested hepatitis B management in the pregnant patient[21,107,108]

Population	Management
First pregnancy visit	Test for HBsAg and anti-HBs
Women who test positive for HBsAg on triple screening	Confirm infection with quantitative measurement of HBV-DNA at baseline and week 28, along with HBeAg status and ALT levels. Patients should also be linked to care for HCC surveillance.[109] 1. If HBV-DNA > 200,000, consider treatment at 28–32 wk of pregnancy to prevent mother-to-child transmission. All infants require HBV vaccination series and HBIG within 12 h of birth. 2. If HBV-DNA < 200,000, No antiviral therapy indicated but monitor closely for every 3 mo for up to 6 mo after delivery for ALT flares and seroconversion. If patient has active disease or cirrhosis: 1. Consider treatment with discussion of shared decision regarding possible risks to fetus with treatment vs the risk of liver decompensation in the mother if untreated. 2. Test household contacts and sexual partners
Women who are HBsAg-negative and anti-HBsAg-negative	Offer vaccination

Abbreviations: ALT, alanine aminotransferase; HBeAg, hepatitis B e antigen; HBIG, hepatitis B immunoglobulin; HBsAg, hepatitis B surface antigen; HBV, hepatitis B virus; HCC, hepatocellular carcinoma.

Adapted from Hepatitis B Foundation Vaccine Schedule https://www.hepb.org/prevention-and-diagnosis/vaccination/guidelines-2/#international.

who are negative for HbsAg and anti-HbsAg should also receive the HBV vaccination series[21] (see **Table 7**). Upon completion of the vaccine course, seroprotection rates to antibodies against HbsAg can be up to 100% in children and almost 95% in healthy, young adults. In patients who are immunocompromised, such as those who are HIV-positive, those who have end-stage renal disease undergoing hemodialysis, those with chronic liver disease, those with diabetes, or those receiving immunosuppressant therapy, the immune response following the vaccination is often reduced, and they will require frequent testing for immunity and eligibility for the booster[103] (see **Table 7**).

Chronic infection with HBV, hepatitis C virus, and MAFLD/MASH is the primary risk factor for HCC. The incidence of HCC and decompensated cirrhosis in individuals infected at birth or early childhood is low in youths but increases exponentially in individuals in their late 30s or early 40s.[98] In order to mitigate these serious complications, programs need to screen all individuals for HBV and identify those infected with HBV early to link them to regular HBV care and treatment. The number needed to screen to identify 1 HBV infection ranged from 32 to 48. HBV is generally incurable, and early identification with screening of unvaccinated individuals is crucial to the control of HBV transmission, morbidity, and mortality.

The vaccine is overall well tolerated, with commonly reported side effects limited to the site of injection, such as erythema, swelling, and induration. Systemic signs of reaction to the vaccine, such as fatigue, fever, headache, nausea, and abdominal pain, are uncommon with only a few reported cases in literature. Fortunately, with the newest 2-dose series vaccine (Heplisav-B), the compliance and completion rate has improved, increasing the number of populations who can be adequately immunized to HBV. HBV vaccination is the most effective measure to control and prevent HBV and its long-term sequelae globally.

SUMMARY

An estimated 2 billion people have been infected with HBV worldwide, with the latest global estimate approximating that around 300 million of these individuals have become chronically infected with HBV.[107] Chronic HBV is the leading cause of liver disease globally, with up to 20% of affected patients at risk of progression to HCC and cirrhosis.[107] The HBV vaccines are proven to be safe and effective, providing immunity to the virus following vaccination for at least 30 years in over 90% of vaccinated individuals.[98] Routine infant vaccination in over 180 countries has resulted in a significant decline in HBV transmission, yet 50 million new cases are reported annually, with most of the new cases spread via vertical transmission in countries with high prevalence.[110]

In the United States, HBV is usually spread either through sexual contact or injection drug use, yet 25,000 infants are at risk of vertical transmission annually. The risk of development of chronic HBV is inversely related to age of exposure, with up to 90% of exposed infants at risk of developing chronic HBV.[107] The American Congress of Obstetrics and Gynecology recommends that every pregnant person undergo HBV screening, and the appropriate vaccination is applied to infants born to infected mothers. In adults, viral clearance after exposure is more common, and only 5% of cases will progress to chronic disease.

Barriers to eradication of HBV transmission include low patient and public understanding of the disease and differing opinions among medical experts on the best clinical management regime.[111] Despite the proven safety and efficacy of the HBV vaccine, adult vaccination coverage rates in the United States remain low overall, likely due to limited awareness of the benefits of the vaccine, inadequate screening for vaccination in routine patient care, poor access to vaccination, payment challenges for patients, and limited stock in outpatient provider offices.[98] Some strategies that have been proposed to improve adult immunization include clinical decision-support tools, standing orders or protocols for vaccination in patient charts, and provider and patient reminders.[98] Fortunately, there has been an improvement in the compliance and vaccination completion rate with the newest and more potent HBV vaccine (Heplisav-B). This simplified 2-dose vaccine series has the 2 doses only 4 weeks apart, compared to the traditional 3-dose vaccine series over a 6-month period. This vaccine has an improved completion rate and a better immune response than previous vaccines. Overall, there is still work to be done in eliminating HBV. Public resources and support will be needed to address common barriers to HBV elimination, such as surveillance for HCC, vaccine tracking, social stigma, provider education, and care coordination in management of chronic infection.

CLINICS CARE POINTS

- The hepatitis B models showed that globally no country is on track to achieve all HBV targets by 2030 or by 2050.
- Global efforts need to be made to improve awareness, screening, access to care, vaccinations, financial resources, political will and commitment, and referral programs.
- Heplisav-B vaccine has improved the completion rate because of its simplified 2-dose vaccine series and higher rate of immune responses in adults than the three-dose regimen, Engerix.
- 5 Pillars toward elimination of HBV:
  1. Test all patients with a "triple panel": HBsAg, anti-HBc antibody, anti-HBs antibody.
  2. Vaccinate all adults who are triple panel negative.
  3. If HBsAg-positive, follow-up with qDNA and anti-HDV testing.
  4. Treat all HBV-DNA-positive patients including those with cirrhosis. Treat until HBsAg loss +12 months consolidation.
  5. Surveillance for HCC and treatment of concomitant liver disease (ie, MAFLD, MASH, HDV, HCV).
- Everyone who are infected with HBV should be evaluated for HIV, HCV, HDV, and MAFLD/MASH. Then the coinfections and/or comorbidities should also be treated.
- Treatment of all who are HBV-DNA-positive will simplify treatment recommendations and:
  ○ Improve quality of life and reduce stigma.
  ○ Reduce the spread of HBV infection.
  ○ Decrease rates of liver cirrhosis and development of HCC.
  ○ Reduce extrahepatic manifestations of HBV.
  ○ Reduce deaths due to HBV.
- Currently, treatment of chronic HBV infection is lifelong with monotherapy. However, with new emerging investigational therapies, we may be closer to finite treatment and improved functional cure rates with combination therapy.
- Chronic HBV infection curative treatments will likely be multi-drug therapy, with up to 4 different drugs with varying mechanisms.

DISCLOSURES

R. Gish consults for VBI, Dynavax, and Gilead and is the Medical Director for Hepatitis B Foundation. C. Brosgart is on the Board of Directors for Galmed, Abivax, Enochian, Eradivir, Hepatitis B Foundation, and Merlin and scientific advisory board for Hepion and Pardes and consults for Dynavax, Mirum, and Moderna.

FUNDING

This research received no specific grant from any funding agency in the public, commercial, or not-for-profit sectors.

ACKNOWLEDGMENTS

The authors thank Kelly Schrank, MA, ELS, of Bookworm Editing Services LLC for her editorial services in preparing the manuscript for publication.

REFERENCES

1. Yardeni D, Ghany MG. Review article: hepatitis B-current and emerging therapies. Aliment Pharmacol Ther 2022;55(7):805–19.
2. Wong RJ, Brosgart CL, Welch S, et al. An updated assessment of chronic hepatitis B prevalence among foreign-born persons living in the United States. Hepatology 2021;74(2):607–26.
3. Kowdley KV, Wang CC, Welch S, et al. Prevalence of chronic hepatitis B among foreign-born persons living in the United States by country of origin. Hepatology 2012;56(2):422–33.
4. Song A, Lin X, Chen X. Functional cure for chronic hepatitis B: accessibility, durability, and prognosis. Virol J 2021;18(1):114.
5. Fung S, Choi HSJ, Gehring A, et al. Getting to HBV cure: the promising paths forward. Hepatology 2022;76(1):233–50.
6. Li X, Zhao J, Yuan Q, et al. Detection of HBV covalently closed circular DNA. Viruses 2017;9(6). https://doi.org/10.3390/v9060139.
7. Candotti D, Boizeau L, Laperche S. Occult hepatitis B infection and transfusion-transmission risk. Transfus Clin Biol 2017;24(3):189–95.
8. de Almeida NAA, de Paula VS. Occult Hepatitis B virus (HBV) infection and challenges for hepatitis elimination: a literature review. J Appl Microbiol 2022; 132(3):1616–35.
9. Dindoost P, Chimeh N, Hollinger BF, et al. The pigeonhole of occult hepatitis B. Acta Med Iran 2014;52(8):582–90.
10. Loomba R, Liang TJ. Hepatitis B reactivation associated with immune suppressive and biological modifier therapies: current concepts, management strategies, and future directions. Gastroenterology 2017;152(6):1297–309.
11. Guo L, Wang D, Ouyang X, et al. Recent advances in HBV reactivation research. BioMed Res Int 2018;2018:2931402.
12. Mast EE, Weinbaum CM, Fiore AE, et al. A comprehensive immunization strategy to eliminate transmission of hepatitis B virus infection in the United States: recommendations of the Advisory Committee on Immunization Practices (ACIP) Part II: immunization of adults. MMWR Recomm Rep (Morb Mortal Wkly Rep) 2006;55(RR-16):1–33, quiz CE1-4.
13. MMWR. Newborn Hepatitis B Vaccination Coverage Among Children Born January 2003–June 2005 — United States. CDC. https://www.cdc.gov/mmwr/preview/mmwrhtml/mm5730a3.htm#:~:text=Hepatitis%20B%20vaccine%20was%20first,the%20United%20States%20(1).
14. Conners EE, Panagiotakopoulos L, Hofmeister MG, et al. Screening and testing for hepatitis B virus infection: CDC recommendations — United States, 2023. MMWR Recomm Rep (Morb Mortal Wkly Rep) 2023;72(1):1–25. https://doi.org/10.15585/mmwr.rr7201a1.

15. Rui F, Yang H, Hu X, et al. Renaming NAFLD to MAFLD: advantages and potential changes in diagnosis, pathophysiology, treatment, and management. Infectious Microbes & Diseases 2022;4(2):49–55.

16. Chan WK, Treeprasertsuk S, Imajo K, et al. Clinical features and treatment of nonalcoholic fatty liver disease across the Asia Pacific region-the GO ASIA initiative. Aliment Pharmacol Ther 2018;47(6):816–25.

17. Azat A, Elmoghazy M. Metabolic dysfunction-associated fatty liver disease from definition to complications Review Article. Medical Journal of Viral Hepatitis (MJVH) 2021;6(1):4–9.

18. Dhamija E, Paul SB, Kedia S. Non-alcoholic fatty liver disease associated with hepatocellular carcinoma: an increasing concern. Indian J Med Res 2019; 149(1):9–17.

19. Yuen MF, Chen DS, Dusheiko GM, et al. Hepatitis B virus infection. Nat Rev Dis Primers 2018;4:18035.

20. Shi Y, Zheng M. Hepatitis B virus persistence and reactivation. BMJ 2020;370: m2200.

21. Terrault NA, Lok ASF, McMahon BJ, et al. Update on prevention, diagnosis, and treatment of chronic hepatitis B: AASLD 2018 hepatitis B guidance. Hepatology 2018;67(4):1560–99.

22. Yip TC, Wong GL. Current knowledge of occult hepatitis B infection and clinical implications. Semin Liver Dis 2019;39(2):249–60.

23. Saitta C, Pollicino T, Raimondo G. Occult hepatitis B virus infection: an update. Viruses 8 2022;14(7). https://doi.org/10.3390/v14071504.

24. Negro F. Hepatitis D virus coinfection and superinfection. Cold Spring Harb Perspect Med 2014;4(11):a021550.

25. KIM TW, KIM MN, KWON JW, et al. Risk of hepatitis B virus reactivation in patients with asthma or chronic obstructive pulmonary disease treated with corticosteroids. Respirology 2010;15(7):1092–7.

26. Pattullo V. Prevention of hepatitis B reactivation in the setting of immunosuppression. Clin Mol Hepatol 2016;22(2):219.

27. Perrillo RP, Gish R, Falck-Ytter YT. American Gastroenterological Association Institute technical review on prevention and treatment of hepatitis B virus reactivation during immunosuppressive drug therapy. Gastroenterology 2015; 148(1):221–44.

28. Reddy KR, Beavers KL, Hammond SP, et al. American Gastroenterological Association Institute guideline on the prevention and treatment of hepatitis B virus reactivation during immunosuppressive drug therapy. Gastroenterology 2015; 148(1):215–9.

29. Thomas HC. Best practice in the treatment of chronic hepatitis B: a summary of the European Viral Hepatitis Educational Initiative (EVHEI). J Hepatol 2007; 47(4):588–97.

30. Smith-Palmer J, Cerri K, Sbarigia U, et al. Impact of stigma on people living with chronic hepatitis B. Patient Relat Outcome Meas 2020;11:95–107.

31. Chen P, Zhu JW, Chen T, et al. [Clinical value of health-related quality of life evaluation in community patients with hepatitis B]. Zhonghua Gan Zang Bing Za Zhi 2017;25(4):313–6.

32. Younossi ZM, Guyatt G, Kiwi M, et al. Development of a disease specific questionnaire to measure health related quality of life in patients with chronic liver disease. Gut 1999;45(2):295–300.

33. Golabi P, Paik JM, Eberly K, et al. Causes of death in patients with Non-alcoholic Fatty Liver Disease (NAFLD), alcoholic liver disease and chronic viral Hepatitis B and C. Ann Hepatol 2022;27(1):100556.

34. Younossi ZM, Stepanova M, Janssen HLA, et al. Effects of treatment of chronic hepatitis B virus infection on patient-reported outcomes. Clin Gastroenterol Hepatol 2018;16(10):1641–1649 e6.

35. Organization WH. Hepatitis: How can I protect myself from hepatitis B? 2023. https://www.who.int/news-room/questions-and-answers/item/hepatitis-b-how-can-i-protect-myself#:~:text=HBV%20is%20spread%20by%20contact,baby%20at%20the%20birth%20(perinatal).

36. Lim JK, Nguyen MH, Kim WR, et al. Prevalence of chronic hepatitis B virus infection in the United States. Am J Gastroenterol 2020;115(9):1429–38.

37. Smith JM, Uvin AZ, Macmadu A, et al. Epidemiology and treatment of hepatitis B in prisoners. Curr Hepatol Rep 2017;16(3):178–83.

38. Cheemerla S, Balakrishnan M. Global epidemiology of chronic liver disease. Clin Liver Dis 2021;17(5):365–70.

39. McGlynn KA, Petrick JL, El-Serag HB. Epidemiology of hepatocellular carcinoma. Hepatology. Jan 2021;73(Suppl 1):4–13.

40. Mazzaro C, Adinolfi LE, Pozzato G, et al. Extrahepatic manifestations of chronic HBV infection and the role of antiviral therapy. J Clin Med 2022;11(21). https://doi.org/10.3390/jcm11216247.

41. Cacoub P, Terrier B. Hepatitis B-related autoimmune manifestations. Rheum Dis Clin North Am 2009;35(1):125–37.

42. Baig S, Alamgir M. The extrahepatic manifestations of hepatitis B virus. J Coll Physicians Surg Pak 2008;18(7):451–7.

43. Li M, Gan Y, Fan C, et al. Hepatitis B virus and risk of non-Hodgkin lymphoma: an updated meta-analysis of 58 studies. J Viral Hepat 2018;25(8):894–903.

44. Dunn R, Wetten A, McPherson S, et al. Viral hepatitis in 2021: the challenges remaining and how we should tackle them. World J Gastroenterol 2022;28(1):76–95.

45. Charuchandra S. Most Countries Not on Track to Eliminate Hepatitis B and C by 2030. https://www.hepmag.com/article/countries-track-eliminate-hepatitis-b-c-2030.

46. Spearman CW. Towards the elimination of hepatitis B and hepatocellular carcinoma. S Afr Med J 2018;108(8b):13–6.

47. Seto W-K, Lo Y-R, Pawlotsky J-M, et al. Chronic hepatitis B virus infection. Lancet 2018;392(10161):2313–24.

48. Observatory CFsP. CDA Foundation's Polaris Observatory. https://cdafound.org/polaris/.

49. Scott J, Fagalde M, Baer A, et al. A population-based intervention to improve care cascades of patients with hepatitis C virus infection. Hepatol Commun 2021;5(3):387–99.

50. Kay ES, Batey DS, Craft HL, et al. Practice transformation in HIV primary care: perspectives of coaches and champions in the southeast United States. J Prim Care Community Health 2021;12. https://doi.org/10.1177/2150132720984429. 2150132720984429.

51. Sehr MA, Joshi KD, Fontanesi JM, et al. Markov modeling in hepatitis B screening and linkage to care. Theor Biol Med Model 2017;14(1):11.

52. Yoo GJ, Fang T, Zola J, et al. Destigmatizing hepatitis B in the asian American community: lessons learned from the san Francisco Hep B free campaign. J Cancer Educ 2012;27(1):138–44.

53. Bailey MB, Shiau R, Zola J, et al. San Francisco Hep B free: a grassroots community coalition to prevent hepatitis B and liver cancer. J Community Health 2011;36(4):538–51.

54. Said ZNA, El-Sayed MH. Challenge of managing hepatitis B virus and hepatitis C virus infections in resource-limited settings. World J Hepatol 2022;14(7): 1333–43.

55. Perz JF, Armstrong GL, Farrington LA, et al. The contributions of hepatitis B virus and hepatitis C virus infections to cirrhosis and primary liver cancer worldwide. J Hepatol 2006;45(4):529–38.

56. Schweitzer A, Horn J, Mikolajczyk RT, et al. Estimations of worldwide prevalence of chronic hepatitis B virus infection: a systematic review of data published between 1965 and 2013. Lancet 2015;386(10003):1546–55.

57. Lok AS. Chronic hepatitis B. N Engl J Med 2002;346(22):1682–3.

58. de Franchis R, Hadengue A, Lau G, et al. EASL international consensus conference on hepatitis B. 13-14 september, 2002 geneva, Switzerland. Consensus statement (long version). J Hepatol 2003;39(Suppl 1):S3–25.

59. Tabor E. Hepatocellular carcinoma: global epidemiology. Dig Liver Dis 2001; 33(2):115–7.

60. Lozano R, Naghavi M, Foreman K, et al. Global and regional mortality from 235 causes of death for 20 age groups in 1990 and 2010: a systematic analysis for the Global Burden of Disease Study 2010. Lancet 2012;380(9859):2095–128.

61. Kawanaka M, Nishino K, Kawamoto H, et al. Hepatitis B: who should be treated?-managing patients with chronic hepatitis B during the immune-tolerant and immunoactive phases. World J Gastroenterol 21 2021;27(43): 7497–508.

62. Organization WH. Hepatitis B. https://www.who.int/news-room/fact-sheets/detail/hepatitis-b. Accessed November 20, 2022.

63. Tang LSY, Covert E, Wilson E, et al. Chronic hepatitis B infection: a review. JAMA 2018;319(17):1802–13.

64. Nassal M. HBV cccDNA: viral persistence reservoir and key obstacle for a cure of chronic hepatitis B. Gut 2015;64(12):1972–84.

65. Martinez MG, Boyd A, Combe E, et al. Covalently closed circular DNA: the ultimate therapeutic target for curing HBV infections. J Hepatol 2021;75(3):706–17.

66. Wang Y, Liu Y, Liao H, et al. Serum HBV DNA plus RNA reflecting cccDNA level before and during NAs treatment in HBeAg positive CHB patients. Int J Med Sci 2022;19(5):858–66.

67. Lin CL, Kao JH. Development of hepatocellular carcinoma in untreated and treated patients with chronic hepatitis B virus infection. Clin Mol Hepatol 2023. https://doi.org/10.3350/cmh.2022.0342.

68. Chen CJ, Yang HI, Su J, et al. Risk of hepatocellular carcinoma across a biological gradient of serum hepatitis B virus DNA level. JAMA 2006;295(1):65–73.

69. Varbobitis I, Papatheodoridis GV. The assessment of hepatocellular carcinoma risk in patients with chronic hepatitis B under antiviral therapy. Clin Mol Hepatol 2016;22(3):319–26.

70. Sinn DH, Kim SE, Kim BK, et al. The risk of hepatocellular carcinoma among chronic hepatitis B virus-infected patients outside current treatment criteria. J Viral Hepat 2019;26(12):1465–72.

71. Nguyen MH, Wong G, Gane E, et al. Hepatitis B virus: advances in prevention, diagnosis, and therapy. Clin Microbiol Rev 2020;33(2). https://doi.org/10.1128/cmr.00046-19.

72. Prasoppokakorn T, Pitisuttithum P, Treeprasertsuk S. Pharmacological therapeutics: current trends for metabolic dysfunction-associated fatty liver disease (MAFLD). J Clin Transl Hepatol 2021;9(6):939–46.

73. Buster EH, Flink HJ, Cakaloglu Y, et al. Sustained HBeAg and HBsAg loss after long-term follow-up of HBeAg-positive patients treated with peginterferon alpha-2b. Gastroenterology 2008;135(2):459–67.

74. Lange CM, Bojunga J, Hofmann WP, et al. Severe lactic acidosis during treatment of chronic hepatitis B with entecavir in patients with impaired liver function. Hepatology 2009;50(6):2001–6.

75. Hann HW, Chae HB, Dunn SR. Tenofovir (TDF) has stronger antiviral effect than adefovir (ADV) against lamivudine (LAM)-resistant hepatitis B virus (HBV). Hepatol Int 2008;2(2):244–9.

76. Hsu YC, Suri V, Nguyen MH, et al. Inhibition of viral replication reduces transcriptionally active distinct hepatitis B virus integrations with implications on host gene dysregulation. Gastroenterology 2022;162(4):1160–70.e1.

77. Martin P, Nguyen MH, Dieterich DT, et al. Treatment algorithm for managing chronic hepatitis B virus infection in the United States: 2021 update. Clin Gastroenterol Hepatol 2022;20(8):1766–75.

78. Smolders EJ, Burger DM, Feld JJ, et al. Review article: clinical pharmacology of current and investigational hepatitis B virus therapies. Aliment Pharmacol Ther 2020;51(2):231–43.

79. Urban S, Bartenschlager R, Kubitz R, et al. Strategies to inhibit entry of HBV and HDV into hepatocytes. Gastroenterology 2014;147(1):48–64.

80. Asselah T, Loureiro D, Tout I, et al. Future treatments for hepatitis delta virus infection. Liver Int 2020;40(Suppl 1):54–60.

81. Kang C, Syed YY. Bulevirtide: first approval. Drugs 2020;80(15):1601–5.

82. Yuen MF, Schiefke I, Yoon JH, et al. RNA interference therapy with ARC-520 results in prolonged hepatitis B surface antigen response in patients with chronic hepatitis B infection. Hepatology 2020;72(1):19–31.

83. Yuen MF, Heo J, Jang JW, et al. Safety, tolerability and antiviral activity of the antisense oligonucleotide bepirovirsen in patients with chronic hepatitis B: a phase 2 randomized controlled trial. Nat Med 2021;27(10):1725–34.

84. Wang J, Lu F. Dual-gRNAs and gRNA-microRNA (miRNA)-gRNA ternary cassette combined CRISPR/Cas9 system and RNAi approach promotes the clearance of HBV cccDNA. Hepatology 2015;62:223A–4A.

85. Shi Y, Tu Z, Duan XD, et al. The combination effects of CRISPR/Cas9 and APOBEC3B editing on HBV cccDNA formation. Hepatology 2017;66:782A.

86. Hui RW-H, Mak L-Y, Seto W-K, et al. Role of core/capsid inhibitors in functional cure strategies for chronic hepatitis B. Current Hepatology Reports 2020;19(3):293–301.

87. Zoulim F, Zlotnick A, Buchholz S, et al. Nomenclature of HBV core protein-targeting antivirals. Nat Rev Gastroenterol Hepatol 2022;19(12):748–50.

88. Yuen MF, Berliba E, Sukeepaisarnjaroen W, et al. Safety, pharmacokinetics, and antiviral activity of the capsid inhibitor AB-506 from Phase 1 studies in healthy subjects and those with hepatitis B. Hepatol Commun 2022;6(12):3457–72.

89. Yuen MF, Gane EJ, Kim DJ, et al. Antiviral activity, safety, and pharmacokinetics of capsid assembly modulator NVR 3-778 in patients with chronic HBV infection. Gastroenterology 2019;156(5):1392–403.e7.

90. Lee HW, Lee JS, Ahn SH. Hepatitis B virus cure: targets and future therapies. Int J Mol Sci 2020;22(1). https://doi.org/10.3390/ijms22010213.

91. Bazinet M, Pântea V, Placinta G, et al. Safety and efficacy of 48 Weeks REP 2139 or REP 2165, tenofovir disoproxil, and pegylated interferon alfa-2a in patients with chronic HBV infection naïve to nucleos(t)ide therapy. Gastroenterology 2020;158(8):2180–94.

92. Lee HW, Park JY, Hong T, et al. Efficacy of lenvervimab, a recombinant human immunoglobulin, in treatment of chronic hepatitis B virus infection. Clin Gastroenterol Hepatol 2020;18(13):3043–5.e1.

93. Gane E, Jucov A, Dobryanska M, et al. Safety, tolerability, and antiviral activity of the siRNA VIR 2218 in combination with the investigational neutralizing monoclonal antibody VIR 3434 for the treatment of chronic hepatitis B virus infection: Preliminary results from the phase 2 MARCH trial. American Association For The Study Of Liver Diseases (AASLD). 2022. https://www.natap.org/2022/AASLD/AASLD_19.htm.

94. Gaggar A, Coeshott C, Apelian D, et al. Safety, tolerability and immunogenicity of GS-4774, a hepatitis B virus-specific therapeutic vaccine, in healthy subjects: a randomized study. Vaccine 2014;32(39):4925–31.

95. Gane E, Verdon DJ, Brooks AE, et al. Anti-PD-1 blockade with nivolumab with and without therapeutic vaccination for virally suppressed chronic hepatitis B: a pilot study. J Hepatol 2019;71(5):900–7.

96. Chen J, Wang XM, Wu XJ, et al. Intrahepatic levels of PD-1/PD-L correlate with liver inflammation in chronic hepatitis B. Inflamm Res 2011;60(1):47–53.

97. Zanetti AR, Van Damme P, Shouval D. The global impact of vaccination against hepatitis B: a historical overview. Vaccine 2008;26(49):6266–73.

98. Nelson NP, Easterbrook PJ, McMahon BJ. Epidemiology of hepatitis B virus infection and impact of vaccination on disease. Clin Liver Dis 2016;20(4):607–28.

99. Control CfD. Heplisav-B® (HepB-CpG) vaccine. US department of Health and Human Services Center for Disease Control and Prevention. 2023. 2023. https://www.cdc.gov/vaccines/schedules/vacc-updates/heplisav-b.pdf.

100. Manley HJ, Aweh G, Frament J, et al. A real world comparison of HepB (Engerix-B®) and HepB-CpG (Heplisav-B®) vaccine seroprotection in patients receiving maintenance dialysis. Nephrol Dial Transplant 2023;38(2):447–54.

101. Amjad W, Alukal J, Zhang T, et al. Two-dose hepatitis B vaccine (Heplisav-B) results in better seroconversion than three-dose vaccine (Engerix-B) in chronic liver disease. Dig Dis Sci 2021;66(6):2101–6.

102. Lee GH, Lim SG. CpG-adjuvanted hepatitis B vaccine (HEPLISAV-B®) update. Expert Rev Vaccines 2021;20(5):487–95.

103. World Health O. Hepatitis B vaccines: WHO position paper, July 2017 - recommendations. Vaccine 2019;37(2):223–5.

104. Prevention CfDCa. CDC guidance for evaluating health-care personnel for hepatitis B virus protection and for administering postexposure management. 2013.

105. Prevention CfDCa. Adult immunization schedule. Center for Disease Control and Prevention 2023. https://www.cdc.gov/vaccines/schedules/hcp/imz/adult.html?CDC_AA_refVal=https%3A%2F%2Fwww.cdc.gov%2Fvaccines%2Fschedules%2Fhcp%2Fadult.html.

106. Hepatitis B Foundation Vaccine Schedule. https://www.hepb.org/prevention-and-diagnosis/vaccination/guidelines-2/#international.

107. Ayoub WS, Cohen E. Hepatitis B management in the pregnant patient: an update. J Clin Transl Hepatol 2016;4(3):241–7.

108. Prevention CDC. Prevention of hepatitis B virus infection in the United States: recommendations of the advisory committee on immunization Practices. MMWR Recomm Rep (Morb Mortal Wkly Rep) 2018;67(1):1–25.

109. Chang CY, Aziz N, Poongkunran M, et al. Serum alanine aminotransferase and hepatitis B DNA flares in pregnant and postpartum women with chronic hepatitis B. Am J Gastroenterol 2016;111(10):1410–5.

110. Williams WW, Lu PJ, O'Halloran A, et al. Surveillance of vaccination coverage among adult populations - United States, 2015. MMWR Surveill Summ 2017; 66(11):1–28.

111. Locarnini S, Hatzakis A, Chen DS, et al. Strategies to control hepatitis B: public policy, epidemiology, vaccine and drugs. J Hepatol 2015;62(1 Suppl):S76–86.

UNITED STATES POSTAL SERVICE® | Statement of Ownership, Management, and Circulation (All Periodicals Publications Except Requester Publications)

1. Publication Title	2. Publication Number	3. Filing Date
CLINICS IN LIVER DISEASE	016 – 754	9/18/2023

4. Issue Frequency	5. Number of Issues Published Annually	6. Annual Subscription Price
FEB, MAY, AUG, NOV	4	$339.00

7. Complete Mailing Address of Known Office of Publication (Not printer) (Street, city, county, state, and ZIP+4®)

ELSEVIER INC.
230 Park Avenue, Suite 800
New York, NY 10169

Contact Person
Malathi Samayan

Telephone (Include area code)
91-44-4299-4507

8. Complete Mailing Address of Headquarters or General Business Office of Publisher (Not printer)

ELSEVIER INC.
230 Park Avenue, Suite 800
New York, NY 10169

9. Full Names and Complete Mailing Addresses of Publisher, Editor, and Managing Editor (Do not leave blank)

Publisher (Name and complete mailing address)

Dolores Meloni, ELSEVIER INC.
1600 JOHN F KENNEDY BLVD. SUITE 1600
PHILADELPHIA, PA 19103-2899

Editor (Name and complete mailing address)

KERRY HOLLAND, ELSEVIER INC.
1600 JOHN F KENNEDY BLVD. SUITE 1600
PHILADELPHIA, PA 19103-2899

Managing Editor (Name and complete mailing address)

PATRICK MANLEY, ELSEVIER INC.
1600 JOHN F KENNEDY BLVD. SUITE 1600
PHILADELPHIA, PA 19103-2899

10. Owner (Do not leave blank. If the publication is owned by a corporation, give the name and address of the corporation immediately followed by the names and addresses of all stockholders owning or holding 1 percent or more of the total amount of stock. If not owned by a corporation, give the names and addresses of the individual owners. If owned by a partnership or other unincorporated firm, give its name and address as well as those of each individual owner. If the publication is published by a nonprofit organization, give its name and address.)

Full Name	Complete Mailing Address
WHOLLY OWNED SUBSIDIARY OF REED/ELSEVIER, US HOLDINGS	1600 JOHN F KENNEDY BLVD. SUITE 1600 PHILADELPHIA, PA 19103-2899

11. Known Bondholders, Mortgagees, and Other Security Holders Owning or Holding 1 Percent or More of Total Amount of Bonds, Mortgages, or Other Securities. If none, check box ▶ ☐ None

Full Name	Complete Mailing Address
N/A	

12. Tax Status (For completion by nonprofit organizations authorized to mail at nonprofit rates) (Check one)
The purpose, function, and nonprofit status of this organization and the exempt status for federal income tax purposes:
☒ Has Not Changed During Preceding 12 Months
☐ Has Changed During Preceding 12 Months (Publisher must submit explanation of change with this statement)

PS Form **3526**, July 2014 [Page 1 of 4 (see instructions page 4)] PSN: 7530-01-000-9931   PRIVACY NOTICE: See our privacy policy on www.usps.com.

---

13. Publication Title	14. Issue Date for Circulation Data Below
CLINICS IN LIVER DISEASE	AUGUST 2023

15. Extent and Nature of Circulation			Average No. Copies Each Issue During Preceding 12 Months	No. Copies of Single Issue Published Nearest to Filing Date
a. Total Number of Copies (Net press run)			115	107
b. Paid Circulation (By Mail and Outside the Mail)	(1)	Mailed Outside-County Paid Subscriptions Stated on PS Form 3541 (include paid distribution above nominal rate, advertiser's proof copies, and exchange copies)	59	66
	(2)	Mailed In-County Paid Subscriptions Stated on PS Form 3541 (include paid distribution above nominal rate, advertiser's proof copies, and exchange copies)	0	0
	(3)	Paid Distribution Outside the Mails Including Sales Through Dealers and Carriers, Street Vendors, Counter Sales, and Other Paid Distribution Outside USPS®	47	32
	(4)	Paid Distribution by Other Classes of Mail Through the USPS (e.g., First-Class Mail®)	8	8
c. Total Paid Distribution (Sum of 15b (1), (2), (3), and (4))		▶	114	106
d. Free or Nominal Rate Distribution (By Mail and Outside the Mail)	(1)	Free or Nominal Rate Outside-County Copies included on PS Form 3541	0	0
	(2)	Free or Nominal Rate In-County Copies included on PS Form 3541	0	0
	(3)	Free or Nominal Rate Copies Mailed at Other Classes Through the USPS (e.g., First-Class Mail)	0	0
	(4)	Free or Nominal Rate Distribution Outside the Mail (Carriers or other means)	1	1
e. Total Free or Nominal Rate Distribution (Sum of 15d (1), (2), (3) and (4))		▶	1	1
f. Total Distribution (Sum of 15c and 15e)		▶	115	107
g. Copies not Distributed (See Instructions to Publishers #4 (page 83))		▶	0	0
h. Total (Sum of 15f and g)		▶	115	107
i. Percent Paid (15c divided by 15f times 100)		▶	99.34%	99.07%

* If you are claiming electronic copies, go to line 16 on page 3. If you are not claiming electronic copies, skip to line 17 on page 3.

PS Form **3526**, July 2014 (Page 2 of 4)

16. Electronic Copy Circulation		Average No. Copies Each Issue During Preceding 12 Months	No. Copies of Single Issue Published Nearest to Filing Date
a. Paid Electronic Copies	▶		
b. Total Paid Print Copies (Line 15c) + Paid Electronic Copies (Line 16a)	▶		
c. Total Print Distribution (Line 15f) + Paid Electronic Copies (Line 16a)	▶		
d. Percent Paid (Both Print & Electronic Copies) (16b divided by 16c × 100)	▶		

☒ I certify that 50% of all my distributed copies (electronic and print) are paid above a nominal price.

17. Publication of Statement of Ownership

☒ If the publication is a general publication, publication of this statement is required. Will be printed in the NOVEMBER 2023 issue of this publication.   ☐ Publication not required.

18. Signature and Title of Editor, Publisher, Business Manager, or Owner	Date
Malathi Samayan	9/18/2023

Malathi Samayan - Distribution Controller

I certify that all information furnished on this form is true and complete. I understand that anyone who furnishes false or misleading information on this form or who omits material or information requested on the form may be subject to criminal sanctions (including fines and imprisonment) and/or civil sanctions (including civil penalties).

PS Form **3526**, July 2014 (Page 3 of 4)   PRIVACY NOTICE: See our privacy policy on www.usps.com

Moving?

Make sure your subscription moves with you!

To notify us of your new address, find your **Clinics Account Number** (located on your mailing label above your name), and contact customer service at:

Email: journalscustomerservice-usa@elsevier.com

800-654-2452 (subscribers in the U.S. & Canada)
314-447-8871 (subscribers outside of the U.S. & Canada)

Fax number: 314-447-8029

Elsevier Health Sciences Division
Subscription Customer Service
3251 Riverport Lane
Maryland Heights, MO 63043

*To ensure uninterrupted delivery of your subscription, please notify us at least 4 weeks in advance of move.

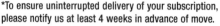

Printed and bound by CPI Group (UK) Ltd, Croydon, CR0 4YY

03/10/2024

01040469-0005